DIVING MEDICINE

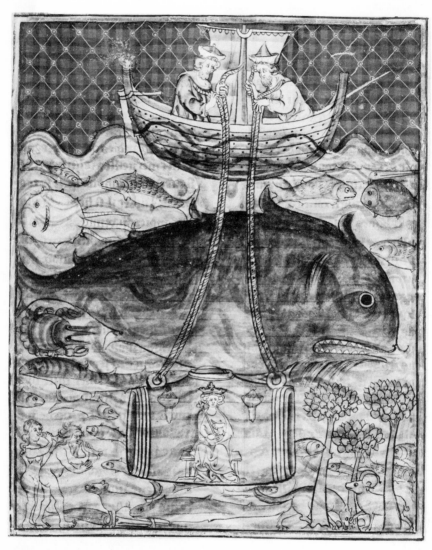

Alexander's Dive. This illumination is from an early fourteenth century French manuscript entitled Histoire d'Alexandre. It depicts Alexander the Great (356-323 B.C.) in what is supposed to be a diving bell, although the vehicle resembles a transparent submarine. Various creatures are shown, some of which are not generally found underwater. (Courtesy of Staatliche Museen Preussischer Kulturbesitz Kupferstich kabineti Berlin-Dahlem, Hs. 78 C 1, fol. 67 r.)

DIVING MEDICINE

Edited by

RICHARD H. STRAUSS, M.D.

Department of Medicine,
Peter Bent Brigham Hospital
and Harvard Medical School,
Boston, Massachusetts;
Department of Physiology,
University of Hawaii School of Medicine,
Honolulu, Hawaii

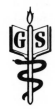

Grune & Stratton
A Subsidiary of Harcourt Brace Jovanovich, Publishers
New York   San Francisco   London

Library of Congress Cataloging in Publication Data
Main entry under title:

Diving medicine.

Includes bibliographical references and index.
1. Submarine medicine. 2. Diving, Submarine
—Physiological aspects. I. Strauss, Richard H.
II. Title. [DNLM: 1. Diving. 2. Submarine
medicine. WD650 D618]
RC1005.D58   616.9'8022   76-10474
ISBN 0-8089-0699-2

Grune & Stratton, Inc.
111 Fifth Avenue
New York, New York 10003

Library of Congress Catalog Number 76-10474
International Standard Book Number 0-8089-0699-2
Printed in the United States of America

CONTENTS

FOREWORD

Albert R. Behnke, M.D.

A relatively new and intriguing challenge to physicians is the need to understand the complexities associated with current widespread diving activity, notably with recreational, scientific, and commercial aspects of scuba diving. During the past 25 years along littoral sea and inland waters hundreds of thousand individuals of both sexes, with varying degrees of aptitude and training, have gone diving. Such persons are in imminent danger of drowning should any mishap occur with equipment or as a result of inclement diving conditions. Too often the scuba diver, in contrast to the professional, is a relatively inexperienced, non-acclimatized amateur. On any particular day he may be in poor physical condition, under the influence of prescribed or other medication, and occasionally on narcotic drugs. Underwater spatial orientation may be greatly impaired by lack of adequate information from visual, proprioceptive, and vestibular systems. As pointed out by Edmonds, the diver's visual cues are virtually abolished in murky water or at night. Proprioceptive information is seriously distorted by zero gravity of neutral buoyancy. Extraordinary significance may be placed on vestibular responses greatly in excess of those customary during terrestrial activity. Impairment of judgment induced by the narcotic effect of hyperbaric nitrogen thwarts the diver confronted by the stresses of an unaccustomed and potentially hostile environment. Confronted with the need for heavy exertion, the scuba diver may be unaware of respiratory inadequacy and hypercarbia. Inexplicably, consciousness may be lost because of blunted recognition underwater of the danger signals which are monitory to protect individuals in a normal environment. Too rapid ascent may precipitate air embolism as a result of general or regional over-expansion of pulmonary tissues. Overstay at depth predisposes to intravascular embolization and gives rise to random symptomatology, remarkable in diversity and intensity.

   The practice of breath-hold diving preceded by hyperventilation is conducive to hypoxic brain and cardiac injury and collapse. Despite the classic investigations of Craig and Scholander and their admonitory repercussion, the lives of adolescents, particularly, are lost in their attempts to establish records.

The physician cognizant of the comprehensive and systematic text dealing with all facets of diving medicine, from advances in physiology to the specific medical examinations and analysis of case histories, is in a highly favorable position not only to prevent diving casualties but to render specific therapy in perplexing situations as well. The early recognition and appropriate therapy for Type II decompression injury involving nervous and cardiovascular systems requires no emphasis. Frequently however, incapacitation is progressive and advanced before the physician is notified. He will need to know the probable benefit or limitations of adjunctive fluid and drug therapy when recompression does not suffice or is not available. He will need to know the value of delayed oxygen recompression in cases of spinal cord involvement. He will require especially the text guidelines in evaluation of hearing loss and vestibular dysfunction. The only proven etiology of inner ear pathology, for example, is fistula of the round window, and immediate reparative surgery has served to prevent chronic invalidism. Likewise, early recognition of juxta-articular bone pathology may forestall crippling disability.

Apart from the exposition of accelerated advances in physiology and diving medicine, the authoritative text has wide ramifications to general medicine. Gas embolism is not solely a diving malady, and the protean manifestations of decompression sickness mimic various clinical entities, notably circulatory shock. Recent knowledge, for example, about the interaction of gas bubbles and blood is pertinent to extracorporal oxygenation of blood and plasma. As a complication of decompression sickness, Philp and his co-workers following a decade of investigation have elucidated the electron-dense layer to which platelets adhere at the interface and interstices between coalesced bubbles and associated lipid masses as well. Biochemical correlates of the hematologic physio-pathology, such as release of serotonin, adenosine diphosphate, and the smooth muscle-constricting kinins, comprise a substantial advance in medicine. Finally, modern technology has brought into quantitative focus such striking entities as compression arthralgia, the high pressure nervous syndrome, and even basic mechanism of anesthesia as revealed by intra- and intermolecular spacing of the physiologically inert gases employed in diving. As Osler's textbook of medicine held the interest of the informed layman, this text reveals the panorama of hyperbaric and undersea medical science, apart from specific elucidation of the measures to prevent and treat diving injuries.

PREFACE

This book is intended for the physician who wishes to become acquainted with the medical aspects of scuba and breath-hold diving. The sport of diving has become so popular that even physicians who practice far from large bodies of water sometimes encounter diving problems. Such problems range from the medical approval for scuba training to cases of air embolism, which can result from scuba diving in a swimming pool and which may be fatal.

In 1974, a one-week course in diving medicine was offered at the University of Hawaii School of Medicine for the first time. It attracted physicians from across the United States and from several other countries. No appropriate text was available, and this book was developed in part to fill such training needs. In addition, divers and diving instructors may find a number of the chapters to be useful references. Each chapter was written by an individual with extensive experience in the subject. The authors come from the United States, Australia, Canada, and England.

The broad range of the subject matter is evident from the table of contents, and the order of the chapters is, by necessity, somewhat arbitrary. Those chapters and sections concerning physiology tend to be among the more technical in nature. The "Medical Examination of the Diver" requires a broad knowledge of diving medicine and is therefore the final chapter. Although the book is oriented toward sport diving, the chapters on saturation diving and diving mammals are of general interest and serve to emphasize specific diving problems. Study questions appear at the end of each chapter so that the reader may test his knowledge if he wishes. The answers are found in Appendix 6.

The ultimate object of this book is to promote safety in diving, through education.

Richard H. Strauss, M.D.

CONTRIBUTORS

Nicholas R. Anthonisen, M.D. Respiratory Division, Department of Medicine, University of Manitoba, Winnipeg, Manitoba, Canada

Arthur J. Bachrach, Ph.D. Behavioral Sciences Department, Naval Medical Research Institute, Bethesda, Maryland

Edward L. Beckman, M.D. Department of Physiology, School of Medicine, University of Hawaii, Honolulu, Hawaii

Peter B. Bennett, Ph.D. Departments of Anesthesiology, Physiology, and Pharmacology, Duke University Medical Center, Durham, North Carolina

Mark E. Bradley, M.D. Commander, Medical Corps, U.S. Navy, Naval Medical Research Institute, Bethesda, Maryland

Robert B. Cook, M.D. Massachusetts Eye and Ear Infirmary, Boston, Massachusetts

K.E. Cooper, M.B., B.S., M.Sc. (Lond.), M.A., D.Sc. (Oxon) Division of Medical Physiology, Faculty of Medicine, The University of Calgary, Calgary, Alberta, Canada

Carl Edmonds, M.D., M.B., B.S., M.R.C.P. (Lond), M.R.C. (Psych), M.A.N.Z.C.P., DipD.H.M. Consultant in Diving Medicine to the Royal Australian Navy; Director, Diving Medical Centre, Mosman, Australia

Glen H. Egstrom, Ph.D. Department of Kinesiology, University of California, Los Angeles, California

Robert Elsner, Ph.D. Institute of Marine Science, University of Alaska, Fairbanks, Alaska

Joseph C. Farmer, Jr., M.D., F.A.C.S. Division of Otolaryngology, Department of Surgery, Duke University Medical Center, Durham, North Carolina

Bruce W. Halstead, M.D. International Biotoxicological Center, World Life Research Institute, Colton, California

Suk Ki Hong, M.D., Ph.D. Department of Physiology, State University of New York at Buffalo, School of Medicine, Buffalo, New York

Eric P. Kindwall, M.D. Department of Hyperbaric Medicine, St. Luke's Hospital, Milwaukee, Wisconsin

Richard H. Strauss, M.D. Department of Medicine, Peter Bent Brigham Hospital and Harvard Medical School, Boston, Massachusetts; Department of Physiology, University of Hawaii School of Medicine, Honolulu, Hawaii

William G. Thomas, Ph.D. Division of Otolaryngology, Department of Surgery, University of North Carolina School of Medicine, Chapel Hill, North Carolina

James Vorosmarti, M.D. Captain, Medical Corps, U.S. Navy, Naval Medical Research Institute, Bethesda, Maryland

D.N. Walder, M.D. Department of Surgery, The University of Newcastle upon Tyne, Newcastle upon Tyne, England

J. Michael Walsh, Ph.D. Behavioral Sciences Department, Naval Medical Research Institute, National Naval Medical Center, Bethesda, Maryland

Walter G. Wolfe, M.D. Department of Surgery, Duke University Medical Center, Durham, North Carolina

David A. Youngblood, M.D. Department of Anesthesiology, Duke University Medical Center, Durham, North Carolina

Eric P. Kindwall

1

A Short History of Diving and Diving Medicine

Man's first entry into the sea was through breath-hold diving, undoubtedly to retrieve lost tools or utensils. From early history, we find that breath-hold divers accomplished prodigious amounts of work and then became economically important. In many areas of the world, commercial pearl and pearl-shell diving still rely on the breath-hold diver to a great extent. Depths of 60 to 80 feet are common and breath-hold diving has been done to depths of 100 feet commercially.

Even the salvage of treasure has been accomplished using the free diver. In 1680, Sir William Phipps recovered some £ 200,000 in sterling silver from a wrecked Spanish galleon in the Caribbean, and the "fishing up of the wrecked plate ships at Vigo Bay" cited by Stevenson in *Treasure Island* was accomplished by naked divers.

The depths that can be reached by the breath-hold diver are dependent on two factors. The first factor is how long the diver can hold his breath without the CO_2 level in the blood forcing him to breathe (breath-hold breaking point). The second factor is the relationship between the diver's total lung capacity and his residual volume. As pressure is increased on the lung, its volume is decreased and even with a thoracic blood shift to fill some of the space, lung squeeze will occur, usually between 100 and 200 feet. However, certain exceptional individuals with a high tolerance for CO_2 and large vital capacities who have practiced breath-hold diving have set extraordinary depth records. A record of 247 feet was set in 1967 by Robert Croft, a U.S. Navy submarine engineman and submarine escape training tower instructor. A more recent record of 330 feet was set by Jacques Mayol, a Frenchman.

BELL DIVING

The use of the diving bell, which consists of trapped air in an inverted container was the next method employed to extend working time on the bottom. Aristotle, in his *Problemata,* mentions that a diver can invert a cauldron over his head to trap air for breathing. In addition, a French manuscript from the Middle Ages contains a fanciful illustration of Alexander the Great descending in a diving bell (frontispiece).

The first modern records of diving bells used in practical salvage start in the 1640s when Von Treileben used a primitive bell for salvaging 42 cannon from the sunken Swedish ship of the line *Vasa* which lay in 132 feet of water in Stockholm Harbor. The bell, shaped like a truncated cone, had no air supply other than that contained within the bell. Bell divers soon learned that the air at the top of the bell was more breathable than that at the bottom, after they had been working for some period under water. Divers would descend in the water in the bell, swim from the bell to the wreck to attach lines to the objects to be salvaged, and then return to the bell for a breath of fresh air between excursions. The reason for the air being better at the top of the bell was that the CO_2 was slightly heavier; as it accumulated, it became more concentrated along the surface of the water toward the bottom of the bell. There is no report of decompression sickness among Von Treileben's submarine workers, but it is extremely possible that working at those depths, especially if they made several dives per day, they could have absorbed enough nitrogen into their systems to cause decompression sickness. It is amazing the amount of work that was accomplished by these early bell divers, as in 1960, when a single remaining bronze cannon was recovered from the wreck by a modern helmeted deep-sea diver, it took the diver $1^1/_2$ days to remove the gun even with all of the advantages of modern equipment and a 150-ton floating crane.

The next recorded note of a diving bell was in 1690 when Halley (discoverer of the comet) devised a successful bell with the first system for renewing air within the bell while it was on the bottom. Lead-weighted barrels carried fresh air down to the occupants of the bell. Halley's bell was somewhat cumbersome and heavy, but we have records that it was used to depths of 60 feet. It is unlikely that any practical salvage was carried out with it.

The first modern practical diving bell was invented by Smeaton in 1790. The reason for its success was that Smeaton devised the first workable force pump for continuously refreshing the air in the bell and this bell, or caisson, was the forerunner of all modern types. It was first used in Ramsgate Harbor,

England, for breakwater construction. Caissons are still used for the construction of bridge piers in much the same manner that Smeaton used his.

SURFACE SUPPLIED DIVING GEAR

The object of having a man free to walk around the bottom without having to hold his breath or return to the safety of a diving bell was first realized when Augustus Siebe invented his diving dress. Siebe was a German coppersmith working in London and, in 1819, he devised a diving rig which consisted of a copper helmet riveted to a leather jacket. The diver entered the dress through the open waist and then thrust his arms into the sleeves with his head protruding into the helmet. There was no control of the amount of air entering the helmet and the excess air bubbled out around the diver's waist. Other inventors had tried their luck at similar designs, but apparently Siebe's diving dress was accepted because of his extremely reliable force pump for producing the necessary compressed air. His original rig was used for successful salvage work on the sunken British war ship, *The Royal George,* and was used by divers on many other important projects. It had one disadvantage in that if the diver were to lie down or turn upside down, the dress quickly filled with water and he was likely to drown. Nevertheless, much useful salvage was accomplished with this primitive apparatus.

Siebe, however, was a constant innovator and, by 1837, he produced an improved design by making a full suit which was waterproofed and could be bolted to a breastplate and helmet. Since the suit covered the diver's entire body, he was enabled to work in any position. Valves were provided for admitting varying amounts of air to the diving suit as needed and an air exhaust valve was provided in the helmet. The 1837 Siebe closed dress design proved itself so successful that it remained essentially unchanged to the present day for classical deep-sea diving. The present U.S. Navy Mark 5 deep-sea diving suit is almost an exact copy of Siebe's original 1837 design, except for some refinements in materials and minor changes in the valves.

The classical deep-sea diving suit remained unchallenged until approximately 1945 when a lightweight diving mask for work down to depths of 90 to 100 feet was introduced. This was designed by Jack Browne and manufactured for the U.S. Navy. It subsequently became widely used among commercial divers, especially on the Gulf of Mexico. It was also at the end of World War II when the self-contained underwater breathing apparatus (scuba) first made its appearance outside of occupied France. It had been invented in 1943 by Emile Gagnon and Jacques Cousteau. The Cousteau-Gagnon patent had at its heart a demand regulator which automatically delivered only the amount of air the diver needed at any depth to which he dived. This simple, but ingenious, device presaged the current boom in sport diving and also was adapted for a number of commercial applications. Since 1960, there have been many advances made in deep-sea diving equipment with the use of more modern helmets made of space-age materials, hot water-heated suits for thermal protection, and the use of the diving bell in combination with the diving suit.

DECOMPRESSION SICKNESS

Our first hint as to the etiology of decompression sickness was provided by Sir Robert Boyle in 1670 when he produced symptoms of decompression sickness in a snake which he had placed in a vacuum cleaner. He was prompted to write: "I once observed a viper furiously tortured in our exhausted receiver which had manifestly a conspicuous bubble moving to and fro in the waterous humor of one of its eyes." Thus, Boyle noted that rapid reduction of ambient pressure may result in the production of bubbles in the tissues of the body.

The first description of the symptoms of decompression in man was provided by Triger in 1841. The victims in this case were coal miners who worked in mines pressurized to keep out the water. Triger noticed that some men suffered cramps and pains in their muscles after leaving the compressed air; apparently, their symptoms were treated vigorously with alcohol given both internally and rubbed on externally. We have no other report as to how they later fared.

Pol and Watelle, in 1854, began to study the phenomenon of decompression sickness and they noticed that this disease was always associated with leaving the compressed air environment. They wrote, "one pays only on leaving." They also noted that return to compressed air alleviated the symptoms. They pointed out that young men of 18 who had "not reached their greatest mature physical strength" suffered less from decompression sickness symptoms than those in their midthirties, "who were in their prime." The first scientific approach to the problem of decompression sickness was begun by the French physiologist Paul Bert, when he published his monumental book "Barometric Pressure" in 1878. Bert was able to demonstrate that bubbles were formed during rapid decompression associated with symptoms of decompression sickness and, furthermore, that these bubbles consisted mainly of nitrogen. Bert also discovered that oxygen was toxic when breathed under pressure. The convulsions that occur when oxygen is breathed for any period of time at pressures greater than 33 ft have been termed the Paul Bert effect.

The word bends as a synonym for decompression sickness came into being during the construction of the piers for the Brooklyn Bridge. The fashionable ladies of the era had an affected posture for walking called The Grecian Bend. Workers emerging from the caisson, limping with symptoms of decompression sickness, were derided by their fellows for "doing the Grecian bend." This was later shortened to simply "the bends" and has become legitimized by use.

By the turn of the century, even though it was known that the etiology of decompression sickness was nitrogen bubbles evolving within the body and that the symptoms could be relieved by returning to increased pressure, there were no decompression schedules that could be followed to minimize the possibility of decompression sickness occurring. Since the Royal Navy consistently used the divers in its routine operations, it commissioned J. S. Haldane to work out a set of decompression schedules that could be written down in tabular form and followed by its fleet divers. In 1908, Haldane published the first set of practical, though empirical, decompression schedules. In his work, Haldane demonstrated that the body could tolerate a two-to-one reduction in ambient pressure without symptoms. All common decompression schedules in use since have been based on Haldane's method. The Haldanian schedules were found to be quite realistic over their middle range; but divers soon found it possible to "cut corners" on short, shallow dives without risking bends, although on long, deep dives the Haldane tables were not conservative enough. Haldane's tables were modified empirically over the years to take care of these problems. To Haldane must also go the credit for developing the concept of half-time tissues. Haldane realized that all of the tissues of the body absorbed nitrogen at varying rates, depending on their vascularity and the types of tissue involved. Recognizing that this was a spectrum which probably went from seconds to hours, he arbitrarily chose to recognize the existence of 5-, 10-, 20-, 40- and 75-minute half-time tissues for mathematical convenience in calculating nitrogen uptake and elimination. He assumed that nitrogen uptake and elimination occurred at equal rates and that the longest half-time tissue in the body was probably 60 minutes. He therefore assumed that the body would be totally saturated in 6 hours. However, he made his longest tissue 75 minutes, just to be on the safe side. Since that time, the U.S. Navy standard air decompression tables have been based on a 12-hour period for total saturation; the exceptional exposure air tables have been based on a 24-hour time period for total saturation. Even longer tissue half-times have been developed for saturation diving.

INCREASING DEPTHS AND EXPERIMENTS WITH HELIUM-OXYGEN BREATHING

In 1915, the U.S. Submarine F-4 sank in 306 feet of water off Honolulu, Hawaii. The U.S. Navy was anxious to recover the submarine and the bodies of its crew and thus diving operations were commenced. Frank Crilley, in that year, set a world depth record of 306 feet by descending to the submarine and attaching a large hawser to it. The pressures at 306 feet are enormous, having been enough to completely crush the sides of the submarine revealing the outlines of the Diesel engines beneath. The fact that Crilley was able to dive to this depth and return to the surface alive by using primitive decompression schedules then employed was an astounding feat. Perhaps Crilley's size had something to do with it, since he weighed only 127 pounds. Three-hundred feet is still about the extreme limit for compressed air diving because the nitrogen narcosis at that depth renders all but the most experienced divers incapable of any kind of useful work. The current U.S. Navy maximum operating depth for compressed air diving is 190 feet.

Because air seemed to have a limit of approximately 300 feet, the physiologist Elihu Thompson wrote a letter to the Bureau of Mines in 1919 suggesting that helium mixed with oxygen might be used as a diving gas. Because helium was so much lighter than nitrogen, he thought that with the decreased breathing resistance permissible, diving depths might be doubled. Nitrogen narcosis was still not understood in 1919. The British Admiralty, along with the U.S. Bureau of Mines, began experimenting with helium/oxygen mixtures and thought that bends might be avoided because nitrogen was no longer in the breathing mixture. However, experiments ceased after Royal Navy divers developed severe decompression sickness when breathing helium, even though decompressed on conservative air decompression schedules. The U.S. Navy Experimental Diving Unit, which had worked with the Bureau of Mines on helium, also abandoned its studies of helium in 1924 since helium seemed to produce decompression sickness more quickly than did compressed air. In Admiral Momsen's words, experimentation with helium diving was "put very much on the back burner." Because of the necessity to dive to great depths on occasion for military operations, Damant extended the original Haldane air schedules to 320 feet in 1930.

NEW DEVELOPMENTS

Occasionally, divers returned to the surface from trivial depths (less than 33 feet) and suffered sudden incapacitation. This was thought to be due to a capricious form of decompression sickness and, indeed, the U.S. Navy reported two cases of "unusual decompression sickness in 16 feet of water" in the mid-1930s. Both of these cases proved fatal, but the mechanism of death was not understood. Submarine escape training began in the U.S. Navy at the beginning of the 1930s and, occasionally, even with the use of the Momsen lung, trainees would develop severe distress or die quickly after surfacing. Further investigation revealed that death in these cases was due to overdistension of the lungs with subsequent rupture and escape of air into the pulmonary veins. From the pulmonary veins, the air bubbles were directed to the left heart and thence to the brain. Cerebral air embolism became recognized for the first time. When it was understood that air bubbles in the brain were the cause of the symptoms and that nitrogen alone was not involved, immediate recompression to 165 feet became the standard treatment and the victims of air embolism were treated as though they had severe decompression sickness. Most of them survived when immediately recompressed and, eventually, a recompression chamber was installed at the top of the submarine escape training towers to handle such cases.

Meanwhile, Albert R. Behnke, a U.S. Navy Submarine Medical Officer and an outstanding scientist, became interested in the problem of mental deterioration when the divers exceeded depths of 150 feet. Using mixtures of gases other than nitrogen, he demonstrated that heavier inert gases produced more narcosis and that it was nitrogen which produced the mental deterioration in air diving. Behnke also demonstrated that high levels of CO_2 contributed to nitrogen narcosis, but that nitrogen itself was the culprit.

HELIUM REVISITED AND NEW DEPTH RECORDS SET

In 1937, Edgar End, a 26-year-old intern at the Milwaukee County General Hospital, thought that helium could be used successfully to avoid nitrogen narcosis. He was undeterred by the fact that both the British Admiralty and the U.S. Navy Experimental Diving Unit had been unable to adapt helium successfully for diving. By doing some original calculations, he developed a set of helium decompression schedules which he believed would be compatible with this rapidly diffusing gas. A friend of End's, Max Gene Nohl, a Milwaukee diver, breathed helium-oxygen with End in an old recompression chamber located at the Milwaukee County Emergency Hospital and together they found that they could surface safely from depths of 100 feet after various exposures to breathing helium. This was followed by a series of open water dives in Lake Michigan to increasing depths. Finally, using Nohl's self-contained suit, Frank Crilley's record was broken and a new world depth record of 420 feet was set in December of 1937 diving from a coast guard cutter off of Port Washington, Wisconsin. Nohl surfaced safely without signs of decompression sickness. After End and Nohl had proved that helium could be used successfully for deep diving, the Navy stepped up its own interests in helium-oxygen experimentation and by 1939 had a series of helium-oxygen decompression schedules ready. These schedules had been developed by Behnke. The helium-oxygen equipment was sent to a warehouse at Kittery, Maine, for field testing in the summer of 1939, when the submarine *U.S.S. Squalus* operating out of Portsmouth, New Hampshire, sank off the Isle of Shoals in 240 feet of water.

The submarine was quickly located and the first dives were made on compressed air. Some 36 men were rescued from the submarine using the Mc-Cann Rescue Bell, but then the actual salvage of the submarine was carried out using the new helium-oxygen schedules and equipment. Over 900 helium dives were made on the Squalus. It is amazing that during this first venture in deep water with a new gas not a single diver was killed. For the next 20 years the U.S. Navy was to be the only user of helium-oxygen diving (as the United States had the only readily available sources of helium) and all U.S. Navy submarine rescue vessels were equipped with helium-oxygen diving gear.

In 1945, Jack Browne, the son of a Milwaukee automobile dealer, had become interested in diving and felt that a practical diving mask could be more useful than the heavy and cumbersome standard deep-sea dress. He devised a triangular shaped mask and in a wet test tank at the Diving Equipment and Supply Company in Milwaukee, Wisconsin, he descended to a new world depth record of 550 feet. The decompression schedules for this dive were worked out by Edgar End with some modifications by Behnke, who was also present.

It was also in 1945 that the Swedish engineer Arne Zetterstrom investigated the possibilities of using hydrogen-oxygen for diving. Hydrogen-oxygen is a nonexplosive mixture when the oxygen percentage is less than 4 percent. Zetterstrom reached a depth of 512 feet in the Baltic Sea in August, 1945, and the hydrogen-oxygen mixture was perfectly satisfactory as a breathing mix. Unfortunately, he was killed on ascent due to a winch accident which had nothing to do with his breathing mixture. Hydrogen diving was not attempted again until the 1970s, when Peter Edel in New Orleans began experimenting with the gas on a contract from the U.S. Navy.

DEVELOPMENT OF TREATMENT TABLES FOR
DECOMPRESSION SICKNESS

There had been many schools of thought as how best to treat a diver stricken with bends. Some felt that the diver should be returned to his original working pressure. Others felt that he should be taken to his depth of relief. Others thought that the treatment pressure should be the depth of relief plus 1 atm. Then there were many schemes for gradually reducing the pressure on the diver so that he would not sustain decompression sickness during his ascent in the treatment chamber. The U.S. Navy, in 1944 and 1945, studied all of these methods and finally promulgated the U.S. Navy Air Recompression Tables I-IV, in 1945. These tables represented a ninefold improvement over previous recompression procedures and became the world standard of treatment for the next 20 years. They embodied the concept that the diver should be taken to the depth of relief plus 1 atm, as a minimum, with a 6 atm maximum as a trade-off between maximally compressing any offending bubbles and causing too much nitrogen narcosis and too much extension of subsequent decompression time. For serious symptoms they provided a "12-hour soak", sometimes known as "the overnight soak", at the 30-foot stop on return to the surface so that all tissues could theoretically be equilibrated to 30 feet. Then, following Haldanian theory, decompression to the surface could be made safely without exceeding a two-to-one ratio for any tissue. However, to be cautious, several more hours were taken to decompress from 30 feet. Tables I through IV proved themselves fairly successful when used to treat decompression sickness stemming from dives carried out on standard Navy schedules. At first, air was used as the breathing medium throughout the tables but, later, oxygen was introduced for use at the shallower stops. The shortest of the air tables, Table 1A, took 6 hours and 13 minutes and Table IV took 38 hours. The length of these schedules did not make them popular with divers; but, on the other hand, they represented the only escape from unbearable pain and/or paralysis.

In 1947, Edgar End, still active in the diving field, began treating caisson workers in Milwaukee with oxygen at pressures of 30 p.s.i.g. (67 feet). He reasoned that nitrogen was the cause of the patient's symptoms and that the addition of more nitrogen to the patient's system, when taken to great depth, only prolonged treatment time. He generally treated his patients for 1 to 2 hours at 30 pounds and then decompressed them. His experience with some 250 cases was excellent, but his data obtained with this method remained unpublished.

Since 1947, no diver or compressed air worker has been treated for bends in the chambers in Milwaukee with compressed air as the breathing gas.

SATURATION DIVING

The first intentional saturation dive was carried out by Edgar End and Max Nohl in Milwaukee, Wisconsin, at the County Emergency Hospital recompression chamber on December 22, 1938, when they spent 27 hours at 101 feet, breathing air. They decompressed fairly successfully taking about 5 hours with only Nohl experiencing decompression sickness. These bends symptoms were treated with moderate pressures of air with complete relief.

Practical saturation diving was first conceived in 1957 by Commander George Bond of the U.S. Navy when working in the Submarine Medical Research Laboratory in New London, Connecticut. Commander Bond (now Captain Bond, USN, Ret.) envisioned undersea laboratories located at various depths down to 600 feet on the continental shelf. He calculated that scientists could work at full sea pressure in these laboratories studying physiology, submarine geology, and marine biology for prolonged periods of time. Then they could be transferred to a shallower habitat where they could continue their studies while decompressing. Several habitats would be used, each one at a shallower depth, so that finally the scientist could emerge with minimal decompression after completing his tour of study which might last weeks.

It was first necessary to demonstrate that animals could tolerate saturation exposures. These research efforts were termed Project Genesis, and after further work at the Experimental Diving Unit in Washington, D.C., under the direction of R. D. Workman, saturation decompression schedules were devised for human beings. These were later tested in the open sea on Projects Sealab 1 and 2. Meanwhile, in 1962, Ed Link saturated a diver for 24 hours at a depth of 200 feet in the Mediterranean. Captain Jacques Cousteau also established saturation habitats in the Con Shelf series.

In 1965, commercial saturation diving was begun when Westinghouse, using their Cachelot diving system, worked on the Smith Mountain Dam in Virginia to replace faulty strainers at a depth of 200 feet. Divers were saturated for periods up to 5 days on this job. Since that time saturation has become commonplace, especially in oil-field work.

COMMERCIAL HELIUM DIVING

With the advent of offshore oil production, diving schedules were required in deep water, and this became an acute problem especially on the West Coast of the United States. Diving companies usually hired local abalone divers to handle various odd jobs associated with drilling rigs. However, when pressures of 250 feet were reached, the compressed air equipment used by the commercial divers caused nearly prohibitive nitrogen narcosis. Dan Wilson, an abalone diver from California, decided that helium-oxygen was necessary. In 1962, using a Japanese abalone deep-sea diving dress and a special oronasal mask, he made the first modern civilian helium dive to a depth of 420 feet. Within a year, Wilson was contracting helium-oxygen diving services to oil companies in the Santa Barbara area.

On the Gulf Coast, the oil rigs were also moving into deeper water and Peter Edel calculated the first helium-oxygen schedules for use in the gulf in 1963. With the demand for deep commercial diving accelerating rapidly, new helium equipment was developed by commercial operators and commercial helium diving capabilities soon outstripped those of the U.S. Navy. Bell diving also came into vogue to deliver the commercial diver to the work site.

In all fairness to the U.S. Navy, it must be stated that in the early 1960s those responsible for Navy budgeting could not identify the operational necessity for deeper helium diving or improved helium diving equipment. It was only in the early 1970s that the U.S. Navy again became active in doing front-line research in this area.

LOW PRESSURE OXYGEN TREATMENT OF
DECOMPRESSION SICKNESS BECOMES WIDESPREAD

By 1964, the Navy noted that the failure rate for bends treatment Tables I through IV began to rise sharply. This was because the Navy was called upon to treat more civilian scuba divers who had failed to observe any kind of standard decompression schedules. In the year 1964 alone, the failure rate on the initial recompression for serious symptoms had risen to 47 percent. Clearly, something had to be done. Workman and Goodman of the U.S. Navy Experimental Diving Unit reinvestigated the use of oxygen under low pressures as the primary treatment modality for decompression sickness. Oxygen had been suggested by Behnke in 1939 as a promising treatment method after starting with a brief excursion to 6 atm absolute. After 3 years of work, enough data had been gathered and the U.S. Navy promulgated the low pressure oxygen Tables 5 and 6 on August 22, 1967. At the same time, treatment Tables 5A and 6A for treatment of air embolism were published. The treatment times required for decompression sickness were drastically reduced and the maximum depth of treatment was only 60 feet (26.7 psig). Table 5 took only 135 minutes and had a failure rate on the initial recompression of only 1 percent. Table 6, for serious symptoms and recurrences, took only 285 minutes and the failure rate on the initial recompression fell to only 3.6 percent. The use of Tables I through IV has now been largely abandoned.

NEW PRESSURE RECORDS

In the mid-1960s, Hannes Keller, a Swiss experimental diver, reached a depth of 1000 feet in the open sea using a "secret" blend of gases and the race of increasing depths was on. In 1970, the British reached a depth of 1500 feet in a dry chamber using helium-oxygen as the breathing mixture at the Royal Navy Physiological Laboratory at Alverstoke, England. A new phenomenon appeared called the high pressure nervous syndrome or HPNS. Helium was the culprit. It was discovered that rapid compression to depths in excess of 500 feet could bring on uncontrollable shaking and nausea in divers breathing helium. Bennett found that slow compressions could be used to minimize or obviate this problem and the British 1970 dive was accomplished using several days to reach maximum depth. Later, he discovered that small amounts of nitrogen mixed with the helium could apparently eliminate HPNS.

The French were in strong competition with the British and, again using slow compression, set a record of 1700 feet in the dry chamber in 1971. The French in 1972 set a new record of 2001 feet in the dry chamber at COMEX in France. The U.S. Navy, using its Mark I deep-diving system set the present open sea depth record of 1148 feet in the Gulf of Mexico in the summer of 1975.

RECENT DEVELOPMENTS

Universities with oceanography programs took an interest in diving, and civilian saturation diving for research purposes gained ascendency in the late 1960s and the early 1970s. The U.S. Navy, along with other agencies of the government, sponsored the Tektite series of saturation dives to depths of 50 feet in the Carribean. The Tektite divers breathed normoxic nitrogen-oxygen mixtures. Hydrolab was established by the Perry Submarine Company off Freeport, Grand Bahama, at a depth of 42 feet. Dozens of scientists have been saturated for periods up to 2 weeks in this habitat breathing compressed air. The Puerto Rican International Underwater Laboratory (PRINUL) was built with saturation capability to 100 feet. The Tektite 2 series saw the first all-woman team of aquanauts carry out scientific research while saturated.

Trigas mixtures became of interest commercially in the 1960s and André Galèrne of International Underwater Contractors pioneered their use. These mixes consist of helium, nitrogen, and oxygen and are being used more and more commercially. Neon and helium are also being used experimentally.

Commercial contracts for deep diving have become more sophisticated and, by 1974, contracts were in existence that called for diving services to depths of 1500 feet in support of offshore oil production, if needed.

FUTURE RESEARCH

Diving depths to 3000 feet are now being considered with trigas mixes. Hydrogen as a diving gas is under active investigation by Peter Edel in New Orleans and William Fife in Texas. The blood changes in decompression sickness are beginning to be quantified. The first symposium on blood changes in bends was conducted in Toronto in 1973.

At the present time, more attention is being paid to the study of the actual elimination curves of inert gas during decompression and for the first time, these are being measured accurately. Future research will undoubtedly provide answers for the exact mechanism of inert gas elimination from the body and what the tolerable limits of tissue trauma may be during this process.

Richard H. Strauss

2
The Physics of Gases

A diver is subjected to elevated water pressures. If he were able to breathe a liquid[1] there would be relatively few medical complications because most problems associated with diving are a consequence of the presence of gas spaces within the body. Tissues are composed mainly of water, which is nearly incompressible and unaffected by pressures within the current diving range.* Gases, however, are compressible and this can lead to problems such as air embolism, decompression sickness, squeeze, and nitrogen narcosis. Even fish are not immune to gas diseases, although those without a swim bladder for buoyancy control can vary depth rapidly over a considerable range. Fish with a gas-filled swim bladder, when forced to surface rapidly, have exhibited a ruptured swim bladder and/or bubble formation in many locations throughout the body.[2] Salmon, swimming in gas-supersaturated water below dams on the Columbia River or in aquaria, develop "gas bubble disease," which is analogous to decompression sickness in humans.[3]

PRESSURE MEASUREMENTS

People normally live at the bottom of a sea of air. The weight of this air impinges on the body surface with a pressure at sea level defined as "one atmosphere." Atmospheric pressure decreases with increasing altitude.

---

*Hydrostatic pressures well beyond those experienced by sport divers are known to alter certain biological processes. Such effects could well limit human penetration into the realm of very high pressures.

Table 2-1
Pressure Equivalents

1 atm	=	33 feet seawater (fsw)
	=	34 feet freshwater
	=	29.9 in. Hg
	=	760 mm Hg
	=	14.7 pounds per square inch (psi)
	=	1 kg/cm^2

A column of liquid exerts a pressure that is proportional to its height, its density, and the acceleration of gravity (Table 2-1). In diving, pressure is often measured in "feet seawater" (fsw). It is useful to remember that 33 fsw exerts a pressure of 1 atm.* Pressure is, by definition, force per unit area and can be expressed as such: for example, 14.7 psi equals 1 atm. An extended table of pressure conversion factors is found in Appendix 1.

Depth gauges and other pressure gauges used in diving indicate zero at the surface. Readings from these instruments are termed *gauge* pressure. Such readings ignore the contribution of air pressure at the surface. To find the *absolute* (total) pressure, atmospheric pressure must be added to the gauge pressure (Fig. 2-1). Since the behavior of gases is determined by the absolute pressure, this conversion is important to remember. At a depth of 33 fsw, the gauge pressure is 1 atm, but the absolute pressure is 2 atm.

Ambient pressure is simply the pressure to which a diver or object is exposed at a given moment. *Hydrostatic* pressure is the pressure exerted by a liquid at rest. For the submerged diver, ambient pressure is the same as hydrostatic pressure.

Sample calculations.   A diver swims at a depth of 99 fsw.

1. What is his gauge pressure in atmospheres?

$$\text{Answer: } \frac{99 \text{ fsw}}{33 \text{ fsw/atm}} = 3 \text{ atm}$$

2. What is his absolute pressure in atmospheres?

$$\text{Answer: } \frac{99 \text{ fsw} + 33 \text{ fsw}}{33 \text{ fsw/atm}} = 4 \text{ atm}$$

or

$$3 \text{ atm gauge} + 1 \text{ atm} = 4 \text{ atm}$$

---

*Abbreviations frequently used include fsw, feet seawater; atm, atmospheres; ata, atmospheres absolute; psi, pounds per square inch.

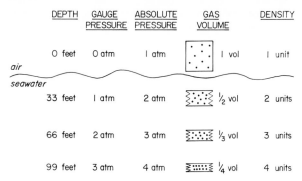

DEPTH	GAUGE PRESSURE	ABSOLUTE PRESSURE	GAS VOLUME	DENSITY
0 feet	0 atm	1 atm	1 vol	1 unit
33 feet	1 atm	2 atm	½ vol	2 units
66 feet	2 atm	3 atm	⅓ vol	3 units
99 feet	3 atm	4 atm	¼ vol	4 units

Fig. 2-1. Gas volume decreases as absolute pressure increases.

KINETIC THEORY OF GASES

Gas molecules are in continuous motion. In a closed container they repeatedly strike the sides causing outward pressure upon the walls. If the container is made smaller, the gas molecules strike the walls more frequently and gas pressure increases. If volume is held constant while gas temperature increases, pressure increases. This is because the addition of energy in the form of heat causes the gas molecules to travel faster and, thus, to strike the walls more frequently and with greater force.

The behavior of gases is well described by the "ideal gas law":

$$PV = nRT,$$

where P is absolute pressure, V is volume, n is the number of moles of gas, R is the universal gas constant, and T is the absolute temperature. Following are several simpler gas laws which stem from the ideal gas law. They are commonly used under conditions associated with diving.

Pressure—Volume Relationship

Boyle's law states that "at a constant temperature, the volume of a given mass of gas is inversely proportional to its pressure." If the absolute pressure P is doubled, the volume V is halved (Fig. 2-1). Stated mathematically:

$$PV = K$$

where K is a constant.

We often wish to know what will happen if we change the pressure on a known volume of gas, for example, in the lungs. The initial conditions P_1 and V_1 are known, the final condition P_2 is known, but V_2 is unknown. Boyle's law is used

$$P_1 V_1 = K = P_2 V_2,$$

so that

$$P_1 V_1 = P_2 V_2,$$

which is a useful equation to remember. Rearranging to solve for V_2,

$$V_2 = \frac{P_1 V_1}{P_2}$$

Sample calculations.   A breath-hold diver leaves the surface with 6 liters of gas in his lungs. What is his total lung volume at a depth of 66 fsw?

Answer: The initial pressure P_1 is 1 atm absolute. The initial volume V_1 is 6 liters. The final pressure P_2 is 66 fsw, gauge pressure. In order to solve the problem, we must convert gauge pressure to absolute pressure, and we often find it convenient to convert pressure measurements from feet seawater to atmospheres.

$$P_1 = 1 \text{ ata}$$
$$V_1 = 6 \text{ liters}$$
$$P_2 = \frac{66 \text{ fsw} + 33 \text{ fsw}}{33 \text{ fsw/atm}} = 3 \text{ ata},$$
$$V_2 = \frac{P_1 V_1}{P_2}$$
$$= \frac{(1 \text{ ata}) (6 \text{ liters})}{3 \text{ ata}}$$
$$V_2 = 2 \text{ liters}.$$

In the above calculation, chest wall forces were assumed to be insignificant as compared to hydrostatic pressure.

Gas volume changes are particularly noticeable near the surface. For example, in going from the surface to 33 fsw, a volume of 1 liter decreases to $1/2$ liter. However, in descending 33 fsw from 99 feet to 132 feet, a volume of 1 liter decreases only to $4/5$ liter. Thus, equalizing ear pressure must be done more frequently at the beginning of descent than at greater depths.

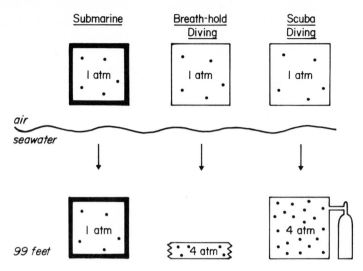

Fig. 2-2. With a submarine, pressure remains at 1 ata (the pressure at sea level). In breath-hold diving, the lungs are compressed and the gas pressure within them is approximately the same as the surrounding (ambient) pressure. In scuba diving, gas is supplied at ambient pressure so that normal respiration can continue.

Breath-hold diving versus scuba diving.   When man goes underwater, he has several choices (Fig. 2-2): (1) He can ride in a submarine, the hull of which is designed to withstand hydrostatic pressure so that passengers remain at 1 ata. (2) He can hold his breath and dive. Gas pressure within the lungs remains approximately the same as the surrounding (ambient) pressure because, within limits, the volume of the thorax decreases readily. Or (3) he can dive while breathing compressed gas, as from scuba (self-contained underwater breathing apparatus). Gas pressure within the lungs then remains close to ambient pressure—as in breath-hold diving—but lung volume remains normal. This occurs because a demand regulator releases gas from a tank to the respiratory tract when respiratory pressure falls below ambient pressure, as during inspiration. Respiration is thus allowed to continue in a relatively normal manner.

With certain types of scuba regulators, inspiration becomes more difficult as depth increases. This is because more molecules of air must flow through the orifice of the regulator for each breath. Similarly, an air tank is exhausted more quickly as depth increases.

Most of the resistance to airflow within the respiratory tract is due to turbulence. This resistance increases with depth because it is proportional to gas density. However, the effect is insignificant under conditions associated with sport diving.

Air embolism.   During ascent, gas within the lungs expands. To avoid overinflation of the lungs, the scuba diver must continue to breathe normally or must exhale during ascent. Failure to do so can lead to air embolism and death. Air bursts from lung spaces into blood vessels of the lung and is carried to various parts of the body where it obstructs circulation. In the brain, emboli of air can mimic the manifestations of stroke. Breath-hold divers are not susceptible to air embolism because, while surfacing, their lungs re-expand only to the volume of their original breath.

Squeeze.   Barotrauma of descent, or "squeeze," is a process in which ambient pressure rises, but pressure within an unventilated gas space does not. The term is also used to describe the results of such a process—usually hemorrhage. For squeeze to occur; (1) there must exist a gas space which is not entirely collapsible; and (2) the gas within the space must not equilibrate fully with gas at ambient pressure.

Middle ear squeeze is a common problem among divers and results from inability to equalize pressure via the eustachian tube. It can result in transudation of fluid, hemorrhage, or rupture of the tympanic membrane. Squeeze has also been found to involve the sinuses, lungs, tissue within the face mask, skin under a fold in a wet suit, the ear canal (from ear plugs), and teeth with recent fillings. The process occurs during descent. Blood within vessels lining the unventilated space is at approximately ambient pressure, so there is a pressure differential across the blood vessel wall tending to rupture the vessel or to cause transudation of fluid. Barotrauma is discussed more fully in Chapters 5 and 9.

Pressure—Temperature Relationships

"At a constant volume, the pressure of a given mass of gas is proportional to its absolute temperature." This is sometimes called the Pressure Law, the formula for which is

$$\frac{P}{T} = K.$$

The pressure within a scuba tank rises when the tank is left in the sun and falls when the tank is placed in cold water.

When gas is forced into a scuba tank or decompression chamber, the gas temperature rises. For this reason, scuba tanks are generally immersed in cool water while being filled. Chambers can be pressurized slowly to permit dissipation of heat and maintenance of a relatively comfortable internal temperature.

Charles' law states that "at constant pressure the volume of a given mass

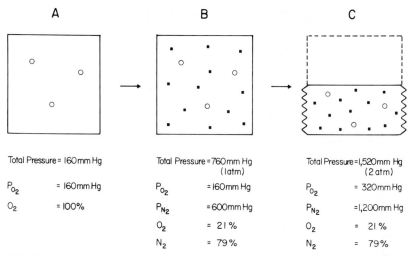

Fig. 2-3. The partial pressure of a species of gas depends upon the number of its molecules per unit volume. The presence or absence of other gas molecules does not matter.

of gas is proportional to its absolute temperature." This law is often cited, but rarely used, in diving.

Partial Pressure

Partial pressure is that pressure which is exerted by a single gas in a mixture of gases. In general, the biological effects of a gas depend upon its partial pressure. This is because both solubility and diffusion are proportional to partial pressure. Thus, supplying the proper amount of oxygen to the body depends upon the partial pressure of oxygen and not merely upon the total gas pressure or the percentage of oxygen. Carbon dioxide balance and nitrogen narcosis are similarly dependent upon the partial pressure of the respective gas.

Dalton's law of partial pressures states: "In a mixture of gases, the pressure exerted by each gas is the same as it would exert if it alone occupied the same volume; and the total pressure is the sum of the partial pressures of the component gases." This law is illustrated in Figure 2-3, which shows a single gas-tight box under three different conditions. In condition A, the box contains only oxygen molecules in a relatively small numbr, so that the total pressure is low: arbitrarily, 160 mm Hg. Since there are no other gases present, the gas is 100 percent oxygen and the partial pressure of oxygen, P_{O_2}, is 160 mm Hg—the same as the total pressure.

In condition B, nitrogen has been added to the box so that the total pressure, P_{total}, is 760 mm Hg. No oxygen has escaped so the P_{O_2} is unchanged. The P_{N_2} is equal to the difference between the total pressure and P_{O_2}:

$$P_{O_2} + P_{N_2} = P_{total}$$
$$P_{N_2} = P_{total} - P_{O_2}$$
$$= 760 \text{ mm Hg} - 160 \text{ mm Hg}$$
$$P_{N_2} = 600 \text{ mm Hg.}$$

The percentage of the total pressure that is contributed by a given gas X is calculated by:

$$\% \ X \ = \frac{P_X}{P_{total}} (100)$$

$$\% \ O_2 \ = \frac{160 \text{ mm Hg}}{760 \text{ mm Hg}} (100)$$

$$= \ 21,$$

$$\% \ N_2 \ = \frac{600 \text{ mm Hg}}{760 \text{ mm Hg}} (100)$$

$$= \ 79.$$

Percentages can be calculated in terms of pressure or number of molecules. The values in condition B are those of air at 1 atm, neglecting the contributions of carbon dioxide (0.04 percent) and inert gases which are present in small amounts.

In condition C, the box has been compressed to one-half its former volume without letting any gas escape. Temperature is held constant. The total gas pressure has doubled. The percentage of each gas has not changed, so the partial pressure of each gas has also doubled.

Calculations are frequently easier if the composition of a gas mixture is expressed in decimal fractions (F_X) instead of percentages:

$$F_X \ = \frac{\% \ X}{100}$$

For example, in air

$$F_{O_2} = \frac{\% \ O_2}{100}$$

$$= \frac{21}{100}$$

$$F_{O_2} = 0.21.$$

Sample Calculations.   (1) What is the partial pressure of oxygen in air breathed at 132 fsw?

Answer:
$$P_{total} = \frac{132 \text{ fsw} + 33 \text{ fsw}}{33 \text{ fsw/atm}}$$

$$= 5 \text{ ata.}$$

$$P_{O_2} = (P_{total})(F_{O_2})$$

$$= (5 \text{ ata})(0.21)$$

$$= 1.05 \text{ atm.}$$

Converting to mm Hg:

$$P_{O_2} = (1.05 \text{ atm})(760 \text{ mm Hg/atm})$$

$$= 798 \text{ mm Hg.}$$

(2) In deep diving, gas mixtures of helium and oxygen are breathed. The use of helium eliminates nitrogen narcosis. The partial pressure of oxygen must be maintained at 160 mm Hg or slightly greater to avoid hypoxia or oxygen toxicity. In a helium-oxygen mixture breathed at 500 fsw, what is the percentage of oxygen that will result in an oxygen partial pressure of 200 mm Hg?

Answer:
$$P_{total} = \frac{500 \text{ fsw} + 33 \text{ fsw}}{33 \text{ fsw/atm}}$$

$$= 16.2 \text{ ata.}$$

Converting to mm Hg:

$$P_{total} = (16.2 \text{ ata})(760 \text{ mm Hg/ata})$$

$$= 12,300 \text{ mm Hg,}$$

$$\% \, O_2 = \frac{P_{O_2}}{P_{total}}(100)$$

$$= \frac{200 \text{ mm Hg}}{12,300 \text{ mm Hg}}(100)$$

$$\% \, O_2 = 1.63.$$

A match will not burn in this atmosphere because its combustibility is dependent more upon the percentage of oxygen in the atmosphere than upon the partial pressure of oxygen.

SOLUTION OF GASES IN LIQUIDS

Henry's law states that "at a given temperature, the mass of gas dissolved in a given volume of solvent is proportional to the pressure of the gas with which it is in equilibrium." Thus, as pressure increases during air breathing, more and more nitrogen is dissolved in the body. During ascent, this nitrogen may come out of solution as bubbles and cause decompression sickness. The physical mechanisms of decompression sickness, and its clinical manifestations, are described more fully in Chapter 6.

REFERENCES

1. Kylstra JA: Liquid Breathing. Undersea Biomedical Research 1:259-269, 1974
2. Strauss RH: Unpublished observations
3. Rucker RR: Gas-Bubble Disease of Salmonids: A Critical Review. Technical Papers of the Bureau of Sport Fisheries and Wildlife 58:1-11, 1972

STUDY QUESTIONS

1. What is the inspired P_{O_2}, in mm Hg, for a patient breathing 40 percent oxygen aboard the hospital ship *Hope*?
2. A scuba diver ditched his gear at a depth of 66 feet and rose to the surface, exhaling continuously. His total lung volume was 6 liters at both the beginning and end of ascent. What volume of gas, measured at the surface, did he exhale?
3. What is the P_{N_2} of air breathed at 99 feet?
4. A patient being treated in a hyperbaric chamber may become uncomfortably warm during
   a. Compression
   b. Decompression
5. Squeeze may occur during
   a. Ascent
   b. Descent

Glen H. Egstrom

3
Diving Equipment

The life support systems used in diving activities vary considerably with the diving circumstances and bottom time requirements. The following discussion will deal with the common types and some considerations for effective use.

Open Circuit Systems

The most common life support equipment is the open circuit self-contained underwater breathing apparatus (scuba). It consists of a tank or tanks for high pressure (1800-4750 psi) air and a regulator that will permit this air to be step-reduced to ambient pressure. Usually two such reduction steps will deliver air to a valve near the mouthpiece where a negative pressure exertion will result in flow of air to the lungs. Figures 3-1 and 3-2 illustrate the two most common open circuit demand systems. The two hose systems are becoming increasingly rare.

These systems are currently designed to deliver air to the diver at inhalation and exhalation resistances of less than $1^1/_2$ inches of water (3 inches maximum) during normal respiration at sea level. The resistance to breathing increases as a function of variables such as respiration rate increase, increased depth of water, temperature variations, etc. Resistance characteristics vary significantly with different regulator designs. Regulators which compensate for changing tank pressure have "balanced" first stage components. Un-

Balanced first stage

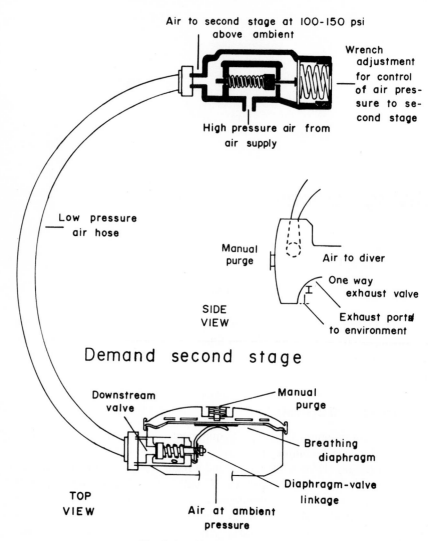

Air to second stage at 100-150 psi
above ambient

Wrench adjustment for control of air pressure to second stage

High pressure air from air supply

Low pressure air hose

Manual purge

Air to diver

One way exhaust valve

Exhaust ports to environment

SIDE VIEW

Demand second stage

Downstream valve

Manual purge

Breathing diaphragm

Diaphragm-valve linkage

TOP VIEW

Air at ambient pressure

Fig. 3-1.   Single hose regulator.

balanced regulators are undesirable because they provide variable resistance as tank pressure becomes low.

The single hose regulator has preempted the field largely because of its relative comfort in breathing and its low maintenance costs. Double hose regulators, due to the location of the first and second stage at the rear of the shoulders, become easier or more difficult to breathe as a result of the depth

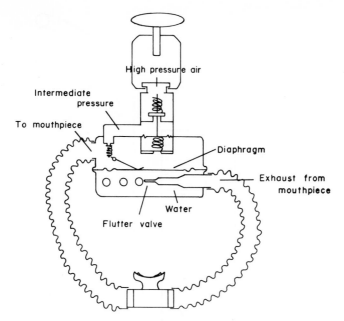

Fig. 3-2.   Double hose regulator.

difference from the mouthpiece to the regulator body. Swimming on the back becomes easier than swimming face down, for example. Surface swimming on the back will usually cause a free flow of air out of the mouthpiece which may cause concern about the resulting air loss. These regulators can free flow underwater in conditions where the mouthpiece is several inches shallower than the regulator body. This can create a hazardous situation for training maneuvers such as buddy breathing and other conditions where the diver removes his tanks and lets his mouthpiece float upward. Single hose regulators are slightly heavier in the mouth and tend to twist slightly to the right due to the hose attachment. This can lead to a tendency to grip the mouthpiece tighter and result in some discomfort in the supporting teeth or the attendant musculature.

Some recent developments in design of moldable mouthpieces permits the diver to spread the load of the regulator over a series of teeth on the top and bottom of both sides of the mouth. The resulting comfort may well relieve jaw fatigue and headaches due to excessive tension.

An inexpensive method for testing the breathing characteristics of a regulator requires a length of 3/16 inch I.D. clear tubing, a ruler, and some masking tape. A simple manometer is made by shaping a "U" with a ruler between the upright ends (see Fig. 3-3). One upright on the "U" should be 12-15 inches longer than the other. The tube should be fixed to a flat vertical surface with the ruler in the center between the uprights. The lower portion

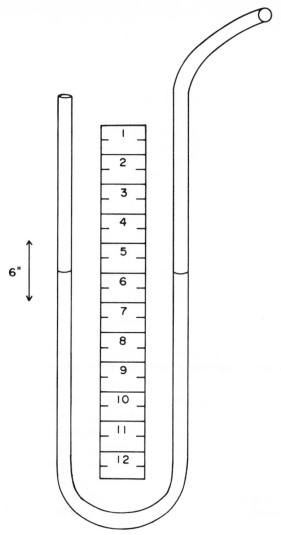

Fig. 3-3.   A simple manometer.

of the "U" is filled approximately one-half full of water and the ruler adjusted so that the tops of the water column are even with the middle of the ruler. With the regulator on a tank, the tube from the manometer is put into the corner of the mouth at the same time the mouthpiece is inserted. The regulator is then breathed normally and the water column will fluctuate with inhalation and exhalation pressure changes. If the fluctuations are excessive, ± 3 inches or more, then the regulator should be taken to a qualified repairman. This apparatus can also provide dramatic insight into the effect of increasing respiration rate upon breathing resistance of the regulator.

It should be remembered that the increased density of air due to depth will result in greater resistances to breathing as well as less effective ventilation in the lung itself, as more energy is required to move the gas during inhalation and exhalation.

Closed Circuit Systems

A typical closed circuit apparatus will consist of a mouthpiece and hoses connected to a breathing bag and CO_2—absorbent canister and an O_2 supply. The diver inhales O_2—enriched gas from the breathing bag and then pushes the exhaled air through the CO_2 absorbent and back into the bag while makeup O_2 is added in preparation for the next inhalation. The flow of oxygen into the breathing bag may be controlled manually by fixed flow or by automatic sensors that monitor oxygen pressure and maintain the partial pressure between preset ranges. These devices do not give off bubbles and are desirable for purposes where bubbles provide a distraction. They do, however, have several requirements for operation that require special training and, therefore, they are generally not considered appropriate equipment for sport divers.

The major concern with the use of closed-circuit apparatus lies in the use of high partial-pressure oxygen. In those systems using 100 percent O_2, the depth restriction is normally 25 fsw or less. Systems that utilize sensors to regulate the partial pressure of oxygen according to depth use an inert gas diluent such as nitrogen or helium as the background for mixing an appropriate breathing gas. The development of these systems is a very complex problem which requires an expensive solution. Full-time technical assistance is necessary for the maintenance and calibration of the systems. Generally several hours of topside effort are required for each underwater hour. A high degree of individual training in their use is also a fundamental prerequisite for safety and effectiveness.

Breathing resistance and large dead spaces are also common to these systems and generally interfere with the diver's ability to perform heavy work at depth.

Carbon dioxide buildup is also a significant threat since the absorbent materials tend to lose efficiency due to channeling of gas through the material, temperature drops, moisture accumulation, and CO_2 saturation.

The systems also require the diver to adjust the volume of gas in the breathing bag during descent. In closed-circuit systems using gas mixtures other than air, it is important to ensure that the oxygen content is not permitted to reach unsafe levels for the depth involved. The controls that permit the addition of inert gas should be clearly different than the controls for oxygen.

Shallow Water Gear

Sometimes referred to as "hookah" gear, this type of equipment is used where extended bottom time or topside communication is necessary. Shallow water gear normally consists of a mask or helmet, air hose, communication line and a surface air supply. It requires a surface tender who is knowledgable about the diving conditions and the divers habits. The diver and tender work as a team using either direct voice signals or pull signals on the umbilical. Since most shallow water systems are continuous flow, there is little chance for CO_2 buildup, although this is a potential hazard in demand-type configurations. A nonreturn valve on the air inlet hose of shallow water gear is a necessary precaution to avert squeeze due to a sudden pressure drop in the hose.

Specialized training is fundamental to working safely with this type of equipment, since umbilical handling procedures, communication techniques, and work methods are significantly different from scuba modes. Somers in his *Research Divers Manual* has a detailed description of this technique.

PERSONAL FLOTATION DEVICES

The use of inflatable devices attached to the diver has been the subject of controversy in scuba diving. The controversy centers on the question of the adequacy of these devices as an emergency measure. It has been generally conceded that the inflatable devices are *tools* to be used to adjust buoyancy for a comfortable dive or a long surface swim. The ditching of the weight belt is still generally held as the first order of action in the event of an emergency requiring a need for positive buoyancy.

There is, however, a trend toward a much more complex system of buoyancy compensation involving inflatable bladders which are connected to the low pressure port on the regulator for inflation directly from the tank. These systems use larger bladders mounted either in a horseshoe fashion around the tank, or in the conventional position on the chest and around the neck. They can be filled by oral inflation methods or directly from tank pressure by opening a valve. They are also equipped with large orifice "dump" valves for deflation purposes permitting rapid inflation and deflation. These more involved systems require additional amounts of training in order to use them effectively. It is believed that the ease of changing buoyancy should eliminate many of the minor emergencies which are felt to be significant contributors to diving accidents. It should be noted, however, that use of these systems does not diminish the need for basic watermanship skills and well-learned emergency procedures.

Basically, a personal flotation device should be easily inflated when using the oral inflator and should be sufficiently buoyant to float the diver in a faceup position, with the face clear of the water. An overpressure valve should be present to prevent overinflation of the vest. Many divers also utilize a crotch strap to hold the vest in position.

The large variation in vest design and placement of oral inflators, CO_2 detonators, inflation valves, hoses, and strapping makes it necessary to thoroughly check the operational procedure for the buddy's gear prior to a dive. It is recommended that groups who dive together develop standards for the types of inflatables to ensure that the placement and operation of inflation and deflation devices are at least similar for the group and appropriate for the diving conditions.

WEIGHT BELTS

Nearly all weights are mounted on a belt that encircles the waist, with a quick release-type buckle located at the front. Weight belts are implicated in many diving accidents, since they are often retained when they should be ditched. Training is obviously implicated in this problem since weight-belt ditching is rarely taught as a skill which must be overlearned. There are, however, several other potential problems:

1. If the weight belt is not snug during the dive, the belt may move, causing the buckle to change location. Some elastic-type belts compensate for the compression of wet suit materials; but, in others, the belt needs readjustment if it was not sufficiently tight on the surface.
2. A clear drop path for the belt is a necessity. Knives located on the outside of the leg have caught ditched belts on several occasions.
3. Adjustable belts, and buckles, in which the belt slides into the buckle, can cause a problem if the end of the belt that goes through the buckle is excessively long. The resulting failure is usually associated with the belt being restricted because of being crooked in the mouth of the buckle. Many programs are using wire buckles that interface with a metal "D" ring. When properly adjusted, they have a positive release and have the added advantage of providing a buckle which can be different from that used on the tank.
4. Weights will usually fail to fall off the body unless the person is nearly upright in the water. It is necessary to learn to pull the belt free of the body when ditching, since there is the possibility that the pressure from the tank may also restrict the free fall of the belt even in the upright position. This is particularly true in well-contoured females.
5. The release location for the belt is well away from the position of the hands of a struggling diver and calls for a rational decision and appropriate action for execution. Persons in a panic state appear to be incapable of such actions.

MASKS

The purpose of the mask is to provide an air pocket which permits the eye to focus, and thus allows the diver to see clearly underwater. The size of the air pocket can vary from that within a special contact lens to the large full-face masks or even helmets. The problems are related to visual distortions, restricted visual fields, and pressure-volume changes with attendant discomfort.

Visual distortion results from variations in the distance from the mask lens to the eye. Most basic diving texts refer to objects being one-quarter to one-third larger and closer. This is fairly accurate for vision directly to the front. As the eye moves across the flat lens, however, the focal length changes and images can be magnified by as much as 50 percent in the peripheral vision. Masks with side windows at corrected angles are somewhat better, but there is always a blind area or distorted area wherever the angle is changed. This can lead to an interesting phenomenon. If the side panel is at right angles to the front lens, a significant "blind area" is developed and a fish seen out of the side lens may disappear while swimming across the side, only to reappear swimming across the front lens.

Comfort with the mask is usually a function of a relatively large surface area for the "seal" and a small dead space.

The field of vision is a function of the distance of the lens from the eye and the obstruction of the nose. A given lens that is close to the eye permits a wider visual field. The length of the nose often becomes a limiting factor in getting the lens close to the eye, so we have masks with nose pockets. These pockets permit an increase in the peripheral visual field, but the somewhat bulky nose pocket increases the masking area of the nose and this significantly restricts the medial portion of the visual field.

Occasionally, the headband on the mask is used improperly, resulting in discomfort. The split at the back of the headband should spread the resistive load of the mask over the upper portion of the back of the skull. Individuals sometimes try to stop water leakage by excessive tightening of the elastic headband when the strap is located improperly at the base of the skull. The poor angle of pull on the mask requires excessive pressure and can result in considerable discomfort. It may also result in an apparent "mask squeeze." However, it should be remembered that mask squeeze occurs as a result of failure to equalize the pressure within the mask by exhaling slightly through the nose on descent. As the diver descends with the nose blocked, water pressure exceeds the gas pressure within the mask, which causes damage to the eye.

Most masks can be fitted with corrective lenses if necessary. These specially ground lenses are usually glued to the faceplate itself. Attempts at installing "glasses" into the mask are usually unsatisfactory.

FINS

Fins are worn to increase the surface area of the foot and are found in a wide variety of configurations and degrees of flexibility.

The criteria for evaluating fins involves comfort, types of activity for which they will be used, and the strength of the user. A study of nine popular fins was conducted at University of California, Los Angeles. Nine subjects were asked to use each fin in random order on two occasions in a blind test under three different work loads. The subjects ranged in size from 6 feet 4 inches to 5 feet 5 inches and were experienced divers. The parameters which were measured included heart rate, respiration rate, thrust level, kick rate, oxygen uptake, CO_2 output, and, in many cases, a filmed recording of the kick style.

As a result of this testing, it was determined that no single fin proved best for all subjects, nor did any fin prove worst. There was evidence that the longer, narrower fins tended to be slightly more efficient than the shorter, wider fins. There was no evidence that the three pairs of fins with vents were superior to those without vents. There was evidence that leg length and strength were more important variables than fin style.

Kicking style was also a critical factor. It is important to apply the resistance of the fin in the direction opposite to the diver's intended swimming path. In Figure 3-4A, the vector of force at 90° of knee flexion is directly to the rear, while at 30° of flexion (Fig. 3-4B) it is nearly directly perpendicular to the desired path of travel. When the legs cross, forward thrust becomes essentially zero. Maximum forward thrust occurs between 90° and 45° of knee flexion. Thus, the widened kicking style is more efficient.

The diver who has insufficient strength and endurance, a poor kick style, or a fin that is not suitable, may suffer discomfort from foot cramps, calf cramps, and/or blisters. It is not unreasonable to expect a novice diver to begin with relatively flexible fins and progressively adapt to larger and more rigid fins as experience is gained and strength and endurance levels improve. Each new pair of fins, however, will require a "breaking-in" period when the diver is adapting. It is not wise to take a new, stronger fin and immediately use it on a strenuous dive.

SNORKELS

Many divers find the adaptation to the use of the snorkel to be one of the most difficult challenges in diving. The evolution of the snorkel in its early phases was based largely on sales appeal, rather than on function. An adequate snorkel should permit the diver to work relatively hard on the surface without encountering resistances that would significantly impair adequate

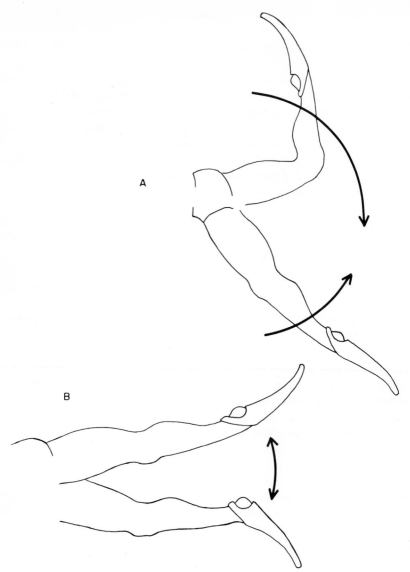

Fig. 3-4. The wide kick (A) is more efficient than the narrow kick (B).

ventilation. Long, small-diameter tubes with unnecessary bends or corruga-
tions are undesirable. Most current snorkels will permit a relaxed diver to lie
on the surface and look about. Few snorkels, however, will permit the diver to
work steadily against a strong current. To double the flow rate, the diver must
overcome four times the resistance to breathing. The snorkel must be considered an extension of the airway and should provide a minimum of resis-

tance. If the diver begins to feel starved for air while snorkeling he should consider swimming on his back with the snorkel and, if necessary, the mask removed from the mouth and nose. An inflated vest is also recommended during long swims.

The snorkel mouthpiece should be placed so that it fits the gums and teeth. Blisters can occur easily if the edges of the mouthpiece are not smoothly aligned in the mouth. Adjustable mouthpieces and moldable tooth grips are desirable.

THERMAL PROTECTION

In most areas, cold is a primary cause of discomfort while diving. The neoprene wet suit was a revolutionary improvement in diver comfort, and diving time can now be extended by a factor of two or three.

Even in tropical waters, it is often desirable to use a thin neoprene top or even a full wet suit, depending on the depth of the dives. Individuals who have adapted to the hot climates are especially susceptible to the cooling effects of water.

Heavier wet-suit materials provide additional restriction to movement and a proper fit becomes increasingly critical. Chafing and blisters are consistent with a poor fit, especially behind the knees and under the armpits. Bulges also provide additional water movement inside the suit which reduces its insulating capacity.

Recently, neoprene dry suits have increased in popularity in colder water areas. These suits permit an insulating layer of air to be kept inside the neoprene envelope. Air, being an excellent insulator, efficiently retains the body heat and greater comfort results. Leaks in such suits result in loss of buoyancy and insulative capacity, but are easily repaired and, therefore, are only a minor problem in contrast to leaks in the thin rubber sheet material used in earlier dry suits.

Significant reductions in mobility and an increased energy cost of work are trade-offs that a diver must adapt to if thermal protective suits are worn.

STUDY QUESTIONS

1. A closed circuit scuba apparatus is potentially dangerous because
    a. The potential for CO_2 buildup is increased
    b. High partial pressures of O_2 can create problems at depth
    c. Breathing resistance can become excessive
    d. All of the above

2. Personal floatation devices are standardized for emergency inflation.
   a. True
   b. False
3. Ditching the weight belt can be complicated by the diver's attitude in relation to the surface.
   a. True
   b. False
4. The magnification by a face mask is consistent as the eye travels across the lens.
   a. True
   b. False
5. A shoulder width flutter kick with the legs held straight without stiffness is recommended for scuba divers.
   a. True
   b. False
6. Increasing the airway resistance in a snorkel by a factor of four is the result of doubling the flow through the tube.
   a. True
   b. False

Nicholas R. Anthonisen

4

Respiratory System in Diving

BOYLE'S LAW, THE LUNG AND BAROTRAUMA

Boyle's law can only be applied easily to gas in the lung when the mass of gas is constant, i.e., when the lung is not free to communicate with a gas source. This of course is a complicated way of defining breath-holding or complete airway obstruction. When a diver holds his breath and changes depth, Boyle's law applies to the gas in his lung—it is compressed or expanded and lung volume changes. Appreciation of the significance of lung volume changes may be enhanced by referring to Figure 4-1 which is a representation of the pressure-volume curves to the human chest wall and lung. These are essentially stress-strain curves indicating the volume attained by each of these structures when a given pressure difference is imposed across it. Conventionally these pressure differences are computed by subtracting pressure outside the structure from pressure inside it. The slope of each curve is the stiffness or compliance of the structure. Increases in lung gas pressure increase lung volume and at 100 percent of total lung capacity (TLC) the lung is very stiff—it has reached the limit of its expansion. Decreases in gas pressure decrease lung volume but do not empty the lungs because at residual volume (RV) the chest wall has approached the limit of its compression and becomes very stiff.

If a diver takes a breath of compressed air at 99 feet (4 ata), breath-holds at 50 percent TLC and ascends, the lung gas expands and at 33 feet (2 ata) his lung volume has doubled—he is at 100 percent TLC. According to Figure 4-1, his lung has reached the limit of expansion; further pressure increases

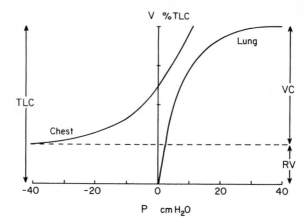

Fig. 4-1. Static pressure-volume curves of the human lung and chest wall. Ordinate: volume as a percent of the maximum (total lung capacity, TLC). Abscissa: pressure, cm H_2O. Pressure is pressure across the lungs (mouth minus pleural surface) or across the chest wall (pleural surface minus ambient). These curves were generated by having a subject go to the requisite volume voluntarily, then relax. Also indicated is the gas volume in the lung at maximal expiration (RV). The difference between TLC and RV is the vital capacity (VC).

will not increase lung volume. Further ascent then increases pressure across the lung to more than 40 cm H_2O. At pressures of 60 to 80 mm Hg, the lung ruptures and gas leaks out either into the pleural space, causing pneumothorax, or into the lung interstitium. From the latter locus it can either dissect into the mediastinum or enter the pulmonary veins and give rise to air embolism.[1] Whether during a given ascent the lung ruptures or not therefore depends on the pressures involved and the lung volume at which the breath is held. If breath-holding commences at TLC, surfacing from a depth of 3 to 4 feet should suffice. Finally, air embolism has been documented in subjects who did not breath-hold. Presumably, this was the result of airway obstruction within the lung with local rupture.

When the breath is held and the subject descends, lung gas is compressed and the lung volume shrinks, until RV is reached. At this point, the chest wall has reached its limit and lung volume can decrease no further. Further descent creates a negative pressure within the thoracic cavity and alveoli, and blood is shifted into the lungs. At some point during descent the pulmonary capillaries become engorged, leak, and rupture with pulmonary edema and hemorrhage. This is termed lung squeeze and was seen in surface-supplied diving with valve failures or when the diver fell from one depth to another faster than the pressure of his air supply could be increased.[2] It has been observed in breath-hold divers. A similar syndrome may be induced by submersion and snorkel breathing if the distance below the surface is great enough (3 feet) that very negative pressures are required to maintain ventilation.

It follows from the above that the potential for lung squeeze must limit the depth attained by breath-hold divers. The normal RV is about 25 percent TLC, so that if the diver started at TLC his lungs should be compressed to RV at about 100 feet. In some young men RV is only 16 percent TLC, so they theoretically could descend to 6 ata or 165 feet before reaching RV. In fact, breath-hold divers have reached depths approximating 250 feet; this depth must have been achieved by shifting blood into the chest. Indeed, at such depths something on the order of 50 percent of the chest volume at surface RV must be filled with blood.[3] This accomplishment pales when compared to that of some diving mammals which descend to more than 1000 feet. Such dives can only be accomplished if these animals have very flexible rib cages and/or intrathoracic vasculature which permit very large blood shifts. Probably both are present.[4,5] Further, at least some diving mammals have cartilage in small airways.[6] This may prevent these airways from collapsing as lung volume is reduced, so that air is expressed from alveoli to airways. Airways, because of their poor blood supply, take up N_2 less efficiently than alveoli so these animals are not susceptible to decompression sickness. In human lungs, small airways collapse as lung volume is reduced, leaving N_2 trapped in alveoli; decompression sickness has been reported in a human after multiple breath-hold dives.[7]

Boyle's law has one final application to the lung in diving. Face masks include the nose so that lung gas may be used to equalize pressures in the mask during descent and avoid facial squeeze, a syndrome of conjunctival capillary engorgement and rupture.

VENTILATION AND GAS EXCHANGE—LIMITATIONS AT DEPTH

Gas Density and Lung Mechanics

Compressed gas diving involves breathing a medium of increased density, a fact that has attracted numerous respiratory physiologists to the diving field. A good deal of elegant experimentation has gone on in this area, with the result that many of the proposed problems are presently at a satisfactory state of resolution.

Dense gas is harder to breathe than light gas because the flow resistive properties of a gas are directly related to its density. To appreciate this and several other points to be considered in this chapter, it is first necessary to briefly review lung mechanics. Lungs have elastic recoil which opposes inflation; to maintain them at a given static volume, tracheal or alveolar pressure

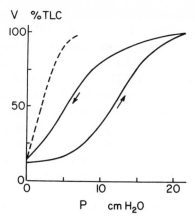

Fig. 4-2. Static pressure-volume curves of an excised lung. Ordinate: volume in percent maximum.
Abscissa: pressure (mouth minus pleural surface).
The solid line was generated by filling and emptying
the lung with air, the dashed one by filling and
emptying the lung with saline.

must exceed lung surface (pleural) pressure by an amount that is related to the
volume chosen. This relationship was shown schematically by the lung
pressure-volume curve of Figure 4-1. A more detailed pressure-volume curve
of the lung is shown in Figure 4-2. Curves like these are generated by inflating
a lung in stepwise fashion and measuring pressure during the pauses (no gas
flow) between steps. It can be seen that the curve demonstrates hysteresis—the
course followed during deflation is different from that followed during inflation. More pressure is required to attain a given volume during inflation. Also
shown in Figure 4-2 is a static pressure volume curve of the same lung when
inflated with saline as opposed to air. Inflation is achieved with much smaller
pressures than was the case with air; much of the elastic recoil of the lung has
vanished. The difference between the saline and air curves simply indicates
that the lung is a liquid-gas interphase and that as such exhibits surface tension which tends to reduce surface area and collapse the lung.[8] Removal of
surface tension by lung inflation with saline deprives the lung of most of its
elastic recoil. It also abolishes hysteresis, indicating that this too is a function
of surface tension. Though most of the lung recoil is the result of forces at the
liquid-gas interphase, it can easily be calculated that the lung does not behave
as if it were lined with normal saline; if it were, much greater pressures would
be required for inflation and there would be no hysteresis. In fact, lungs are
lined by lipoprotein (surfactant) that reduces surface tension, especially during deflation from high lung volumes (Fig. 4-2). The presence of surfactant
maintains alveoli in the gas-filled state, even at low lung volumes. Its absence
results in massive atelectasis.

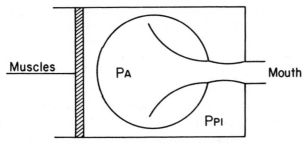

Fig. 4-3. Model of respiratory system. The lung is a balloon inside a boxlike thorax. Respiratory muscular movements are symbolized by a piston in the thorax. The airway has in intrapulmonary segment, an extrapulmonary intrathoracic segment, and an extrathoracic segment. Breathing is accomplished by the respiratory muscles changing pleural pressure (P_{pl}), which changes alveolar pressure (P_A); the two pressures are related by the elastic recoil of the lung (Pel).

The lung-chest system is depicted schematically in Figure 4-3. Ventilation is achieved by changing pressure in the pleural space. During lung inflation, some of this pressure is used to increase lung volume as indicated in Figures 4-1 and 4-2. However, to breathe it is also necessary to cause gas to flow from mouth to alveoli, and part of the pressure generated by the respiratory muscles is used in overcoming flow resistance in the airways between these two points. Flow resistance (R) is analogous to electrical resistance and, in the case of gas flowing through a tube, relates flow (V, liters/second) to the pressure drop (P, cm H_2O) from one end of the tube to another; for example, $VR = P$. The flow resistance of small tubes is obviously higher than that of large tubes; but, in the lung, the total cross-sectional area of the small airways is greater than that of the large airways so that the total bronchiolar resistance is much less than that of the trachea.[9] For this reason the peripheral airways of Figure 4-3 are drawn to indicate a large cross-section and low resistance. During quiet breathing, only inspiration is active—inspiratory muscles decrease pleural pressure and lung volume increases. Expiration is achieved by simply stopping inspiration; with muscle relaxation, the elastic recoil of the lung returns the system to its starting point—the functional residual capacity (FRC). Most of the pressure generated by the respiratory muscles during quiet breathing is therefore used to overcome the elastic recoil of the lung. However, as ventilation is increased, as in exercise, flow resistance becomes a much more important factor and necessitates that expiration be achieved by contraction of expiratory muscles. Indeed, maximum ventilation is limited by flow resistance, specifically flow resistance during expiration. With forced expiration, pleural pressure is increased to as much as 100 to 200 cm H_2O. Alveolar pressure, which is the pressure driving gas out of the lungs, is equal to pleural pressure plus the pressure due to the elastic recoil of the lung at the particular volume considered (see Figs. 4-1 and 4-2), so that there is a very large pressure difference between mouth and alveolus. However, the pleural pressure is also applied to the intrathoracic, extrapulmonary airways. If the flow resistance of the intrapulmonary airways is high enough for pressure loss in them to equal the elastic recoil pressure of the lung, then the pressure inside the extrapulmonary intrathoracic airways (i.e., trachea) is less than the pressure outside them and they collapse, limiting the expiratory flow rates. This dynamic collapse of airways occurs in practice at lung volumes of less than 70 percent VC in normal men and limits both forced expiration and maximum ventilation.[10]

Thus, in examining ventilatory capability in normal men, determinations of maximum expiratory flow at 50 percent VC measure fundamentally the same thing as do determinations of maximum voluntary ventilation. Both depend on flow resistance, and flow resistance is dependant on gas density. The nature of this relationship depends on the kind of flow being dealt with. In humans, at virtually all levels of exercise, flow in large airways is turbulent and, under these circumstances, flow is inversely proportional to the square root of gas density.

$$V = \frac{K}{\sqrt{\text{density}}}$$

That is to say, if flow through a given tube were 8 liters/second at 1 ata, when the gas density was increased fourfold (4 ata), flow would be halved. This prediction, which would be entirely accurate for stainless steel pipes, holds remarkably well for intact humans,[11,12] whether maximum flow at a given lung volume or maximum voluntary ventilation is measured (Figure 4-4). One feature of this relationship perhaps not apparent from Figure 4-4 but obvious from Equation 1 is that while gas density need only be quadrupled to halve ventilation, it must increase 16-fold to limit ventilation to one-quarter of its original value.

What does all this mean in terms of the diver? Is the kind of ventilatory limitation shown in Figure 4-4 of significance, and if so, to whom? Let us consider the simplest case first, that of the exercising air-breathing diver. At 1 ata, even at maximal exercise, normal humans utilize only 50 to 60 percent of their maximum voluntary ventilation (Figure 4-4), which is roughly equal to maximum voluntary ventilation at 4 ata (100 feet). At this depth, however, exercising subjects regularly approach 100 percent of their maximum voluntary ventilation (Anthonisen, unpublished data); so that to depths of 100 feet there should be virtually no ventilation-imposed exercise limitation in the air-breathing diver. At greater depths nitrogen narcosis is probably as important

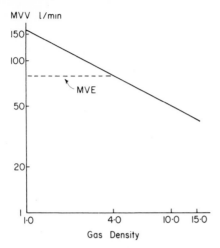

MVV l/min

Fig. 4-4. Ventilation (ordinate) as a function of gas density (abscissa). Both ordinate and abscissa are logarithmic scales. Maximum voluntary ventilation is symbolized by the solid line and maximum exercise ventilation by the dashed line.

a factor in limiting exercise as is increased flow resistance. Because of nitrogen narcosis, helium is used as the inert gas in virtually all deep diving. In addition to its nonnarcotic property, helium has the advantage of extremely low density—1/7 that of nitrogen. Breathing helium, gas densities equivalent to air at 100 feet are approached at depths of 600 feet. Indeed, it is almost certain that useful physical exercise can be performed by divers breathing helium at depths greater than 2000 feet.[12]

This discussion has assumed that all the resistance to breathing is within the lungs. Practically speaking, this is not the case. All scuba gear has discernible resistance, and this resistance probably obeys the rules just outlined. The double-hose (7/8-inch internal diameter) open circuit scuba used so long by the U. S. Navy constitutes a formidable load on the respiratory system. Fortunately, modern single-hose rigs and semiclosed systems have considerably better flow-resistive properties. Finally, the human respiratory system is not very sensitive to moderate external resistance because dynamic airway collapse during forced expiration remains the limiting factor.[3] Thus we feel that if good equipment is used, gas density should not limit the scuba divers activities.[12]

Gas Density and Pulmonary Gas Exchange

A second effect of increased gas density which has interested respiratory physiologists is the fact that increased density slows gas-in-gas diffusion. This process is vital in human respiration: during normal breathing the tidal

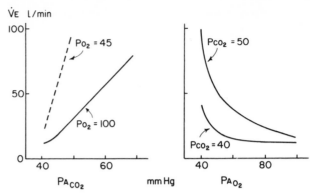

Fig. 4-5. Ventilatory responses to CO_2 (left) and hypoxia (right). Ordinates: minute ventilation. Abscissae: alveolar CO_2 (left) and O_2 (right) tensions. These curves were generated by having the subjects inhale gas mixtures containing appropriate amounts of O_2 and CO_2 and measuring minute volume of ventilation and alveolar (end-tidal) O_2 and CO_2 tensions. Shown are curves in which CO_2 was varied at two fixed O_2 tensions (left) and in which O_2 was varied at two fixed CO_2 tensions (right).

volume is 0.5 to 0.7 liters, while the volume of gas in the lungs before the breath (functional residual capacity, FRC) is 3.0 to 3.5 liters. For optimum O_2 and CO_2 exchange between alveoli and pulmonary capillaries, there must be adequate mixing between alveolar FRC-gas and the fresh inspirate of the tidal volume. There is ample evidence that this mixing occurs through gas-in-gas diffusion, O_2 diffusing from the inspirate to the alveolar wall and CO_2 diffusing in the reverse direction. Seriously slowing the diffusion process would have the same general effect as increasing the respiratory dead space—gas would be inhaled and exhaled, but relatively little exchange with capillary blood would occur. This problem has been investigated in both animals and man; and while there are some discernible density dependant effects on gas exchange, they are not important. There is no evidence that breathing dense gas significantly limits O_2 and CO_2 exchange.[14,15]

Diving and Ventilatory Control

An area of respiratory physiology of particular relevance to divers is that of ventilatory control. Early reports indicated that some working divers showed striking elevations of end-tidal CO_2 tension,[16] which is usually equivalent to alveolar or arterial CO_2 tension. This, in the presence of a normal metabolic output of CO_2, indicates alveolar hypoventilation (alveolar ventilation times alveolar CO_2 equals metabolic CO_2 output). As has been

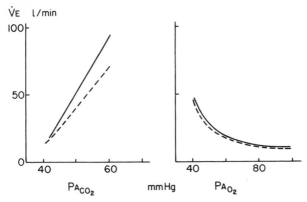

Fig. 4-6. Ventilatory responses to CO_2 (left) and O_2 (right) at 1 and 4 ata. Ordinates and abscissae as in Figure 4-5. Dashed lines are data at 4 ata, solid lines are data at 1 ata. The CO_2 response curves were generated at alveolar O_2 of 200 mm Hg; the O_2 responses were generated at alveolar CO_2 of 40 mm Hg. At 4 ata the CO_2 response is depressed, but the hypoxic response is not.

discussed, density dependant increases in flow resistance do not limit ventilation under most circumstances; so the observed hypoventilation was not due to an absolute inability to increase ventilation, but was due to a choice made by the diver, which, in turn, implies an alteration of the normal ventilatory control system.

In simplified form, the ventilatory control system may be considered as a system concerned with error detection and minimization. The errors detected are those of arterial O_2 and CO_2 tension, specifically hypercapnia and hypoxia. There are two sensing sites, one in or about the medulla oblongata which is sensitive to CO_2. The other receptors are located chiefly in the carotid bodies; they are sensitive to hypoxia and also to CO_2, but are probably responsible for a relatively minor share of the total CO_2 response. Hypercapnia is a powerful stimulus to ventilation, while hypoxia is a relatively feeble one (Fig. 4-5). When both hypoxia and hypercapnia are present simultaneously, the ventilatory response is greater than that seen when the two stimuli are presented individually and the responses summed by the investigator (Fig. 4-5). Increases of external airway resistance depress the ventilatory response to CO_2, probably because true response to hypercapnia is one of increased effort on the part of the respiratory muscles and resistance decreases the amount of ventilation resulting from a given augmentation of effort.[17] The same is true to a lesser extent in the case of hypoxia.[18] The increases in internal flow resistance attendant on increases in gas density have the same effect:[19] CO_2 response is depressed, the O_2 response much less so (Fig. 4-6). As indicated in Figure 4-5, CO_2 responses at high O_2 levels are less than at low. High O_2 levels and

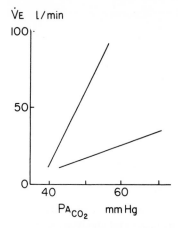

Fig. 4-7. Normal variation in ventilatory response to CO_2. Ordinate: minute ventilation. Abscissa: alveolar CO_2 tension. Shown are two curves representing extreme responses of normal subjects to inhaled CO_2 at alveolar O_2 of more than 200 mm Hg.

increased gas density prevail in many underwater situations; so CO_2 retention due to decreased CO_2 sensitivity might be a rational thing to expect.

However, these observations were made in resting nondivers, while CO_2 retention was observed in working divers. When nondivers exercise at 4 ata, no diminution of ventilation or CO_2 retention is observed; at greater depths, CO_2 retention should be observed only during very heavy exercise. It is possible that divers have different ventilatory control systems from nondivers. Normal variations in the ventilatory response to CO_2 are wide (Fig. 4-7), and it has been repeatedly stated that divers as a group tend to exhibit relative sluggish CO_2 responses.[16] Divers also tend to ventilate less during exercise than nondivers.[20] Whether these findings are learned responses or the result of diver selection is an interesting and unanswered question.

A further problem in ventilatory control and its assessment is the breathing pattern employed by many divers at depth. This consists of employing very large tidal volumes and low frequencies with end-inspiratory breath-holds. Use of low breathing frequencies per se decreases ventilatory response to CO_2, and prolonged inspiratory breath-holds have the effects of maximizing pulmonary gas exchange per unit ventilation and causing end-tidal CO_2 to be an overestimate of arterial CO_2.[21]

To summarize, respiratory sensitivity to CO_2 is reduced by a number of conditions which prevail at depth, such as low breathing rates, high O_2, and increased gas density. Experienced divers appear to have reduced ventilatory responses to both CO_2 and exercise. These may well be adequate explanations for the tendency of working divers to retain CO_2. This CO_2 retention tends to conserve breathing gas and limit ventilatory effort, but it is doubtful that these benefits outweigh the dangers of CO_2 narcosis.

LIQUID BREATHING

Theoretically, any medium that can be moved in and out of the lungs, contains enough O_2, and will remove CO_2 is a suitable breathing medium. If a liquid could be found that qualified, it would represent an enormous advance in diving. Liquids are not compressible, so air embolism and lung squeeze would not exist. Liquids could contain O_2 at nontoxic levels without containing inert gases, so decompression sickness would be impossible. In theory, a liquid could be equilibrated with O_2 at 1 ata and supplied to the diver who could descend as far and as fast as he wanted, stay as long as his liquid lasted, and surface immediately. Diving would be revolutionized.

Animal liquid-breathing experiments have been conducted which have proven these advantages and outlined the problems that will have to be solved to realize the benefits. Dogs and mice have breathed oxygenated saline.[22] Because O_2 is not very soluble in water, the saline had to be oxygenated hyperbarically. Though some animals survived, it was clear that this was not the system of the future. Saline is very dense and viscous compared to gas; pulmonary saline flow resistance was very high. In addition, use of saline as a breathing medium eliminated the lung recoil due to surface tension. While this may have facilitated inspiration, static lung recoil—the tendency for the lung to collapse—is an important factor in maintaining expiratory flow rates and therefore ventilation. Indeed, under conditions of dynamic airway compression, the elastic recoil of the lungs is the driving pressure for intrapulmonary flow (see Fig. 4-3). For these reasons, it was immediately clear that intact humans would never be able to move enough saline in and out of their lungs to support useful activity.

Further, O_2 and CO_2 diffusion are 1000 times slower in saline than in air. Because of this diffusion, "mixing" of O_2 and CO_2 between the tidal breath and the saline FRC was grossly impaired—the respiratory dead space was enormously increased. Because of this effect plus the fact that the animals could not be hyperventilated, there was progressive, severe CO_2 retention during saline breathing. Finally, saline lavage of lungs is one of the commonly used methods to obtain pulmonary surfactant; and though it has not been proven, one must suspect that saline ventilation tended to wash surfactant out of the lung.

A major advance in the liquid breathing field was the development of fluorocarbon liquids.[23] Both O_2 and CO_2 are remarkably soluble in these liquids. Equilibrated with O_2 at 1 ata fluorocarbons contain enough O_2 to ensure adequate exchange in the lung. Fluorocarbons are more dense than saline, are immiscible in water, and have a lower surface tension than saline. They therefore do not wash surfactant out of the lung, do not totally deprive the lung of its surface dependant elastic recoil, but may be more flow resistive than saline. Artificial ventilation has succeeded in maintaining normal levels of arterial CO_2 in animals.[24] However, moving fluorocarbon is not easy and most animal studies have shown CO_2 retention. We are unaware of studies of the dead space effect due to limitation of O_2 and CO_2 diffusion in fluorocarbon, but this is likely to be significant.

In summary, liquid breathing offers major theoretical advantages in diving. Unfortunately, because liquids are extremely difficult to move in and out of the lung and because they are poor vehicles for O_2 and CO_2 diffusion, it appears that further breakthroughs will have to be made in this area before human liquid breathing can be attempted.

CHEST MEDICINE RELEVANT TO DIVING

Diving medicine is not a branch of chest medicine or any other conventional specialty. However, diving and chest medicine do overlap in some areas. Diagnosis and treatment of lung rupture without air embolism are similar in the two areas. Pneumothorax and pneumomediastinum present with chest pain, cough, and dyspnea. Palpable air may be present in the neck in pneumomediastinum; breath sounds may be decreased over pneumothoraces; and, in both syndromes, a variety of crunching, crackling noises may be associated with the heart beat. Pneumomediastinum is treated by watchful waiting while pneumothorax associated with diving is usually treated by pleural suction. Both are usually diagnosed by x-ray, but in the diving situation it may be necessary to put a needle in the pleural space for diagnostic purposes. Concern about diagnosis and treatment should never delay treatment of associated air embolism which should be suspected.

As chest physicians and divers, we are frequently asked to comment on the physical qualifications of other divers. Individuals will not be passed with abnormal chest x-rays, especially those with blebs or bullae, since these may predispose to lung rupture. For the same reason, subjects with significant obstructive lung disease, either bronchitis or asthma, are also rejected. Beyond this, there are no pulmonary qualifications for diving. Good general physical shape and experience are the most precious assets.

REFERENCES

1. Lanphier EH: Overinflation of lungs, in Fenn WO, Rahn H (eds): Handbook of Physiology, Sect. 3: Respiration, vol. 11, Washington, D.C., American Physiological Society, 1965, p 1189

2. US Navy, US Navy Diving Manual, NAVSHIPS, 250:538, Part 1, Washington, D.C., Navy Dept, 1963, 1.6.8

3. Schaefer KI, Allison RD, Dougherty JH Jr, et al: Pulmonary and circulatory adjustment determining the limits of depths in breath-hold diving. Report Naval Department 531, Submarine Medical Research Laboratory, 1968

4. Andersen HT: Cardiovascular adaptations in diving mammals. Am Heart J 74:295, 1967

5. Harrison RJ, Tomlinson JDW: Normal and experimental diving in the common seal *(Phoca vitulina)*. Mammalia 24: 386, 1960

6. Denison DM, Warrell DA, West JB: Airway structure and alveolar emptying in the lungs of sea lions and dogs. Respir Physiol 13:253-160, 1971

7. Paulev P-E: Decompression sickness following repeated breath-hold dives. J Appl Physiol 20:1028-1031, 1965

8. Radford EP Jr: Static mechanic properties of mammalian lungs, in Fenn WO, Rahn H (eds): Handbook of Physiology, Sect 3: Respiration, vol 1, Washington, D.C., American Physiological Society, 1964, p. 429

9. Weibel E: Morphometrics of the lung, in Fenn WO, Rahn H (eds): Handbook of Physiology, Sect 3: Respiration, vol. 1. Washington, D.C., American Physiological Society, 1964

10. Pride NB, Permutt S, Riley RL, Bromberger-Barnea B: Determinants of maximum expiratory flow from the lungs. J Appl Physiol 23:646-662, 1967

11. Wood LDH, Bryan AC: Effect of increased ambient pressure on the flow-volume curve of the lung. J Appl Physiol 27:4-8, 1969

12. Anthonisen NR, Bradley ME, Vorosmarti J, et al: Mechanics of breathing with helium-oxygen and neon-oxygen mixtures in deep saturation diving, in Lambertsen CJ (ed): Underwater Physiology, Proceedings of the Fourth Symposium on Underwater Physiology. New York and London, Academic Press, 1971, p 339

13. Demedts M, Anthonisen NR: Effects of increased external airway resistance during steady-state exercise. J Appl Physiol 35:361-366, 1973

14. Wood LDH, Levison H, Bow SK, et al: Effect of helium on gas exchange and lung mechanics in asthma. Fed Proc 29:269, 1970

15. Martin RR, Zutter M, Anthonisen NR: Pulmonary gas exchange in dogs breathing SF_6 at 4 ata. J Appl Physiol 33:86-92, 1972

16. Lanphier EH: Pulmonary function, in Bennett PB, Elliott DH (eds): The Physiology and Medicine of Diving and Compressed Air Work. London, Balliere, Tindall, and Cossell, 1969, p 84

17. Milic-Emili J, Tyler JM: Relation between work output of respiratory muscles and end tidal CO_2 tension. J Appl Physiol 18:497-504, 1963

18. Barnett JB, Rasmussen B: Ventilatory responses to hypoxia and hypercapnia with external airway resistance. Acta Physiol Scand 80:538-551, 1970

19. Doell D, Zutter M, Anthonisen NR: Ventilatory responses to hypercapnia and hypoxia at 1 and 4 ata. Respir Physiol 18:338-346, 1973

20. Lally DA, Zechman FW, Tracy RA: Ventilatory responses to exercise in divers and non divers. Respir Physiol 20:117-129, 1974

21. Nye RE Jr: Influence of the cyclical pattern of ventilatory flow on pulmonary gas exchange. Respir Physiol 10:321-337, 1970

22. Kylstra JA, Paganelli CV, Lanphier EH: Pulmonary gas exchange in dogs ventilated with hyperbarically oxygenated liquid. J Appl Physiol 21:177-184, 1966
23. Clark LC Jr: Proceedings of a symposium on inert organic liquids for biological oxygen transport. Fed Proc 29:1695, 1970
24. Sass DJ, Ritmann EL, Caskey PE, et al: Liquid breathing: prevention of pulmonary arteriovenous shunting during acceleration. J Appl Physiol 32:451-455, 1972

STUDY QUESTIONS

1. Lung squeeze is seen in one or more of the following:
   a. Scuba diving
   b. Breath-hold diving
   c. Aviators
   d. Hard-hat divers
2. Patients with air embolism usually become symptomatic on arrival at the surface. Why?
3. At 265 feet breathing air, a diver's maximum voluntary ventilation is reduced by how much?
4. Does dynamic compression of airways occur during inspiration?
5. Give four factors that tend to cause CO_2 retention in divers.
6. List the most important advantages of fluorocarbons over saline as breathing liquids.

Carl Edmonds

5

Barotrauma*

Barotrauma is probably the commonest occupational disease of divers. It refers to the tissue damage resulting from expansion or contraction of gas spaces that are found within, or adjacent to, the body. It is a direct effect of the gas volume changes that cause tissue distortion. The normal relationship between changes of volume of gas and the pressure applied to it is described by Boyle's Law. This states that if the temperature remains constant, the volume of a given mass of gas is inversely proportional to the absolute pressure; i.e., as the pressure increases, gas is compressed and its volume diminishes; whereas if the pressure decreases, then that volume of gas is allowed to expand. When this contraction and expansion of gases occurs within the body tissues, then damage to these tissues is likely. Because descent in the water results in an increased pressure applied to the body and all its contents, the contraction of enclosed gas spaces will result in barotrauma of descent. With ascent in the water and the associated reduction in pressures applied to the body and all its contents, enclosed gas spaces will expand and result in barotrauma of ascent. As these two physiological and pathological changes are opposite, it is easy to understand why the clinical symptoms related to descent and ascent are often dissimilar, even though they affect the same organs.

Some of the gas spaces within the body are surrounded by distensible tissues, e.g., the gut; therefore, these are not commonly the site of barotrauma.

*This chapter has been modified with approval from *Diving and Sub-aquatic Medicine (1976)* by Edmonds, Lowry and Pennefather, a Diving Medical Centre Publication, 6 Hale Road, Mosman 2088 Australia.

Other gas spaces are surrounded by solid structures such as the sinus and middle ear; here, unless the openings to these cavities are patent, barotrauma is common. Other gas spaces involve tissues with limited distensibility, e.g., the lungs. Some gas spaces may be artificial or pathological, e.g., the space within the face mask or between the diver's suit and his body, or cavities within carious teeth. These spaces are equally likely to involve body tissue with changes of pressure and are therefore potential sites of barotrauma.

As an example of this disorder,[1] one maxillary sinus with a blocked ostium may be used to illustrate the pathophysiology. At the surface, both the cavity within the maxillary sinus and the diver's body tissues are both at 1 ata as he descends underwater to 33 feet or 10 meters; according to Boyle's Law, the gas volume within the sinus will be reduced to approximately 50 percent of the predive volume. If the sinus cavity was a rigid pressure-resistant canister, this would not happen, and the air within the sinus would remain at 1 ata.

In practice, the bony wall of the sinus is penetrated by multiple apertures for the transmission of tissue and blood vessels. These apertures enable pressure changes within the body of the diver, occurring outside the sinus, to be transmitted to the internal lining of the sinus. There is thus a potential gradient of 2 atm outside the sinus to 1 atm inside the sinus. As the pressure is transmitted through the blood vessels and the apertures, there is a movement of tissue and fluid into the sinus mucosa. This leads to vascular congestion and edema within the mucosa. The swelling of the mucosa is limited, and once its limit is exceeded, hemorrhage will occur either into the mucosa itself, the submucosal space, or the lumen of the sinus. It is this compensatory element which occupies space and allows the air to contract to the expected volume according to Boyle's Law. Under these circumstances, the sinus will eventually become pressurized to 2 ata.

From this example, it can be seen that the main cause for pathology is a pressure difference between the body tissues and the enclosed gas spaces. In the same example, when ascent commences, the pressure differential is reversed. The expanding gas will distend the sinus, together with its congested edematous and hemorrhagic mucosa, and is likely to cause pain prior to an explosive release of pressure—usually through the sinus ostium, with blood and gas escaping into the nasal cavity.

The sinus is only given as an example. Exactly the same will occur in other gas spaces surrounded by relatively rigid containers. With the increased pressure, the contracting gas space must be taken up by some volume-replacing substance. In the case of the middle ear, this substance may be either blood and edema of the middle ear mucosal lining, air transmitted through a perforated tympanic membrane, perilymph flowing from a round window fistula, or, more commonly, equalization by air transmitted through the eustachian tube while performing the Valsalva or other similar maneuver.

Table 5-1
Classification of Barotrauma

I   Barotrauma of Descent ("Squeeze")
    Ear
        External ear
        Middle ear
        Inner ear
    Sinus
    Dental
    Mask, suit, and helmet
    Pulmonary
II Barotrauma of Ascent
    Ear
    Sinus
    Dental
    Suit
    Pulmonary
    Gastrointestinal
III Miscellaneous Effects of Barotrauma
    Surgical emphysema
    Orbital, mandibular, etc

During ascent, the reverse process may result in problems, although less common, with the expulsion of air and fluid either through a perforated tympanic membrane or through the eustachian tube. It can thus be seen that the analogy of the sinus can be applied to other gas spaces (see Table 5-1). These will now be discussed in further detail, with a description of the clinical features, prevention and treatment of the various forms of barotrauma.

For simplicity, it has been decided to combine the barotraumas of descent and ascent under the one anatomical section with which they deal. It is not uncommon for barotrauma of descent to be followed by barotrauma of ascent, as often the underlying pathological conditions predisposing to these are similar. It is nevertheless important that they be differentiated in the student's mind, as the symptoms are often considerably different. The use of the term squeeze—which is far too prevalent in medical literature on this subject—implies a gross oversimplification, and refers only to the barotraumas of descent, but not the barotraumas of ascent.

EAR AND SINUS BAROTRAUMA[1-5]

For a detailed coverage of these topics see Chapter 9 *Ear and Sinus Problems in Diving.*

DENTAL BAROTRAUMA[6]

Gas spaces may exist at the roots of infected teeth or beside fillings that have undergone secondary erosion. During descent, this space is filled with the soft tissue of the gum or with blood. Pain may prevent further descent. If symptoms are not noticed on descent, then gas expansion on ascent may be restricted by blood in these spaces, which results in pain.

Another form of dental barotrauma occurs in cases involving a carious tooth with a cavity and very thin cementum. As pressure differences across the cementum develops, the tooth may cave in (implode) on descent, or explode on ascent, and cause considerable pain. Fast rates of ascent or descent will be more likely to precipitate this disorder.

A third form of dental barotrauma involves the tracking of gas into tissues through interruptions of the mucosa, e.g., after oral surgery, dental extractions, or manipulations. Gas may pass from the oral cavity into the dental area during Valsalva maneuvers, present as surgical emphysema.

Preventive measures include biannual dental checks (including x-ray) and avoidance of all diving after dental extractions or surgery until complete tissue resolution has occurred, i.e., until the mucosal surface is intact. Descent and ascent should be slow.

Treatment consists of analgesia and dental repair. The differential diagnosis of pain in the upper bicuspids or the first and second molars, if sporadic or constant, but not localized in one tooth, must include referred pain from the maxillary sinus. This may also present as a burning sensation along the mucobuccal fold.

MASK, SUIT AND HELMET BAROTRAUMA[3,5]

Facial Barotrauma of Descent (Mask Squeeze)

The use of a face mask is a necessity for good underwater vision. This creates an additional gas space external to, but in contact with, the face. Unless pressure is equalized by exhaling gas through the nose, facial tissues will be forced into this space during descent.

Clinical features include puffy edematous facial tissues, especially under the eyelids, purpuric hemorrhages, conjunctival hemorrhages, and, later, generalized bruising of the skin underlying the mask.

This condition is rarely serious and prevention involves exhaling into the face mask during descent. Treatment involves abstinence from diving until all forms of tissue damage are healed.

Skin Barotrauma of Descent (Suit Squeeze)

This condition is usually encountered only in association with dry suits, or poorly fitting wet suits. In these cases, pockets of air are present between the skin and the suit; during descent, this air is reduced in volume and trapped in folds in the suit. The skin tends to be sucked into these folds which leaves linear weal marks or bruises. The condition is usually painless and clears within a few days.

Head and Body Barotrauma of Descent (Diver's Squeeze)

The use of a rigid helmet, common to standard diving, predisposes the diver to this complication. If extra gas is not added during descent to compensate for the effects of Boyle's Law, the suit and occupant may be forced into the helmet, which may cause bizarre injuries or death. This sequence of events may present dramatically if the heavily weighted diver falls off his stage. There is a similar result when the diver loses his compressed air pressure, e.g., due to a compressor or supply line failure. To prevent this, a non-return valve is now required in supply line connections.

The clinical features include dyspnea and a heavy sensation in the chest; a bulging sensation in the head and eyes; swelling in the areas associated with rigid walls, e.g., the helmet, and then edema; hemorrhages within the skin of the face, conjunctiva, neck, and shoulders; and bleeding from the lungs, gastrointestinal tract, and nose, and into the ears and sinuses. These pathological changes are due to the effects of barotrauma on the enclosed gas spaces and to a pressure gradient forcing blood from the abdomen and lower extremities into the thorax, head, and neck because of the negative pressure differential in the helmet. Similarly induced hemorrhages occur in the brain, heart, respiratory mucosa, and other soft tissues.

Suit Barotrauma of Ascent ("Blowup")

During ascent in a standard diving suit, the expanding gas must be able to escape. If it does not, then the whole suit will expand like a balloon and cause a rapid and uncontrolled ascent to the surface. The associated problems include barotrauma of ascent, decompression sickness, imprisonment of the diver, and physical trauma. With the decreasing use of standard diving, this emergency is not now encountered very often; but a less impressive manifestation is probable with divers who use an inflatable object, such as a buoyancy vest, dry suit, or counterlung, and inflate it accidently.

A clinically dissimilar and relatively minor symptom is noted by divers in an upright position using equipment which has a counterlung, or breathing bag, positioned below the head and neck. The pressure gradient from the bag to the diver's head results in a sensation of head and neck distension and bulging of the eyes.

PULMONARY BAROTRAUMA

This is the most serious of the barotraumas and causes the most concern in all types of diving operations. It is a clinical manifestation of Boyle's Law as it affects the lungs.

Pulmonary Barotrauma of Descent (Lung Squeeze)[9,11]

Descent barotrauma is not common in breath-hold diving, and very rare with open-circuit diving apparatus. The actual depth limit for breath-hold diving is probably determined by two factors:

Residual lung volume. The total lung volume decreases with increasing depth, in accordance with Boyle's Law. Once the actual volume approximates the residual volume, lung compressibility ceases and subsequent descent results in pressure gradients that are equalized by pulmonary congestion, edema, and hemorrhage. Further descent may also result in collapse of the chest wall.

Individual variations in the dilatory response of the pulmonary vascular bed to an increased pulmonary vascular to alveolar pressure gradient. It has been found that in deep breath-hold dives, the pulmonary venous bed dilates and blood displaces air in the thorax, which decreases the effective residual volume. This extends the depth that can be reached in safety.

Breath-hold dives in excess of 80 meters have been possible because of a combination of increased dilatation of the pulmonary venous bed, a large vital capacity, and a small residual volume. The minimal residual volume, which if further reduced will result in pulmonary damage, has not been determined. An average full lung contains 6 liters of air at the surface, but this is compressed to 1.5 liters at 30 meters. This approximates the normal residual volume, and further descent may be hazardous. The individual pulmonary vascular response will determine the final volume limitation.

In diving with open-circuit apparatus, inhaled gases are at the same pressure as the surrounding environment and the diver, which prevents pulmonary barotrauma of descent.

Pulmonary barotrauma of descent is possible in the following situations:

Breath-hold diving
Loss of surface pressure supply with failure or absence of a nonreturn valve. This may occur with surface supply and standard diving.
Failure of the gas supply to compensate for the rate of descent. This is more common with standard diving in which there is no automatic relationship between the gas supply and the ambient pressures and in which the diver is overweighted and has negative buoyancy.

Clinical aspects are poorly documented and include chest pain, hemoptysis with hemorrhagic pulmonary edema and death. Treatment is based on general principles. Intermittent positive pressure respiration may be needed. Initially, 100 percent oxygen should be used with replacement of fluids, treatment of shock, etc. The use of positive end-expiratory pressure would seem hazardous due to predisposition to subsequent gas embolism, but may be necessary if hypoxia cannot be corrected.

Pulmonary Barotrauma of Ascent (Burst Lung) [3,7,8,10,12]

This is the result of overdistension and rupture of the lungs by expanding gases during ascent. Normally, intrapulmonary and environmental pressures are equalized by exhalation during ascent. Pressure gradients necessary to cause pulmonary barotrauma are approximately 80 mm Hg near the surface, but greater pressure gradients may be recorded with the use of abdominal or thoracic binders. Barotrauma may result when the ambient water pressure falls by 80 mm Hg or more below the intrapulmonary pressure, i.e., with an ascent from a depth of just over 1 meter, to the surface. It is more likely to occur after full inspiration before ascent. A diver whose total lung volume is 6 liters at 10 meters will need to exhale 6 liters of gas during ascent to maintain his normal 6 liter lung volume at the surface. Once the total lung capacity is reached, the lung tends to stretch against an increasing resistance until the elastic limit of the pulmonary tissues is exceeded and tearing results.

Precipitating factors include internal air trapping and inadequate exhalation caused by panic, faulty apparatus, or water inhalation. This is encountered in free ascents and submarine escape training, or emergency ascents.

Although many cases of pulmonary barotrauma may be due to voluntary breath-holding during ascent, or to the pathological lesions and techniques just mentioned, attitudes toward these etiologies are changing. A number of divers have been observed to carry out correct exhalation techniques and still develop pulmonary barotrauma. These divers were also passed as medically fit before the dive and showed none of the previously mentioned pathology afterward. A consistent finding with these subjects is a reduction of compliance at maximum inspiratory pressures, i.e., the lungs are stiffer and are exposed to more stress than normal divers' lungs when distended.

There are four manifestations of pulmonary barotrauma of ascent which may occur singly or in combination: pulmonary tissue damage, surgical emphysema, pneumothorax, and air embolism.

Pulmonary tissue damage. After the diver surfaces, exhalation of expanded gases may be accompanied by a characteristic sudden high-pitched cry. Dyspnea, cough, and hemoptysis are symptoms of the lung damage, and widespread alveolar rupture may result in respiratory death.

Investigations include arterial gas measurements, hematological assessment, and serial chest x-ray examinations. These tests are usually not possible during the all-important few minutes after ascent.

Surgical emphysema. After alveolar rupture, gas escapes into the interstitial pulmonary tissues. This gas may track along the loose tissue planes surrounding the airways and blood vessels, into the hilar regions, and thence into the mediastinum and neck. It may also extend to produce a pneumopericardium.

Symptoms may appear immediately in severe cases, or may be delayed several hours in lesser cases. They may include a voice change into a hoarseness or brassy monotone, a feeling of fullness in the throat, dyspnea, dysphagia, retrosternal discomfort, syncope, shock, or unconsciousness.

Clinical signs include surgical emphysema of neck and upper chest wall, i.e., crepitus under the skin, decreased areas of cardiac dullness to percussion, faint heart sounds or crepitus related to heart sounds; i.e., Hamman's sign, left recurrent laryngeal nerve paresis, and cardiovascular embarrassment with cyanosis, tachycardia, and hypotension. There may be radiological evidence of an enlarged mediastinum with air along the cardiac border or in the neck.

Pneumothorax. If the visceral pleura ruptures, air enters the pleural cavity and expands during ascent. This may be accompanied by hemorrhage and then form a hemopneumothorax.

Symptoms usually have a rapid onset and include sudden unilateral or pleuritic pain, dyspnea, and tachypnea. Clinical signs include diminished chest wall movement, displacement of trachea and apex beat, hyperresonance in the affected side, diminished breath sounds on the affected side, signs of shock, x-ray evidence of pneumothorax, and arterial gas and lung volume changes.

Air embolism. This is a dangerous condition and is the result of gas passing into the pulmonary veins and then into the systemic circulation where it can cause vascular obstruction and infarction.

During overdistension of the lung, the capillaries and small vessels are stretched and may tear, along with other tissues. Since these vessels are small and often compressed by distended air sacs, air embolism does not result until overdistension is relieved by exhalation. Only a small volume of gas in the systemic arterial system is necessary to produce severe disturbances, and serious effects may result from blockage of cerebral or coronary vessels by bubbles in the order of 30 μ to 2 mm in diameter. Death may follow coronary or cerebrovascular occlusion. Other tissues affected may include spleen, liver, kidney, or limb.

Air embolism is more commonly encountered in cases of mediastinal emphysema than in cases of pneumothorax.

Serious symptoms that develop immediately after ascent may be regarded as air embolism and treated accordingly until a definitive diagnosis has been made. The manifestations are usually acute and include loss of consciousness; other neurological abnormalities such as confusion, asphasia, visual disturbances, paraesthesia, vertigo, convulsions, or varying degrees of paresis; cardiac-type chest pain; Liebermeister's sign, a sharply defined area of pallor on the tongue; gas bubbles in retinal vessels; and abnormal electrocardiograms (ischemic myocardium, arrhythmias, or cardiac failure) and electroencephalograms (generalized slowing or flattening of waves).

Autopsy techniques. Recommended to facilitate the pathological diagnosis include postmortem radiography of the chest and soft tissue supraclavicular and neck areas. Bubble traps are employed for carotid perfusions, or the thorax and brain are opened underwater. These are discussed in detail in Chapter 23, Investigation of Diving Accidents.

Treatment. Once pulmonary barotrauma has resulted in the liberation of gas within body tissues, it may be aggravated by other factors. Further ascent in a chamber or under water, or ascent to altitude during air transport, will expand the enclosed gas and cause deterioration in the clinical state of the patient. Physical exertion, increased respiratory activity, or coughing may also result in further pulmonary damage or in more extraneous gas passing through the tissues. If the diver has exposed himself to depths and times resulting in tissue supersaturation of inert gas, this gas will have a pressure gradient between the tissue and the bubbles, which results in transport by diffusion into the latter. The result is that a situation develops which has factors of both pulmonary barotrauma and decompression sickness and may require more energetic recompression therapy. Another way in which the entrapped gas from pulmonary barotrauma may be temporarily increased in volume is by breathing a lighter, more rapidly diffusible, gas, e.g., helium, in the correct belief that this may improve ventilation.

Treatment of the *pulmonary tissue damage* involves the maintenance of adequate respiration with 100 percent oxygen to ensure acceptable arterial gas levels. Positive pressure respiration could increase the extent of lung damage and should be used only if absolutely necessary. Support for the cardiovascular system may be required, and attention should be paid to the electrolyte and fluid balance.

Treatment of the *surgical emphysema* may not be urgent for these cases; however, exclusion of air embolism or pneumothorax is necessary; if in doubt, treatment for these should take precedence. Management of surgical emphysema varies according to the clinical severity. If the patient is asymptomatic, only observation with rest is necessary. With mild symptoms, 100 percent oxygen administered by mask without positive pressure will increase the gradient for removal of nitrogen from the emphysematous areas. If symptoms are severe, therapeutic recompression using oxygen is necessary. Tables 5, 5A, 6 or 6A of the U.S. Navy Diving Manual are often employed (see Appendix 2 and Chapter 7). Cannulation to remove a localized pocket of retrosternal air has been proposed, but this is rarely, if ever, indicated.

Treatment of *pneumothorax* depends on the degree of clinical severity. The possibility of associated air embolism must be excluded. Mild cases require only intermittent administration of oxygen, without positive pressure. The patient may also need bed rest, analgesics, and physiotherapy at a later stage. Serious cases, often with more than 20 percent lung collapse, require intercostal cannulation and suction or underwater drainage. This may be needed while the patient is undergoing recompression therapy. Therapeutic recompression performed for other manifestations of pulmonary barotrauma gives rapid initial relief from the pneumothorax. Because the pneumothorax is likely to be reexpanded during ascent, thoracentesis and/or the use of 100 percent oxygen is indicated. A pneumothorax may be converted into a tension pneumothorax during decompression and thus requires immediate thoracentesis. Ascent must be halted until this is completed, and then recommenced with great care.

Treatment of *air embolism* is urgent, must be instituted immediately, and must take precedence over treatment for all other manifestations of pulmonary barotrauma. Immediate recompression is necessary and a recompression chamber should always be available near surfacing positions of all free ascent or submarine escape training. The techniques of therapy often rely on the facilities available. Immediate recompression to 50 meters (6 ata) reduces the gas bubbles to one-sixth of their volume. This allows them to pass through most vessels, which thereby limits their effect to smaller areas. Once moving, bubble dissipation and absorption are expedited. Ascent and reversion to oxygen therapeutic tables are begun when possible.

Cardiopulmonary resuscitation before and during recompression may be necessary. The highest safe oxygen concentration, without positive pressure, should be used. Reduction of cerebral and pulmonary edema may be achieved by cooling and by intravenous administration of mannitol or steroids. In the absence of a recompression chamber, the patient should be positioned head down and lying on his left side to reduce the risk of further cerebral air embolism. Circulatory and respiratory support with 100 percent oxygen by mask is necessary, while the recompression facilities are acquired. Prevention and/or treatment of secondary complications such as myocardial infarction, renal failure, cerebral hemorrhage, and infections should be carried out.

Heroic measures such as reimmersion to 30 meters in water should be avoided in all but the most exceptional circumstances, and then only if (a) sea conditions are suitable; (b) adequate air supply is available; (c) several experienced support divers are present; and (d) the patient is fully conscious, or equipment is suitable for sustaining the unconscious patient. An alternative or complementary regime to the water recompression on air from 30 meters is the water recompression on oxygen from 9 meters—this is discussed elsewhere.

GASTROINTESTINAL BAROTRAUMA[3, 4]

Gas expansion occurs within the intestines on ascent and may result in eructation, flatus, abdominal discomfort, and colicky pains. This is rarely severe, but it has been known to cause syncopal and shock-like states. Inexperienced divers are more prone to aerophagia, predisposing to this condition. Carbonated beverages and heavy meals are best avoided before and during exposure to hyperbaric conditions. Treatment involves either slowing the rate of ascent, stopping ascent, or even recompression. The simple procedure of releasing tight-fitting restrictions such as belts and girdles may give considerable symptomatic relief.

LOCALIZED SURGICAL EMPHYSEMA

This may result from the entry of gas into any area where the integument skin, or mucosa is broken and in contact with a gas space. Although the classical site involves the supraclavicular area in association with tracking mediastinal emphysema from pulmonary barotrauma, other sites are possible. Orbital surgical edema, severe enough to completely occlude the palpebral fissure, may result from diving with facial skin, intranasal, or sinus injuries. Surgical emphysema over the mandibular area is common with buccal and dental lesions. The surgical emphysema, with its associated physical sign of crepitus and its radiological verification, tends to occur in the loose subcutaneous tissue. Treatment is by the administration of 100 percent oxygen by a nonpressurized technique, and usually complete resolution will occur within hours. Otherwise, resolution may take a week or more. Recompression is rarely indicated, but abstinence from diving is mandatory until this resolution is complete and the damaged integument has completely healed.

REFERENCES

1. Fagan P, McKenzie B, Edmonds C. Sinus barotrauma in divers. *Ann Otol, Rhinol, Laryngol* 1975 (in press)
2. Edmonds C, Fereman P, Thomas R, et al: Otological Aspects of Diving. Australasian Medical Publishing Co, Sydney, 1973
3. Edmonds C, Thomas R, Medical aspects of diving. Med J Aust. 2:1300, 1972
4. Hill L: Caisson Sickness. London, Edward Arnold, 1912
5. Hoff EC: A Bibliographical Sourcebook of Compressed Air, Diving and Submarine Medicine, vol I. Washington, D.C., BuMed Dept. of Navy, 1948
6. Hoff EC, Greenbaum LJ Jr: A Bibliographical Sourcebook of Compressed Air, Diving and Submarine Medicine, vol. II. Washington, D.C., ONR and BuMed, Dept. of Navy, 1954
7. Miles S: Underwater Medicine. London, Staples Press, 1969
8. Polak IB, Adams H: Traumatic air embolism in submarine escape training. US Navy Med Bull 30:165, 1932
9. Schaefer KE, Allison RD, Dougherty JH, Parker D: Pulmonary and circulatory adjustments determining the limits of depths in breathhold diving. Science 162:1020, 1968
10. Schaefer KE, McNulty SP, Carey CR, Liebow AA: Mechanism in development of interstitial emphysema and air embolism on decompression from depth. J Appl Physiol 13:15-29, 1958
11. Strauss MB, Wright PW: Thoracic squeeze diving casualty. Aerosp Med 42(6):673-675, 1971
12. Colebatch HJH: The mechanical properties of the lungs in healthy divers. Royal Australian Navy School of Underwater Medicine Project 4/70, 1970

STUDY QUESTIONS

1. If the ostium of a sinus is occluded, external pressure is transmitted to the sinus mucosa through what structures?
2. Pulmonary barotrauma is thought to be possible during ascent from a depth as small as
   a. 1 meter
   b. 3 meters
   c. 10 meters
3. Name three pathological conditions which may result from breath-holding during ascent following the respiration of compressed air.

4. A scuba diver who is known to be approaching the end of his air supply makes a sudden, rapid ascent. Two seconds after reaching the surface, the diver becomes unconscious and is quickly pulled into the boat where he remains semiconscious. What is the most likely diagnosis?
5. What is the primary treatment for air embolism?

Richard H. Strauss

6
Decompression Sickness

Decompression sickness is sometimes called the bends or caisson disease. Its primary cause is the formation and growth of bubbles within tissues or blood. Bubbles can occur when the body, or part of it, becomes supersaturated with gas. Supersaturation is the condition in which the total pressure of all gases dissolved in a tissue is greater than the ambient (surrounding) pressure. For example, a descending scuba diver breathes air at higher and higher pressures. The elevated air pressure forces increasing amounts of gas into solution in the blood and tissues. Once the diver begins to ascend toward the surface, the water pressure may fall below the total pressure of the gases dissolved in a given tissue. The tissue is then said to be supersaturated with gas, and bubbles may occur in a manner that is somewhat analogous to the appearance of bubbles in a Coke bottle when the top is removed. Supersaturation is a necessary condition for the occurrence of stable bubbles, but some degree of supersaturation is tolerated by the body without causing apparent decompression sickness. Supersaturation, bubble formation, and bubble growth are treated more rigorously later in this chapter (see Physiology of Decompression).

INCIDENCE

The incidence of decompression sickness among sport divers is unknown, although attempts have been made to document sport-diving accidents.[1] U.S. Navy dives requiring decompression have a 0.69 percent incidence of decompression sickness.[2] Symptoms may appear during or immediately following decompression, or after a delay of several hours. The delay may be due, in part, to evolution of a gas phase and perhaps, more importantly, to the gradual progression of pathological processes, such as edema, following the original insult. In general, more severe damage is associated with an earlier onset of symptoms. In a study of 935 cases of decompression sickness in divers, 54.7 percent had symptoms or signs within 1 hour of surfacing and 92.8 percent had manifestations within 12 hours.[2] A history of diving within the past 24 hours with compressed gases for breathing, should alert the physician to the possibility of decompression sickness. Decompression sickness also can occur following exposure to pressure in chambers, in tunnel work, or during high-altitude flights in unpressurized aircraft.

PATHOGENESIS

In severe cases of decompression sickness in which the diver or experimental animal has died, bubbles have been reported almost everywhere: within blood vessels, presumably having impeded circulation; extravascularly, distorting tissues; and possibly within cells.[3] The pathogeneses of the more common, nonlethal signs and symptoms are less clear. Following some dives, bubbles can be detected in the venous circulation using the Doppler bubble detector,[4] even though decompression sickness has not occurred. There appears to be a correlation between the number of bubbles detected and the occurrence or severity of decompression sickness. Obstruction to blood flow in arterioles or venules[5,6] has been proposed as a major mechanism of pathology.

Numerous changes in the blood have been noted following decompression[7]: clumping of red cells, rouleau formation, sludging of blood in small vessels, and a decrease in number of platelets. Hematological changes may be due in part to the gas-blood interface of bubbles and to damaged endothelium of vessels.[8] Hemoconcentration occurs, possibly from increased capillary permeability. In addition, the osmotic activity of dissolved gases has been suggested as a mechanism for fluid shifts.[9] The higher concentration of gas in tissues, as compared to blood, is hypothesized to draw water from blood to tissue. Decompression sickness is associated with release into blood of a "Smooth Muscle Acting Factor" (SMAF) which causes constriction of blood vessels and bronchi and potentiates bradykinin.[10] Numerous other biologically active substances associated with stress have been observed in decompression sickness. Pharmacological agents that will help prevent or treat decompression sickness are being sought.

CLINICAL MANIFESTATIONS

Decompression sickness is sometimes classed as Type II, which includes serious manifestations such as those resulting from neurological damage, and Type I, which includes less serious manifestations such as "pain-only bends" and "skin bends."

Central Nervous System Manifestations

Among sport divers, central nervous system "bends" is the most significant type of decompression sickness because it can result in permanent neurological deficit. About half of 100 cases of decompression sickness studied in Hawaii involved the central nervous system.[11] These cases were among sport and civilian divers.

Neurological lesions often involve the spinal cord, particularly the thoracic segments, but also the upper lumbar and lower cervical segments. The white matter of the cord, rather than the gray matter, is generally affected. Early lesions consist of petechiae and hemorrhage, followed by perivascular degeneration of nerve fibers, edema, and cavity formation.[12]

It is important that both the diver and his physician recognize the early manifestations of spinal cord decompression sickness because immediate treatment in a decompression chamber may result in complete recovery, whereas delay decreases the chances of a good outcome. Soon after surfacing, the diver's first symptom may be transient back pain with radiation to the abdomen. However, he often attributes this pain to the lifting of air tanks. Therefore, the first manifestation noticed by the diver is usually a feeling of "pins and needles" in his legs, that is, paresthesias and hypesthesias (Fig. 6-1). The diver thinks his legs are asleep and he tries to increase their circulation by walking, but the symptoms do not improve. Next, the legs become weak and the gait ataxic, at which point the diver usually realizes that something is clearly wrong. He often cannot initiate urination, although his bladder may be distended. Finally, paralysis below the waist or neck may ensue.[14]

Cerebral damage may occur among sport divers, particularly following an unusually rapid ascent. It is also seen among saturation divers. Manifestations include visual disturbances, hemiparesis, and unconsciousness. Among aviators, the cerebrum is involved more commonly than the spinal cord. Vertigo ("the staggers") may result from cerebellar or vestibular damage.

When decompression procedures have been violated badly, symptoms may appear immediately and progress to paralysis within minutes. Injury to the central nervous system is often associated with marginal decompression and an *unusually rapid rate of ascent* (greater than 60 feet/minute) in an emergency situation such as running out of air during a dive.

Even when standard practices are used, decompression sickness occurs

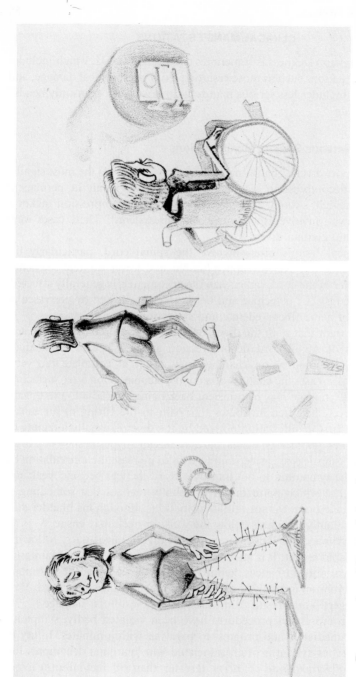

Fig. 6-1. Decompression sickness of the spinal cord may evolve over a period ranging from minutes to hours. It often begins with paresthesias and hypesthesias of the legs (left) and may progress to ataxia (center) and then to paralysis (right). (From *Skin Diver Magazine*.[13])

occasionally and may progress over several hours. For example, an East Coast diver made a single dive to less than 110 feet for 14 minutes to investigate a sunken ship. He ascended directly to the surface at his normal rate because no decompression was indicated; shortly thereafter, he experienced generalized abdominal pain briefly and tingling of the legs which lasted for 1 hour. Three hours after the dive, he noted paresthesias and numbness below the waist. These symptoms became more pronounced over several hours and were followed by progressive ataxia of gait and difficulty initiating urination, at which time the diver sought treatment. He had experienced no extremity pain.[14]

Decompression sickness involving the central nervous system is a medical emergency and the syndrome should be recognized before paralysis is present. When treated immediately with hyperbaric oxygen, the symptoms may disappear without residua. Conversely, when treatment is delayed for several hours, permanent neurological damage may occur. It is postulated that therapy can quickly reduce bubble size and improve tissue oxygenation, but it cannot reverse hemorrhage, thrombosis, or severe edema. Results of treatment cannot be predicted with certainty, but the sooner recompression is begun, the better the outcome. The victim should be transported immediately to a decompression chamber, by air if that is the fastest mode of transportation, while continuously breathing oxygen by mask. The cabin pressure of the aircraft should remain as close to 1 atm as possible. The time saved by air transportation is felt to more than compensate for a moderate decrease in ambient pressure.

It should be noted that some patients have shown considerable improvement following recompression as late as 24 hours or more after the onset of decompression sickness. Therefore, hyperbaric therapy should be performed even if considerable delay has occurred.

Extremity Pain

The term the bends was first applied at the end of the last century to the joint pain and damage of caisson workers. The bends is now used loosely as a synonym for decompression sickness.

Although pain may occur in many extremity locations, shoulder and elbow joints are more commonly involved in divers, as contrasted to hip and knee joints in tunnel workers. The pain is usually steady and boring, similar to a toothache; but occasionally, it may be throbbing. It reaches a peak in minutes or hours and often subsides spontaneously a number of hours later, even if left untreated. The mechanism of pain production is not clear. Treatment by recompression helps to relieve the pain and may possibly decrease subsequent tissue damage.

The extremity usually looks completely normal, there is little tenderness, and moderate joint motion is well tolerated. Extremity pain may also result from local injury unnoticed in the excitement of the dive. Such injuries bear characteristics of trauma, e.g., swelling, discoloration, tenderness, and exacerbation of pain upon motion.

Aseptic necrosis of bone is an occupational hazard among divers and compressed air workers which may not become evident for months or years after diving. It is probably a consequence of "inadequate" decompression and can result in chronic joint deformities (see Chapter 8).

Other Manifestations

The "chokes" is a severe form of decompression sickness characterized by chest pain, dyspnea, and sometimes cough. Pain and cough are aggravated by deep inspiration and by smoking. These symptoms are thought by some to be caused by obstruction of the pulmonary vessels by bubbles. Without recompression, circulatory collapse and death may follow.

"Skin bends" are sometimes seen in scuba divers, but more often follow simulated dives in chambers. The affected skin, usually on the back or elsewhere on the trunk, itches, burns, and becomes mottled. If it is the only manifestation of decompression sickness, skin bends is frequently left untreated or is treated by oxygen breathing at 1 atm. The rash disappears spontaneously over a few hours or days. Persons with such signs should remain available for chamber treatment for 12 to 24 hours after the dive in the event that further manifestations of decompression sickness appear.

Fatigue much greater than that expected from the work performed sometimes follows marginal or inadequate decompression. It may or may not be associated with other signs of decompression sickness.

PREDISPOSING FACTORS

Susceptibility to decompression sickness varies among individuals and even in the same diver from day to day. Predisposing factors include obesity, exertion, poor physical conditioning, aging, cold, dehydration, and injury. Some acclimatization may occur, in that tunnel workers and divers appear to be less susceptible to decompression sickness when working daily than after an inactive period.

BREATH-HOLD DIVING

During breath-hold diving, air within the lungs is at a pressure close to that of the surrounding water. It is therefore "compressed" air and conceivably could lead to decompression sickness if the depths, and total time spent at depth, were sufficient during repeated, frequent dives. No such cases have been reported among sport divers. One case was reported following repeated dives in a submarine escape training tank.[15]

In the past, breath-holding to depths greater than 100 feet was practiced by pearl divers of the Tuamotu Archipelago. After an unusually strenuous series of dives, persons occasionally surfaced and became unconscious or paralyzed. Death or permanent brain damage (called taravana, to fall crazily) sometimes followed.[16] This syndrome may be a form of decompression sickness.

PREVENTION OF DECOMPRESSION SICKNESS

Decompression Tables

In practice, decompression sickness is avoided by following schedules, generally called decompression tables, which have been tested for safety. The tables most respected and used among experienced sport divers in the United States are the Standard Air Decompression Tables of the U.S. Navy.[17] These tables are reproduced in Appendix 2. Although certain instructions are included in the appendix, their actual use must be covered in a basic scuba course. Other nations and certain industries have developed their own decompression schedules. The section entitled Physiology of Decompression is devoted to the principles underlying decompression techniques.

Decompression Meters

A decompression meter is a device worn or carried by a diver to indicate his decompression status. It is sometimes used as an alternative to consulting the tables. At present, such devices involve the slow transfer of gas from a compartment exposed to ambient pressure into a second compartment to which an indicator of gas pressure is attached. A diffusion barrier such as silicone rubber, or some other barrier to gas flow, separates the two compartments. Gas passes into or out of the indicator compartment in proportion to ambient pressure, presumably in a manner somewhat analogous to that of the body. Since the body consists of more than one type of tissue, in terms of gas uptake and loss, a decompression meter with several diffusion units, rather than one, can mimic the body more effectively. Decompression meters are generally designed to approximate an accepted set of tables. Clearly, quality control is important in the production of these devices. The diver should know the reputation and peculiarities of a decompression meter before relying on it. A small electronic computer that integrates time, depth, and possibly other factors could become the best decompression meter.

Diving at Altitude

Diving is done in mountain lakes and other bodies of water which exist at altitudes well above sea level. The use of sea-level decompression tables becomes less safe as altitude increases. Various decompression methods for altitude diving have been proposed, but few have been tested extensively and some are dangerous. In Switzerland, Buhlmann et al[18] calculated new altitude decompression tables and reported no cases of decompression sickness in 214 test dives. These tables appear in Appendix 3. They are an extension to altitude of the Buhlmann sea level tables which, in turn, are based upon modifications of the Haldane principles.

Flying after Diving

In 1961, several members of the crew of a commercial airliner incurred decompression sickness on an intercontinental flight.[19] They had been scuba diving the morning and afternoon prior to their evening flight. Other incidents of decompression sickness aboard commercial and private aircraft following diving have been reported. Studies by Edel et al[19] led to the following conclusions:

Scuba divers who stay strictly within the limits (depth-time) of the standard U.S. Navy's *no-decompression limits* and repetitive group designation table for no-decompression dives for a period not exceeding 12 hours will not develop decompression sickness if, after diving, they allow a minimum *two-hour surface interval* before flying in a pressurized commercial aircraft (maximum cabin altitude 8,000 feet). Divers who make dives beyond these no-decompression limits should allow a surface interval of 24 hours before decompression to a commercial aircraft's cabin altitude pressure if they are to avoid the risk of bends.

PHYSIOLOGY OF DECOMPRESSION*

General Principles of Decompression

Early work at elevated air pressure, as in caissons and the construction of tunnels beneath rivers, frequently resulted in pain and crippling. In an attempt to avoid such consequences, J. S. Haldane and his associates[20] set forth a number of principles for decompression procedures. These principles, although modified to some extent, form the basis for much of current decompression practice, including the U.S. Navy decompression tables. Following are four main principles. They involve several assumptions which have not been verified experimentally.

*The clinician who has little interest in the basis of decompression practice may wish to omit the remainder of this chapter.

The uptake or loss of gas by a given tissue is exponential in form.   Let us assume for the moment that a person has breathed air at sea level for a number of days. The P_{N_2} (partial pressure of nitrogen) within his tissues will be equal to the P_{N_2} in the alveoli of his lungs. His body is said to be "saturated" at 1 ata because there is no net exchange of inert gas between the body and the surrounding atmosphere.† If the ambient pressure is raised and maintained for several days, all tissues in the body will become saturated with inert gas at the new pressure. However, tissues do not become saturated instantly, for two reasons: (1) At equilibrium, each tissue has a capacity for dissolved gas that is determined by the solubility of the gas in the tissue. (2) Gas molecules must travel from the alveoli, via the bloodstream, to tissue, and then must diffuse from the capillaries to all parts of the tissue.

The rate-limiting step, or bottleneck, in the saturation process is thought to be the tissue's rate of blood flow in most cases. Gas uptake in such tissues is said to be "perfusion limited." In a few tissues, such as the vitreous humor of the eye, where diffusion distances are great, gas transfer may be "diffusion limited." In either case, as the inert gas pressure of the tissue approaches that of the alveoli, the driving force for transfer of gas into the tissue becomes less and less, and the rate of gas transfer decreases. Thus, the P_{N_2} of a tissue rises rapidly at first and then slows down. This sort of change is "exponential" with respect to time and is found frequently in nature, e.g., in radioactive decay. Figure 6-2 shows the change in nitrogen pressure in two hypothetical tissues following an increase, and later a decrease, in alveolar nitrogen pressure. The tissue P_{N_2} at time t is described by the equation

$$P_{N_2}(t) \; = \; P_{N_2}(0) \; + \; \left(P_{N_2}(1) \; - \; P_{N_2}(0) \right) \; (1 - e^{-kt}).$$

In this equation, $P_{N_2}(0)$ is the initial tissue P_{N_2} and $P_{N_2}(1)$ is the tissue P_{N_2} at equilibrium at the new ambient pressure. The term e is the base of natural logarithms (2.72) and k is a constant characteristic of a given tissue and gas.

It is often assumed that when ambient pressure decreases, gas is lost from tissue in a manner analogous to gas uptake. This assumption is not true if significant bubble formation has occurred, because part of the gas then diffuses into bubbles within the tissue rather than providing a gradient for diffusion of gas into blood.

The rate of saturation varies from tissue to tissue.   As noted above, the rapidity with which a given tissue becomes saturated at a new pressure de-

---

†Actually, this is a state of equilibrium and not true saturation because the tissue gas pressure remains a little below ambient pressure. See the section on *Inherent Unsaturation* in this chapter.

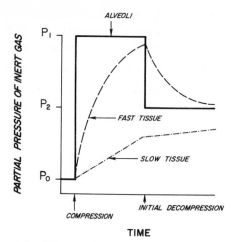

Fig. 6-2. When ambient pressure is increased during compression with air breathing, alveolar P_{N_2}
changes immediately. However, the P_{N_2} of various
tissues increases gradually, at a rate which becomes
less as saturation is approached. The initial
decompression results in supersaturation of the "fast"
tissue shown. Such supersaturation is intended to
cause rapid loss of gas but, hopefully, no significant
bubble formation. The "slow" tissue continues to ab-
sorb gas, but at a lesser rate.

pends upon (1) the solubility of the gas in the tissue, and (2) the rate at which
gas is transported to or from the tissue. For example, nitrogen is more soluble
in fat than in aqueous tissue. Fat is poorly perfused, but has a high capacity for
nitrogen storage, so it saturates slowly and is known as a "slow" tissue. In
contrast, the brain is a well-perfused "fast" tissue.[21]

Because of the exponential form of the saturation curve, the time necessary for completion of saturation is difficult to determine. Therefore, the term
tissue half-time is often used. This is the time required for the partial pressure
of an inert gas to reach one-half its saturation value. It is rarely possible to
assign precise half-times to real tissues. However, several theoretical half-time
tissues are assumed in the calculation of decompression tables.

During decompression, the inert gas that is lost through the lungs comes
from many tissues simultaneously. During a single decompression stop, much
gas is lost initially. As time progresses, only the slower tissues retain a significant amount of dissolved gas above the equilibrium pressure, and only they
contribute to further gas loss.

*Decompression should be initiated by a relatively large drop in ambient
pressure.* The object of decompression is to reach the surface as rapidly as

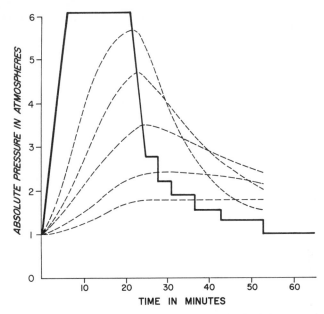

Fig. 6-3. Decompression of several hypothetical tissues such that no tissue P_{N_2} (broken lines) is ever greater than about twice ambient pressure (solid line). (After Haldane.[20])

possible without causing decompression sickness. This is a bit like approaching the edge of a cliff as closely as possible, for the view, without falling over. Early decompression was often linear; that is, ambient pressure was decreased at a constant rate from beginning to end. Haldane suggested that an initial step of rapid decompression would quickly cause supersaturation of fast tissues, and thus speed their gas loss; it would also decrease the gradient driving gas into slow tissues (see Fig. 6-2). The initial pressure decrease is limited by the amount of supersaturation estimated to be tolerable for the tissues involved. This principle is currently under debate.

Tissue gas pressure should never be greater than about twice ambient pressure. Haldane[20] found that men could spend several hours at approximately 2 ata and then be decompressed rapidly to 1 ata without incurring decompression sickness. Upon reaching 1 ata, the inert gas pressure in many tissues would have been about twice ambient pressure. He reasoned that decompression would be safe if tissue supersaturation were controlled so that the inert gas pressure of any tissue was never more than about twice ambient pressure. Figure 6-3 is redrawn from Haldane's original paper, showing the decompression of several hypothetical tissues by pressure increments that decrease as the surface is approached. Decompression by steps is called stage decompression, as opposed to continuous decompression. In diving, stage decompression is generally more convenient, but the principles discussed in this chapter can be applied to either stage or continuous decompression.

As divers were subjected to greater and greater pressures it was found that the ratio

$$\frac{\text{tissue gas pressure}}{\text{ambient pressure}} \leq \frac{2}{1}$$

had to be reduced progressively to avoid decompression sickness. However, reduction of pressure by some value of this ratio is still the basis for much of decompression practice in diving. Linear decompression is still used in tunnel work.

Additional Factors in Decompression

Inherent Unsaturation.[22]   Under normal conditions, any isolated collection of gas within the body will be resorbed spontaneously in a matter of hours or days. This applies to a pneumothorax which no longer has air leaking into it, or to gas injected under the skin. To understand this process, gas saturation must be defined more carefully. True saturation is the condition in which the total gas pressure within a liquid or tissue is equal to the surrounding (ambient) pressure. During air breathing, total gas pressure within a part of the body is the sum of the partial pressures of nitrogen, oxygen, carbon dioxide, and water vapor. For saturation then,

$$P_{N_2} + P_{O_2} + P_{CO_2} + P_{H_2O} = P_{\text{ambient}}.$$

Arterial blood is nearly saturated, but venous blood and tissues are not (Fig. 6-4). As dry air is inspired at 1 ata (760 mm Hg), it is diluted with water vapor. In the alveoli, oxygen is lost and carbon dioxide is gained,* but the total pressure remains 1 ata because open airways connect the alveoli with ambient pressure. Within the pulmonary capillaries, blood normally equilibrates with alveolar gas. Subsequently, a small amount of deoxygenated venous blood from the heart and lungs mixes with the oxygenated blood so that arterial blood has a slightly lower P_{O_2} than does alveolar gas.

As blood passes through the capillaries of systemic tissues, it loses oxygen and picks up carbon dioxide. Carbon dioxide is more soluble in blood than is oxygen. For this reason, P_{O_2} falls about 50 mm Hg, but P_{CO_2} rises

---

*On the average, 4 molecules of CO_2 are gained by the alveoli for every 5 molecules of O_2 lost. This is because some O_2 contributes to the formation of H_2O rather than CO_2.

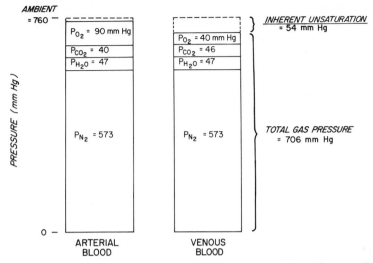

Fig. 6-4.   Arterial blood is nearly saturated with gas. Venous blood is normally (inherently) unsaturated, since the total gas pressure within it is significantly less than ambient pressure.

only about 6 mm Hg. Thus, the total gas pressure in blood leaving the systemic capillaries is less than ambient pressure, and the venous blood is unsaturated (Fig. 6-4). Tissue is in approximate equilibrium with venous blood and is also unsaturated. Any collection of gas, such as a bubble, within soft tissue remains at approximately ambient pressure, even as it is being absorbed. This is because external pressure is readily transmitted to the gas through soft tissue. Ultimately, all of the trapped gas diffuses into the unsaturated capillary blood and the gas phase disappears.

During decompression, the body's inherent unsaturation can provide a margin of safety for prevention of supersaturation.[22] In addition, breathing oxygen at a higher than normal partial pressure can increase the degree of unsaturation. This effect, sometimes called the oxygen window, is used to speed decompression and to increase the rate of inert gas loss from bubbles within the body during treatment of decompression sickness.

Bubble Growth.   For a bubble to grow from "nothing" to a finite size, it must go through two distinct phases: (1) formation of a small bubble where nothing was previously observable; and (2) growth of a small bubble to a larger one. Bubble growth is well understood and will be discussed first.

For a bubble to grow, the total gas pressure within the bubble (P_{bubble}) must be greater than the pressures tending to constrict or crush it. There are several constricting pressures. Most important is the ambient pressure ($P_{ambient}$). In addition, because of its structure and osmotic balance, tissue tends to resist being deformed and thus causes tissue pressure (P_{tissue}). Finally, surface tension (γ) tends to make a bubble smaller. The pressure due to surface tension (P_γ) is given by the equation

$$P_\gamma = \frac{2\gamma}{r}$$

where r is the radius of the bubble. For large bubbles, P_γ is negligible. However, as r gets smaller, the pressure due to surface tension increases. Indeed, it is difficult to imagine how very small bubbles can exist at all.

The necessary condition for bubble growth is

$$P_{bubble} > P_{ambient} + P_{tissue} + P_\gamma.$$

Gas within the bubble tends to equilibrate with gas in the surrounding tissue. Therefore, following decompression from a dive using air, the necessary condition for bubble growth can be rewritten in terms of gas pressures within the tissue:

$$P_{N_2} + P_{O_2} + P_{CO_2} + P_{H_2O} > P_{ambient} + P_{tissue} + P_\gamma.$$

This condition can also be called supersaturation. Conversely, bubbles will shrink if the above inequality is reversed.

Bubbles in tissue may be stable for a while when tissue resistance prevents further growth in spite of existing supersaturation. In contrast, bubbles are essentially unstable in liquids because there is no tissue resistance to limit their growth. Bubbles below a critical size will shrink and disappear because of the strong effect of surface tension.

Bubble Formation.   The mechanism of bubble formation in animals is poorly understood, although certain studies in simple systems may be helpful. The reason for wishing to understand bubble formation is that better methods of decompression might result.

It appears that some sort of nuclei for bubble formation exist in animals, since bubbles form when supersaturation is in the range of a few atmospheres or less, as in decompression. Bubbles can form without nuclei ("de novo"), but in pure water this is thought to require supersaturation in the order of 1000 atm. One conceivable type of nucleus is a small pocket of gas which is stabilized as shown in Fig. 6-5.[3,23] The gas is trapped within a crack or irregularity on a solid. The walls of the irregularity can have any shape, but must be nonwetting to prevent water from creeping in and obliterating the gas cavity. The gas-liquid interface in vitro is flat. Therefore, the surface tension does not tend to make the gas cavity smaller, as it would in a true bubble, because the volume of the gas is independent of the area of the gas-liquid interface.

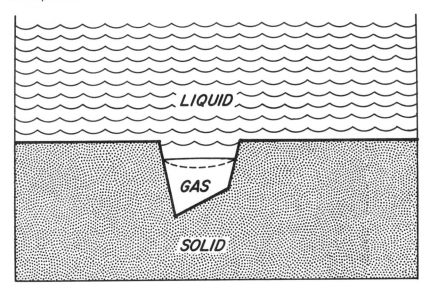

Fig. 6-5. Model of a gas nucleus at equilibrium. A small pocket of gas is stabilized by association with a nonwetting solid surface. The gas-liquid interface is flat in a closed, nonliving system (solid line). In animals, the interface bulges into the gas cavity due to "inherent unsaturation" (broken line).

At equilibrium, gas pressure within the nucleus would equal the dissolved gas pressure in the liquid. In animals, because of inherent unsaturation, the gas pressure of the nucleus would be a little less than the hydrostatic pressure of the tissue fluid. The gas-liquid interface would therefore bulge into the gas cavity until being sufficiently restrained by surface tension.

When supersaturation occurs, the surface of the nucleus tends to bulge outward. This outward bulge is opposed by surface tension; but, if the critical gas pressure is exceeded, a bubble will form and grow. Large nuclei probably form bubbles more readily than small ones. In a liquid, such as blood, the bubble may break away from the solid and leave the nucleus to generate more bubbles. Conversely, in tissue, the bubble would be held in place. Application of high hydrostatic pressures may cause gas nuclei to become smaller and to remain so, or to be eliminated entirely, possibly due to wetting of the wall.

Work with transparent shrimp[24] suggests that gas nuclei exist in these animals. Studies of bubble formation in gelatin[25] have elucidated the behavior of gas nuclei. They suggest that instead of decompressing a tissue by the Haldane ratio, the *difference* between tissue gas pressure and ambient pressure (rather than the ratio) should remain constant to minimize bubble formation. If these findings are shown to be applicable to humans, decompression profiles would become somewhat more linear than at present, with a smaller initial step ("first pull"). Earlier work[22] suggested that supersaturation should be avoided entirely until shallow depths are reached. This work followed observations on divers in Australia who decompressed rapidly by spending more time at deeper decompression stops than at shallow ones—the converse of the Haldane ratio.

Bubble Detection. Several devices are helpful in detecting bubbles inside the human body without causing damage. The Doppler flow meter can detect bubbles moving within venous or arterial blood.[4] An ultrasonic signal is passed through a blood vessel and is reflected much better by a bubble than by the normal elements of blood. The frequency of the reflected signal is shifted in proportion to the bubble's velocity.* The reflected signal is picked up and modified so that a bubble passing by can be heard as an audible "chirp." Stationary bubbles cannot be detected by the Doppler device, but can be detected, if large enough, by pulsed ultrasound as used in echocardiography. The gas-tissue interface is a good sound reflector that can be localized in terms of distance from the transducer.

Alternative Inert Gases

A physiologically inert gas is the major component of most breathing mixtures because oxygen becomes toxic at high pressures (see Chapter 11). The inert gas most commonly breathed is nitrogen, usually as compressed air. However, breathing nitrogen at elevated pressures leads to nitrogen narcosis (see Chapter 12). Helium is physiologically inert and does not lead to narcosis at any pressure tested, thus far, in man. It is generally used in dives deeper than about 190 fsw. It has the disadvantages of being expensive, of reducing intelligibility of speech, and of rapidly conducting heat away from the body. Helium results in decompression sickness in much the same way that nitrogen does. It is less soluble in water and fat than is nitrogen and diffuses more readily. Helium saturates and desaturates the body more rapidly than does nitrogen, so that decompression from a helium saturation dive is more rapid than from a nitrogen saturation dive to the same depth. A nonsaturation dive on helium may or may not lead to faster decompression than the same dive on nitrogen, depending upon depth and duration.

Following a helium-oxygen dive, decompression time may be shortened by breathing nitrogen-oxygen during the latter part of decompression.[26] This is thought to be the case because helium leaves the body more rapidly than nitrogen enters it, which results in decreased total gas pressure within tissue. Conversely, it may be unwise to breathe helium-oxygen during the treatment of decompression sickness which followed a dive with compressed air, since inward diffusion of helium may cause existing nitrogen bubbles to grow.[27, 28]

---

*The Doppler shift in frequency can be heard as the change in pitch of the whistle of a train as it speeds past an observer.

In a helium environment, breathing a mixture containing nitrogen or neon may result in bubble formation within the skin, without decompression. This is due to counterdiffusion of gases through the skin and results in itching, wheals, and skin damage.[29]

Other physiologically inert gases can be breathed, but are not used commercially for diving at present. Neon is less narcotic than nitrogen, but more narcotic and more expensive than helium. Hydrogen is under investigation for diving despite its potential explosiveness in mixtures with oxygen. Xenon is narcotic even at 1 atm. Sulfur hexafluoride is an unusually dense gas. Its density results in increased airway resistance, which is useful in respiratory experiments but is to be avoided in diving.

REFERENCES

1. Schenck H Jr, McAniff J, Schenck ML, Schenck H: Diving accident survey, 1946-1970, including 503 known fatalities. Scuba Safety Report Series, Report No. 5. Kingston, R.I., University of Rhode Island, 1972
2. Rivera JC: Decompression sickness among divers: An analysis of 935 cases. U.S. Navy Experimental Diving Unit Research Report 1-63. Washington Navy Yard, 1963
3. Harvey EN, et al: Bubble formation in animals. J Cell Physiol 24:1-22, 23-34, 117-132, 1944; Harvey EN, et al: The effect of mechanical disturbance on bubble formation in single cells and tissues after saturation with extra high gas pressures. J Cell Physiol 28:325-337, 1946
4. Smith KH, Spencer MP: Doppler indices of decompression sickness: Their evaluation and use. Aerosp Med 41:1396-1400, 1970
5. Buckles RG: The physics of bubble formation and growth. Aerosp Med 39:1062-1069, 1968
6. Bove AA, Hallenbeck JM, Elliott DH: Circulatory responses to venous air embolism and decompression sickness in dogs. Undersea Biomed Res 1:207-220, 1974
7. Ackles KN (ed): Blood-bubble interaction in decompression sickness. DCIEM Conference Proceedings No. 73-CP-960. Ontario, Canada, Department of National Defense, 1973
8. Smith KH, Stegall PJ, D'Aoust BG: Pathophysiology of decompression sickness, in Hong SK (ed): International Symposium on Man-in-the-Sea, Honolulu, 1975 (in press)
9. Kylstra JA, Longmuir IS, Grace M: Dysbarism: Osmosis caused by dissolved gas? Science 161:289, 1968
10. Chryssanthou CP: Humoral factors in the pathogenesis of decompression sickness (DS), in Ackles KN (ed): DCIEM Conference Proceedings No. 73-CP-960. Ontario, Canada, Department of National Defense, 1973, p 165

11. Erde AE, Edmonds C: Decompression sickness: A clinical series. J Occup Med 17: 324-328, 1975
12. Haymaker W, Johnston AD: Pathology of decompression sickness. Milit Med 117:285-306, 1955
13. Strauss RH: Spinal cord bends. Skin Diver Mag, September 1973, p 50
14. Strauss RH, Prockop LD: Decompression sickness among scuba divers. JAMA 223:637-640, 1973
15. Paulev P: Decompression sickness following repeated breath-hold dives, in Rahn H (ed): Physiology of Breath-hold Diving and the Ama of Japan. Washington, D.C., Publication 1341, National Academy of Sciences, 1965, p 221
16. Cross ER: Taravana diving syndrome in the Tuamotu diver, in Rahn H (ed): Physiology of Breath-hold Diving and the Ama of Japan. Washington, D.C., Publication 1341, National Academy of Sciences, 1965, p 207
17. US Navy Diving Manual. Washington D.C., Navy Department, 1973
18. Buhlmann AA, Schibli R, Gehring H: Experimentelle untersuchungen uber die dekompression nach tauchgangen in bergseen bei vermindertem luftdruck. Schweiz Med Wochenschr 103:378-383, 1973
19. Edel PO, Carroll JJ, Honaker RW, Beckman EL: Interval at sea-level pressure required to prevent decompression sickness in humans who fly in commercial aircraft after diving. Aerosp Med 40:1105-1110, 1969
20. Boycott AE, Damant GCC, Haldane JS: The prevention of compressed-air illness. J Hyg 8:342-443, London, 1908
21. Kety SS: The cerebral circulation, in Field J (ed): Handbook of Physiology, vol 3. Washington, D.C., American Physiological Society, 1960, p 1751
22. Hills BA: Thermodynamic decompression: An approach based upon the concept of phase equilibration in tissue, in Bennett PB, Elliott DH (eds): The Physiology and Medicine of Diving and Compressed Air Work. Baltimore, Williams & Wilkins, 1969, p 319
23. Yount DE, Strauss RH: Bubble formation in gelatin: A model for decompression sickness (in preparation)
24. Evans A, Walder DN: Significance of gas micronuclei in the aetiology of decompression sickness. Nature 222:251-252, 1969
25. Strauss RH: Bubble formation in gelatin: Implications for prevention of decompression sickness. Undersea Biomed Res 1:169-174, 1974
26. Keller H, Buhlmann AA: Deep diving and short decompression by breathing mixed gases. J Appl Physiol 20:1267-1270, 1965
27. Van Liew HD, Passke M: Permeation of neon, nitrogen and sulfur hexafluoride through walls of subcutaneous gas pockets in rats. Aerosp Med 38:829-831, 1967
28. Strauss RH, Kunkle TD: Isobaric bubble growth: A consequence of altering atmospheric gas. Science 186:443-444, 1974
29. Graves DJ, Idicula J, Lambertsen CJ, Quinn JA: Bubble formation in physical and biological systems: A manifestation of counterdiffusion in composite media. Science 179:582-584, 1973

STUDY QUESTIONS

1. The primary pathogenic mechanism of decompression sickness is
   a. Agglutination of formed elements in the blood
   b. Shifts of fluid due to the osmotic activity of gases
   c. Bubble formation and growth
   d. Smooth muscle acting factor
2. Even a slight supersaturation of tissue by gas generally results in decompression sickness.
   a. True
   b. False
3. More than half of the manifestations of decompression sickness occur within 1 hr of surfacing.
   a. True
   b. False
4. Manifestations of decompression sickness may include
   a. Paralysis from the neck down
   b. Difficulty initiating urination
   c. Numbness and tingling of the legs
   d. Shoulder pain
   e. All of the above
5. Decompression sickness involving the central nervous system generally clears spontaneously within a few hours, and recompression therapy is optional.
   a. True
   b. False
6. Rapid ascent rates (faster than 60 feet/minute) may contribute to the cause of decompression sickness.
   a. True
   b. False
7. List three factors that predispose a diver to decompression sickness.
8. Using current decompression meters is safer than using the U.S. Navy standard decompression tables.
   a. True
   b. False
9. A scuba diver has remained within the no-decompression limits of the U.S. Navy tables. What is the minimum time he should allow between his last dive and flying in a commercial, pressurized aircraft?
10. It is safe to use standard decompression tables in mountain diving.
   a. True
   b. False

11. Some tissues of the body take up and lose gas more rapidly than other tissues.
    a. True
    b. False
12. Breathing oxygen at sea level causes the body's "inherent unsaturation" to
    a. Increase
    b. Decrease
    c. Remain unchanged
13. Helium causes decompression sickness in much the same way that nitrogen does.
    a. True
    b. False

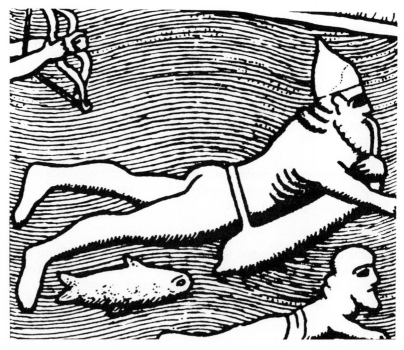

Assyrian frieze (900 BC). From *History of Diving*, U.S. Navy Diving Manual, 1973.

Eric P. Kindwall

7

Hyperbaric and Ancillary Treatment Of Decompression Sickness, Air Embolism, and Related Disorders

When a diver is suffering from decompression sickness or air embolism, the sine qua non is to place him once again under pressure as quickly as possible. Regardless of what the patient may be suffering from, have him lie down. If he has pulmonary symptoms (hemoptysis, cough) or central nervous system (CNS) symptoms or signs (seizures, coma, unequal pupils, blindness, or paralysis), he should be kept in a position with his buttocks elevated approximately 30° above his head. Since it will not be immediately known whether or not the patient has air embolism, it is best to turn him slightly toward the left at about a 10° to 15° angle from the prone position, or onto his left side. Once this maneuver has been carried out, it should be definitely determined that the patient has a free airway. Cardiopulmonary resuscitation should be started, if indicated; and throughout the period of diagnosis and transportation to the ultimate treatment center, the patient should be kept in this relative position and all measures taken to support or restore cardiopulmonary action. Instruct all scuba personnel *never to give up any resuscitative attempts until the patient is pronounced dead by a licensed physician.*

When shifting the patient with cerebral symptoms from the boat to the dock and then to the ambulance, it is important that the head be kept lower than the feet at all times. This position can be maintained in the ambulance with suitable blocks under the stretcher. Keep the patient warm to help combat possible shock. If oxygen is available, it must be given during transportation to the treatment center. Scuba instructors and others can be taught to feel

83

the patient's neck and the area below the jaw for subcutaneous emphysema or a "rice crispies" feeling under the skin. If these signs are present, the information can be relayed ahead to the facility which will treat the patient and, indeed, it may determine which facility is used.

TRANSPORTATION

Having observed the rules for positioning of the patient during transportation, the most important factor in moving the victim is speed. It would be wise to establish radio contact with the coast guard if many hours must be spent reaching the shore by boat. The use of *a pressurized aircraft or low altitude air transportation may prove lifesaving.* The Lear jet aircraft can maintain sea level cabin pressure up to an altitude of 23,000 ft.

If an automobile must be used for transporting the patient, he should be placed in the back seat with his buttocks above the level of his head and held in place by an attendant on the way to the medical facility. Again, cardiopulmonary support must be carried out if necessary.

TREATMENT OF MEDIASTINAL EMPHYSEMA AND PNEUMOTHORAX

Occasionally, the only signs of lung rupture occurring during ascent may be subcutaneous emphysema, a fullness in the throat, or distortion of the voice. This indicates that the patient has suffered mediastinal emphysema with dissection by air from the lung into the mediastinal space. Often there is pneumopericardium which can be seen on x-ray. The patient may or may not have concommitant cerebral air embolism and/or pneumothorax. However, if mediastinal emphysema, even with pneumopericardium, is the only problem, treatment in the hyperbaric chamber is rarely, if ever, necessary. The patient should simply be put to bed and observed carefully to be sure he does not develop any respiratory or cardiac embarassment. The air will generally resolve spontaneously after 3 to 4 days of bed rest. Intermittent oxygen breathing may speed the process.

Pneumothorax is an extremely frightening complication of lung rupture, especially if it occurs during ascent either in the water or in the decompression chamber. A patient presenting with pneumothorax is not a candidate for treatment in the chamber until his pneumothorax is managed with standard surgical methods. A convenient way of relieving the pneumothorax is to insert a Clagget needle into the second intercostal space with a one-way condom check valve attached to the end of the needle. This will permit air to escape from the chest, but will prevent its entrance. As an alternative, constant suction can be applied over a 20 cm water seal. In cases where continuous suction is used on a pneumothorax, the tube should be clamped during compression in the chamber. Suction is continued during time at depth and during decompression.

DEFINITIVE TREATMENT

Today, oxygen recompression is the treatment of choice for most cases of decompression sickness, with the maximum treatment depth being 60 feet. In air embolism, a brief excursion to 165 feet is indicated before returning to 60 feet for oxygen treatment. The initial deep excursion is used only when a chamber capable of this 6 ata is available.

Historically, air recompression was used for the treatment of both bends and air embolism, and the old U.S. Navy Air Tables I through IV, promulgated in 1945, became the standard of the world for over 20 years. These tables represented a ninefold improvement over previous procedures. For many years, they were quite acceptable (despite their being very lengthy, taking between 6 and 38 hours), with the overall failure rate on the initial recompression for the period 1946 to 1964 being only 14.3 percent. However, for the single year 1963, the failure rate was 21.9 percent. By 1964 it had climbed to 26.7 percent. Even more disconcerting was the fact that the failure rate on initial recompressions for serious symptoms using Tables III and IV had jumped from 29.7 percent in the period from 1946 to 1964 to 46.4 percent in 1963 and 47.1 percent in 1964.[1]

The reason for the increasing failure rate was that more civilian scuba divers who had failed to observe any sort of standard decompression schedule were being treated at Navy facilities, and the cases being treated were much more serious.

As an answer to these increasing problems in treatment, the U.S. Navy, under the aegis of Goodman and Workman, reinvestigated the use of oxygen breathing at relatively low pressures for bends treatment. Yarbrough and Behnke had originally experimented with treating compressed air illness by utilizing oxygen in 1939 after an initial excursion to 6 ata and reported good results;[2] but further investigation along these lines was dropped by the Navy at the time.

Between 1964 and 1966, Goodman and Workman developed two new treatment schedules and tested them in the field on over 50 cases. The failure rate for all initial recompressions in the experimental group was only 2 percent as compared with 26.7 percent for Tables I through IV in the year 1964. The failure rate in the "serious symptom" cases was only 3.6 percent in the oxygen-treated group. If one compares the data, the experimental case load was composed of older divers who had been exposed for longer bottom times at deeper depths. Analysis of the results showed them to be statistically valid.[1]

Thus, if oxygen recompression is available, it is now the treatment of choice. Oxygen treatment (Tables 5 and 6) was approved in 1967.

Air embolism treatment also changed at the time of the introduction of the oxygen treatment tables, when the Navy promulgated Tables 5A and 6A, (the "embolism tables") developed by Waite. Previously, air embolism had always been treated on Tables III or IV. Waite demonstrated in dogs that only a *brief recompression* with air to 6 ata was necessary to restore circulation and function, even if followed by immediate decompression to the surface.[3] In humans, however, oxygen is used from 60 feet to the surface as a safety factor and to reduce cerebral edema.

Table 5 (Appendix 2) is only 135 minutes in length and is for mild or "pain only" cases of bends. This form of bends, which does not present with neurologic or pulmonary symptoms but only with pain, is termed Type I bends. Table 5 may be used for Type I bends if the patient gets complete relief of all his symptoms within 10 minutes while breathing oxygen at 60 feet. Should his pain not disappear within 10 minutes, Table 6 should automatically be used.

Table 6 is for "serious symptoms" (Type II cases) referrable to the central nervous or pulmonary systems and for recurrences of previously treated decompression sickness of any kind. It is also used for "pain only" cases which do not respond with complete relief within 10 minutes at 60 feet and for cases of decompression sickness which begin their onset while the diver is still decompressing from his original dive. This latter situation is termed bends occurring under pressure. The Table is 285 minutes in length, (Appendix 2), but may be lengthened an additional 100 minutes if necessary.

Table 5A (Appendix 2) is for cases of air embolism that show complete resolution of all symptoms within 15 minutes of breating air at 165 feet (6 ata). If symptoms are still present at 15 minutes Table 6A (Fig. 4) is used, which provides for a maximum of 30 minutes at 165 feet for recovery. Previously, it was mandatory that if the patient had not recovered completely or was not rapidly recovering after 30 minutes at 165 feet, he was then committed to Table IV (38 hours in length). In the experience of the author, this is not necessary, and maximum benefit of compression to 6 ata will have been realized within a few minutes of reaching 165 feet. It is more important at this point to decompress to 60 feet and start the patient on oxygen.

If, after adequate treatment on the appropriate table, the patient still has neurological symptoms remining, it may be useful to re-treat him once or twice a day for 90 minutes at 2.5 ata with 100 percent oxygen for several days following the initial treatment.

CHOICE OF DECOMPRESSION CHAMBER

Decompression chambers come in two basic types:"walk-in" types which have room for more than one person and are pressurized with air (Fig. 7-1); and one-man chambers which are for the patient only. In one-man chambers, no inside attendant can accompany the patient. One-man chambers usually are pressurized with pure oxygen. The larger walk-in chambers frequently are equipped with an inner and an outer lock so that people or supplies may be locked in or out during the course of treatment.

In handling a case of decompression sickness or air embolism, one seldom gets to "choose" a chamber, but usually must "make do" with whatever kind of chamber is nearest at hand. As a rough rule of thumb, the nearest chamber that is operational and competently manned is usually the best chamber.

No additional instruction will be given here for treating decompression sickness in the standard large walk-in chamber equipped with oxygen masks. However, there are a number of Vickers, Sechrist or Bethlehem 3-atm one-man hyperbaric chambers available in hospitals, but they are pressurized with pure oxygen.These chambers may be used for the treatment of decompression sickness and can be used for the treatment of air embolism if a 165-foot (6 ata) chamber is not available.[4]

It is impossible to take the patient off and on oxygen while at pressure in the one-man chamber. The following treatment regimen is suggested for use with the one-man chamber since Tables 5 and 6, with their periods of air breathing, cannot be used.

1. *Pain only, Type I cases.* Flush the chamber with oxygen to remove air, then raise pressure to 26 psig (1.8 kg/cm²). If all symptoms are gone within 10 min, hold the patient at 26 psig for 1/2 hr and then slowly decompress to a pressure of 14.7 psig (1 kg/cm²) over a 15-min period. Keep the patient at 14.7 psig for 1 hour, then slowly decompress to the surface over a 15-min period.

2. *"Serious symptoms", Type II bends, or cases of air embolism.* If a patient has serious symptoms or does not achieve relief within 10 minutes at 26 psig on pure oxygen, hold the patient at that pressure for 1/2 hour and then decompress to 14.7 psig over a period of 1/2 hour. Hold the patient at 14.7 psig for 1 hour, and then decompress to the surface taking an additional 30 minutes. If the symptoms are not completely relieved using this treatment schedule, it may be repeated after a 1/2 to 1 hour's surface interval of breathing air. One-man chambers pressurized with oxygen are available at increasing numbers of hospitals because of their use in treat-

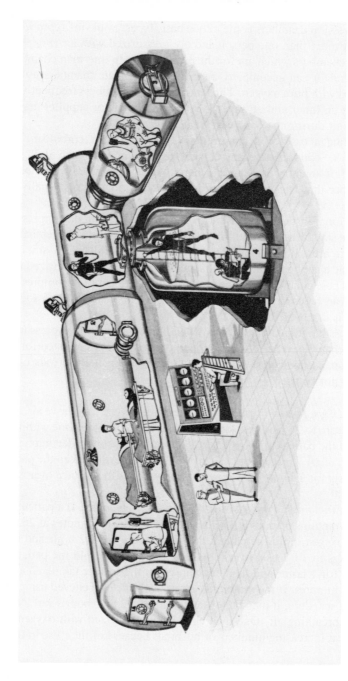

Fig. 7-1. A large hyperbaric chamber complex used for both treatment and research. (Courtesy of C. J. Lambertsen, M.D., Institute for Environmental Medicine, University of Pennsylvania.)

ing carbon monoxide poisoning, gas gangrene, chronic osteomyelitis, some forms of decubitus ulcer, and other nondiving medical conditions. However, the whole area of nondiving hyperbaric medicine is too large to be included in the scope of this text.

DRUG THERAPY OR MEDICAL ADJUNCTS TO RECOMPRESSION

If one assumes that the patient has been or is about to be recompressed and that the nitrogen bubbles present in his body have been or will be quickly obliterated, the damage to the body caused by their having been present must be reckoned with.

Thus far, it appears that damage from bubbles includes increased sludging of the blood, increased platelet aggregation and microthrombi, and hemo-concentration with loss of volume from the vascular compartment and spinal cord and brain edema. Drug therapy would be appropriate for correcting any of these conditions.

In the following sections, some drugs are discussed that have been used in treating decompression sickness (and/or air embolism) as adjuncts to recompression. Because every case of decompression sickness is different, careful drug selection is necessary on the part of the physician.

Low Molecular Weight Dextran (Dextran 40, Rheomacrodex)

Low molecular weight dextran has been a useful plasma expander; but, in nondiving diseases, there is now some question as to whether it is superior to, or even as good as, its heavier analog dextran 80.

In decompression sickness, however, low molecular weight Dextran *in saline* is extremely useful as it appears to alter the charge on the surface of the red cells and tends to prevent rouleaux formation. Even though it is rapidly excreted by the healthy kidney, it is useful in immediately expanding blood volume, the loss of which is a problem in severe bends shock. In a normal individual, 500 ml given twice a day for a maximum of 5 days is usually safe. If a patient has had symptoms for more than 2 hours prior to treatment, the author gives 500 ml intravenously as a matter of routine. The agent should not be continued if the patient is asymptomatic after chamber treatment. In cases of severe shock, dextran 40 *alone* should not be relied upon.

Plasma (Reconstituted Plasma, Plasmanate)

This is a useful volume expander which can be given in cases of shock due to decompression sickness. Cockett[5] has shown that it alone could prevent death in a group of experimental dogs where the controls untreated with plasma died. This agent should be reserved only for *shock* due to decompression sickness.

Heparin

Despite its common use as an anticoagulant in hospitals, heparin appears to exert its beneficial effect in decompression sickness because of its lipemia-clearing ability and not its anticoagulant effect. Cockett[6] has demonstrated that heparin can prevent death from decompression sickness in dogs while their untreated controls died. Reeves and Workman,[7] however, were not able to demonstrate any beneficial effect in mild to moderate cases of decompression sickness in experimental dogs. The author's feeling is usually to reserve it for cases of bends shock. However, there is some recent evidence that it may be quite useful in spinal cord bends. A suggested dosage is 7500 international units intravenously followed by 5000 unit doses at intervals later if necessary.

Steroids

Steriods are chiefly useful in those cases where one suspects central nervous system involvement or edema of the spinal cord or brain. Theoretically, steroids will tend to exascerbate oxygen toxicity, although Workman (personal communication) claimed that he has never heard of a case of oxygen convulsions occurring on Tables 5 or 6 when the patient had been pretreated with steroids. However, it is the author's practice to sometimes withhold steroids until the 30-foot stop has been reached, especially if the patient is showing signs of incipient oxygen toxicity.

Hyperbaric oxygen itself has very strong vasoconstrictive properties and for this reason, tends to reduce intracranial pressure by about 50 percent within 2 minutes of commencement of oxygen breathing at 3 ata. However, one should use steroids to continue control of edema after the patient has left the chamber, especially with spinal cord or cerebral damage. The customary dose has been Dexamethazone phosphate 10 mg intravenously followed by 4 mg intramuscularly every 6 hours up to 72 hours. If given for no longer than 72 hours, the steroid can be discontinued abruptly and need not be tapered. If continued for longer than 72 hours, tapering of the dose is necessary. Even during the short 72-hour regimen recommended here, however, steroid ulcer is a very real possiblity; and should the patient have any type of ulcer history at all, he ought to be placed on prophylactic antacids.

Digitalis

Digitalis can be quite useful in bends shock if the heart rate is high. In one case treated by the author, it appeared to be the drug that saved the patient's life when everything else had been used. The digitalizing drug can be one of the quick-acting intravenous cardiac glycosides such as Cedilanid-D 0.8 mg intravenously.

Aminophyllin

If a patient suffers from "chokes" due to decompression sickness and does not experience relief upon immediate recompression, it may be tempting to use this drug. However, the author's experience has not been encouraging in treating chokes with Aminophyllin.

Use of Blood Pressure Cuff

The author is unsure if Edgar End taught him this trick or if he learned it from someone in the U.S. Navy. However, if one is treating a diver for a mild case of "pain only, Type I" bends and only one sore spot persists in a knee or elbow, one may become committed to Table 6, as the stopwatch approaches 10 minutes. In such a situation, it may be worthwhile to try applying a blood pressure cuff over the sore spot and rapidly pumping it up to 300 mm. Hg. The cuff then is immediately released. In about half the cases, the pain will vanish even after the blood pressure cuff has been removed. If it does not, nothing is lost.

PRECAUTIONS TO BE OBSERVED DURING CHAMBER TREATMENT

It is important to bear in mind that the laws of physics are immutable, and if one does not observe them continuously, the patient may suffer dire consequences. Be sure that all glass intravenous bottles are vented while being used in the chamber. If a vent tube does not extend from the air-vent needle opening in the bottle, all the way up to the air-filled space at the bottom of the bottle when hanging, the air above the fluid will expand during decompression, driving the entire contents of the intravenous container into the patient to be followed by a bolus of air—depending upon how empty the bottle is at the time decompression is started. Using flexible plastic bags as containers for intravenous fluids in the chamber will obviate the need to ever be concerned about this problem.

The most common error in treating decompression sickness is failure to recognize the seriousness of the patient's condition. Even if the patient complains only of subjective pain, do as thorough a neurologic examination as possible. If any neurologic signs are present, even if the patient is not aware of them, it will automatically mean he must be treated on a longer table. Be sure to check for subcutaneous emphysema in the neck and, of course, listen and percuss for pneumothorax. A diver presenting with mild symptoms may sometimes get worse (especially if it is a spinal cord case) while undergoing oxygen treatment. This could be due to the development of spinal cord edema and/or thrombosis of the venous system surrounding the cord. Don't panic if this occurs, but simply administer steroids, low molecular weight dextran, and, perhaps, in such cases, heparin.

During compression, the diver occasionally complains of increasing pain. This is often referred to as a "bone bubble," which has no scientific meaning other than identifing a sometimes-seen clinical occurrence. It has been postulated that a tiny bubble of nitrogen under the periostium is compressed, returning the periostium to its normal position, which then causes intense pain. Regardless of the cause, the only solution is to slow down the compression rate until it is tolerable for the diver, but persist until treatment depth is reached. Then, the pain will eventually disappear.

HANDLING THE DOUBTFUL CASE

Occasionally the diving doctor may be faced with a dilemma when a patient who has just surfaced from a dive complains of pain, perhaps in a knee or shoulder. This is especially perplexing if the patient acknowledges a recent sprain in the area or if an obvious bruise is present. If the pain continues to get worse, one might suspect decompression sickness. Mild symptoms of bends are often referred to as "air pains" or "niggles" (British). Air pains or niggles persisting longer than 30 minutes *should be considered bends and treated.* People often refer to niggles and air pains saying that they "can feel the bubbles running."

Test of Pressure

When faced with the problem of deciding whether or not to treat a patient for possible decompression sickness, a test of pressure is the method of choice. Take the patient in the dry chamber to a pressure of 60 feet for 20 minutes breathing oxygen. If the pain is *unchanged* in *intensity, nature, position,* or *quality,* it is usually safe to assume it is not decompression sickness. Should the pain later intensify or turn out to be true decompression sickness, nothing has been lost. Never recompress the symptomatic diver in the water, even as a "test of pressure," except under extremely isolated conditions where special preparations have been made (see Chapter 21).

MISSED DECOMPRESSION

Occasionally, the situation may arise where a diver is making a decompression dive but, for some reason, cannot make the required decompression stops. This may be due to running out of air or losing the descending line. Under these circumstances, where there is no chamber available, the diver may reenter the water to make up for his decompression, only if he remains completely asymptomatic and his surface interval is no longer than a few minutes. If the diver can obtain another set of air tanks, or if he has air remaining in his own tank, he should return to the water and repeat any decompression stops deeper than 40 feet. It is highly unlikely that, in making a scuba dive, a stop at such a depth would be required. The diver should then proceed as follows, taking 1 minute between stops.

A. Remain at the 40-foot stop (if called for in the table) for one-quarter of the length of the 10-foot stop designated for the particular dive.
B. Remain at the 30-foot stop (if called for in the table) for one-third of the length of the scheduled 10-foot stop designated for the particular dive.
C. Remain at the 20-foot stop (if called for in the table) for one-half of the length of the 10-foot stop designated.
D. Remain at the 10-foot stop for one and one-half times its normal length. The diver may then surface.

This schedule is included in the September 1973 U.S. Navy Diving Manual vol. I, Air Diving, Section 8, pp. 35-36.

If the diver has symptoms or signs of decompression sickness following his decompression he must never be recompressed in the water. In such case, *take him to the nearest recompression chamber, no matter how far away it is.*

REFERENCES

1. Goodman MW, Workman RD: Minimal Recompression, Oxygen-breathing Approach of Treatment of Decompression Sickness in Divers and Aviators. BU-SHIPS Project SF0110605, Task 11513-2, Research Report 5-65. Washington, D.C., Bureau of Medicine and Surgery, November, 1965
2. Yarbrough OB, Behnke AR: The treatment of compressed air illness utilizing oxygen. J. Ind Hyg Toxicol 21 (6) 1939
3. Waite CL, Mazzone WF et al: Cerebral Embolism, 1, Basic Studies. US Naval Submarine Medical Center Research Report, No 493, April, 1967
4. Hart GB: Treatment of decompression sickness and air embolism with hyperbaric oxygen. Aerosp Med 45 (10) 1190-1193, 1974
5. Cockett ATK, Nakamura RM: A new concept in the treatment of decompression sickness (Dysbarism). Lancet 1:1102, 1964.
6. Cockett ATK, Pauley SM, Roberts AP: Advancements in treatments of decompression sickness: An evaluation of heparin, Proceedings of the Third In-

ternational Conference on Hyperbarics and Underwater Physiology. Editor, X. Fructus, *DOIN Editeurs*, Paris, 1972

7. Reeves SE, Workman RD: Use of heparin for the therapeutic/prophylactic treatment of decompression sickness, Aerosp Med 42 (1) 20-23, 1971

8. Sukoff MH, Hollin SA, Jacobson JH II: The protective effect of hyperbaric oxygenation in the experimentally produced cerebral edema and compression. Surgery 62 (1) 40-46, 1967

STUDY QUESTIONS

1. Oxygen breathing by mask is of value in handling the pressure related diving casualty even if it is not given under pressure.
   a. True
   b. False

2. A diving casualty with pulmonary or CNS symptoms or signs should be kept in Fowler's position during transportation to a treatment facility.
   a. True
   b. False

3. A patient with "pain only" decompression sickness is treated on Table 5 with immediate relief of all his symptoms. Four hours later, his symptoms of "pain only" recur. He is then diagnosed as a Type II case.
   a. True
   b. False

4. Mediastinal emphysema and pneumothorax do not usually require treatment in the chamber.
   a. True
   b. False

5. Table IV is more successful in the treatment of air embolism than Table 6A.
   a. True
   b. False

6. Oxygen recompression is superior to air recompression even though it presents the problems of potential oxygen toxicity.
   a. True
   b. False

7. A diver experiences the onset of pain in one knee while decompressing at the 10-foot stop having made a 130-foot dive. On surfacing, he should be treated on
   a. Table 5A
   b. Table 6A
   c. Table IV
   d. Table 5
   e. Table 6

8. Type II bends cases unfortunately cannot be treated in the one-man chamber.
   a. True
   b. False
9. The greatest value of low molecular weight dextran is that it
   a. tends to prevent rouleaux formation.
   b. it is an optimal plasma expander.
   c. prevents blood clotting.
   d. reduces spinal cord edema.
   e. is reserved for air embolism cases.
10. Dextran 40 is better than plasma or plasmanate for expanding volume in severe cases of bends shock.
    a. True
    b. False
11. Heparin can be given to patients suffering from severe decompression sickness as it has a lipemia clearing effect.
    a. True
    b. False
12. Steroids tend to protect against oxygen toxicity.
    a. True
    b. False
13. Steroids should be given in conjunction with hyperbaric oxygen because, under pressure, oxygen breathing tends to raise intracranial pressure.
    a. True
    b. False
14. Inflating a blood pressure cuff over a "sore spot" remaining during bends treatment in the chamber is sometimes of value even though bends symptoms may sometimes be due to blood sludging.
    a. True
    b. False
15. Glass bottles are superior to plastic bags for containing intravenous solutions in the chamber as plastic bags will tend to deform as pressure is built up.
    a. True
    b. False
16. If pain gets *worse* during compression, recompression therapy must be halted and the patient treated with plasma and steroids.
    a. True
    b. False
17. A "test of pressure" involves taking the patient to 60 feet and having them breathe oxygen for 20 min.
    a. True
    b. False

18. If the nearest recompression facility is more than 100 miles away, it is usually best to treat a diver's symptoms of bends in the water.
    a. True
    b. False.

D.N. Walder

8

Aseptic Necrosis of Bone

Introduction

Aseptic bone necrosis is one of the many terms used to describe the changes seen in the bones of some men following exposure to increased barometric pressure. Therefore, it is a condition seen both in compressed air workers and divers. It does not affect every bone in the body or indeed all of any one bone, but rather seems to be limited to a few specific and circumscribed sites.

The most important sites are those adjacent to the joint surfaces of the shoulder and hip (juxta-articular lesions). The normal load carried at such sites may result in collapse of the dead bone and the disruption of the bearing surfaces that are usually smooth (Fig. 8-1). This, in turn, can lead to nonspecific compensatory changes in and around the joint surfaces to result in the secondary condition commonly called arthritis. From the patient's point of view, such a sequence of events eventually results in a state in which some movements are painful and some limited. In the early stages, prior to collapse of the articular surface, the condition is usually symptom free and, at present, can only be detected by radiography.

In addition to these juxta-articular lesions are the shaft lesions that characteristically affect the lower end of the femur and the upper end of the tibia. Unfortunately, there is a lack of human histological material illustrating this type of lesion, but it is believed that the necrosis affects the tissues of the marrow cavity.[1] Thus fat is involved and, as this breaks down, fatty acids are released which combine with calcium to give the diffuse calcified marking typical of these lesions (Fig. 8-2).

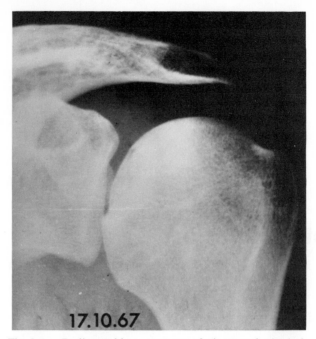

Fig. 8-1.   Radiographic appearance of a juxta-articular lesion
affecting head of left humerus. Collapse of the articular surface
has occurred.

Classification

To standardize the systems used by different centers to describe the
radiographic appearances of bone lesions seen in compressed air workers and
divers, the Medical Research Council (M.R.C.) Decompression Sickness
Panel has drawn up a classification (Table 8-1) which has proved to be extremely useful. To assist radiologists in recognizing the various lesions mentioned in the classification, a limited number of radiological atlases[2] were distributed from the M.R.C. Decompression Sickness Team in Newcastle. Many
of the x-rays from it have been reproduced and are to be found in a publication by Ilford.[3] It is recognized that as time passes any lesion may progress
into a more serious type, so that it is necessary to keep a running record of an
individual's bone lesion state.

Radiography and Other Methods of Diagnosis

It must be realized that the only changes that can be seen by x-ray examination are changes in the amount of calcium salts present in the bone.
There is no difference in the radiographic appearances of a bone examined

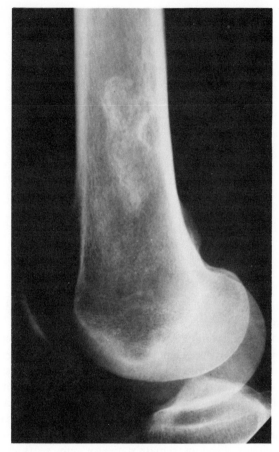

Fig. 8-2. Radiographic appearance of a shaft lesion in lower
end of femur.

today when alive and tomorrow when dead. Neither does the time after death
of the examination make any difference. The bones of a man x-rayed many
years after death may be practically indistinguishable from those x-rayed on
the day of death. As the amount and distribution of calcium salts are seen to
change after a bone is damaged, it is clear that there must be some form of circulation surrounding that damage and perhaps extending into it at places.

When, for example, aseptic bone lesions affecting the head of the
humerus are examined by histology, it is found that in some parts of the lesion
the trabeculae no longer contain living osteocytes in their lacunae, but in
other regions the dead trabeculae are covered by a layer of new bone with living osteocytes (Fig. 8-3).

These changes are slow; it is thought from the evidence available; at pres-

Table 8-1
Classification of Bone Necrosis
in Compressed Air Workers and Divers

Juxta-articular Lesions
A1. Dense areas, with intact articular cortex
A2. Spherical segmental opacities
A3. Linear opacity
A4. Structural failures:
    a. Translucent subcortical band.
    b. Collapse of articular cortex.
    c. Sequestration of cortex.
A5. Osteoarthritis.

Head, Neck, and Shaft Lesions
B1. Dense areas
B2. Irregular calcified areas
B3. Translucent areas.

---

ent, that a lesion cannot be detected radiologically until some 3 to 4 months after the causal incident.

This is not the only limitation of radiological studies. When it has been possible to compare the histological state of a bone with previous radiographs it has been found,[4] as might be expected from the previous discussion, that the radiograph does not always reveal the full extent of the lesion (Fig. 8-4). Furthermore, it is not yet possible to predict from the radiological appearance whether a specific early juxta-articular lesion will progress to give collapse of the articular surface in a few months as illustrated in Figure 8-1 or whether it will, like the majority of lesions, remain stable for many years and never cause any further involvement of the bone or any signs or symptoms.

Occasionally, the radiographic appearance of a diver's bones give rise to the suspicion that a lesion may exist, but the evidence is not conclusive. In such cases, further radiographic studies in 6 months or a year should be undertaken to confirm whether a lesion is developing or not. If it is important to make an earlier diagnosis, special techniques such as tomography may be helpful. If a suspected lesion is accompanied by pain on movement there may well be a breakdown of articular surface continuity which may only be revealed by tomography.

A further diagnostic technique is the use of bone-seeking isotopes. These have been employed very successfully in the detection of other bone abnormalities,[5] and there is some evidence of their potential value in the early diagnosis of aseptic necrosis of bone.[6] Before such a technique could be adopted as a widespread alternative to radiological surveillance of divers, it would be essential to confirm that the body dose of irradiation to each man was no

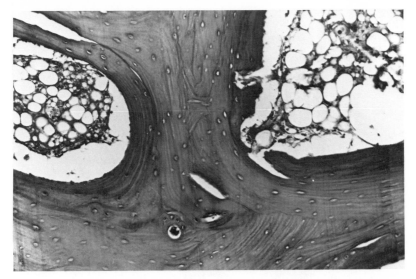

Fig. 8-3.   Photomicrograph (×125) showing dead trabeculum with empty lacunae onto which a layer of appositional new bone has formed with vital osteocytes in its lacunae.

greater. Zinn[7] has pointed out that pertrochanteric bone biopsy and bone phlebography are both useful additional methods that may assist in the early diagnosis of these lesions. Fortunately, simple radiological surveys, such as are recommended here, seem to be sufficient to make a diagnosis in the vast majority of cases.

The Size of the Problem

It is important to put into perspective the problem of aseptic necrosis of bone as it affects divers. There can be no doubt that men exposed to a pressurized environment, such as in civil engineering compressed air work and diving, run a risk of damage to their bones. In one study,[8] a bone radiographic survey was carried out on two groups of manual laborers employed on tunneling work. One group of men worked in compressed air many times over a period of years, whereas the other group did similar jobs at atmospheric pressure. There was eventually a 26 percent incidence of bone lesions in the 171 compressed air workers, but none of the 120 men in the other group developed a lesion.

For divers there have been widely differing reports of the incidence of bone necrosis. Ohta and Matsunaga[9] reported an incidence as high as 50 percent in Japanese diving fishermen. A survey by Harrison and Elliott[10] of British Navy clearance divers showed an overall figure of 5 percent though most

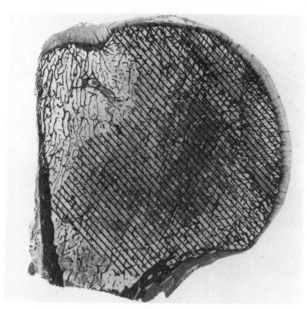

Fig. 8-4.   Photomicrograph ($\times$2) of head of humerus showing aseptic necrosis. Beneath the articular cartilage is an area of necrotic bone bounded by a line of fibrous tissue. The hatched area beyond this line shows evidence of dead trabeculae which have been covered by living bone and this represents the full extent of the original damage.

of the lesions were found in divers who had engaged in experimental diving (dives in which the decompression schedules used were not of proven adequacy[11]). Adams and Parker's recent report[12] on U.S. Navy divers suggested that the incidence might be as high as 30 percent, though it is possible that these figures included bone islands and other minor bone changes so that the true incidence may be more in line with that of the British Navy. The figure for the 1830 North Sea commercial divers x-rayed in Great Britain is approximately 2 percent.

The Distribution of Bone Lesions in Divers

The lesions of aseptic necrosis of bone are found at the same sites in compressed air workers and divers, but the frequency with which the sites are affected seems to differ from one report to another. In the British experience, the commonest site for lesions is the lower end of the femur, but the head of the femur is rarely affected in divers. Such observations have lead to speculation as to why this should be so and, if it is, whether it can provide some additional clue as to the aetiology of aseptic necrosis of bone.[13] Unfortunately, the

Japanese experience[14] is more like that seen in British compressed air workers, where the hip lesions occur with just about half the frequency of the shoulder lesions.

Radiographic Monitoring of Divers' Long Bones

Not only is it important for the individual diver to know that his bones are free from necrosis, but it is also important for an employer to be aware of any preexisting bone abnormalities in a man about to be taken onto his staff.

Obviously there is a radiation hazard associated with every radiographic examination, and this must be kept to an acceptable limit. It has been calculated that the long bone survey recommended by the British M.R.C. Decompression Sickness Panel may be carried out safely every 6 months, though it is emphasized that a gonad protector must be used.

Experience so far at the M.R.C. Decompression Sickness Central Registry in Newcastle Upon Tyne Great Britain indicates that bone necrosis is very rare in air diving (i.e., nonsaturation diving to depths of up to 50 meters). In fact, the author has only seen the condition in two divers who have never been deeper than 50 meters, so bone studies are not carried out on amateur and sport divers.

The extent of the radiological examination recommended by the M.R.C. Decompression Sickness Panel to study bone lesions in divers is shown in Table 8-2. The full survey should be carried out before starting work, and thereafter annually, unless the presence of a suspect lesion requires more frequent monitoring.

Differential Diagnosis

There are many conditions in addition to hyperbaric exposure which can lead to aseptic necrosis of bone in man (Table 8-3). Most of them can be identified by specific tests. For example, alcaptonuria is associated with the presence of homogentisic acid in the urine, sickle cell anemia by the presence of abnormal hemoglobin S. in the blood, and so on. The presence of "chronic alcoholism" is rather more difficult to establish, but in any case the evidence is tenuous that alcoholism is a significant factor which has to be excluded in divers with bone lesions.

Bone Islands

The bone island is seen radiographically as an isolated area of increased density. The shape is usually round or oval, the longer diameter varying between 2 and 15 mm and the margins may be well defined or irregular and indistinct.

Table 8-2
The Radiography of the Bones of
Compressed Air Workers and Divers

---

1. Good definition of the trabecular structure of the bone is essential.
2. The gonads must be protected from ionizing radiation by the use of a lead shield.
3. *Projections required*
    a. *Anteroposterior projection of each shoulder joint.*
    The patient is placed in a supine position with the trunk rotated at an angle of
    approximately 45°, to bring the shoulder to be radiographed in contact with the
    table. This arm is partially abducted and the elbow is flexed. Center 1 inch
    below the coracoid process of the scapula and come to show as much humerus as
    possible; bring in the lateral diaphragms to show only the head and shaft of the
    humerus. This view should show a clear joint space and the acromion should not
    overlap the head of the humerus.
    b. *Anteroposterior projection of each hip joint.*
    The patient is placed in a supine position with the feet and 90° to the table top.
    The edge of the gonad protector should be as near the femoral head as possible,
    but not in any way obscuring it. Center the cone over the head of the femur, that
    is 1 inch below the midpoint of a line joining the anterior superior iliac spine
    and the upper boarder of the pubic symphysis.
    c. *Anteroposterior and lateral projections of each knee.*
    Center at the level of the *upper* border of the patella. The field should include the
    lower third of the femur and the upper third of the tibia and fibula.

Conti and Sciarli[15] have suggested that bone islands are more common in
divers than others and indeed it is possible that some authors have classified
them as bone lesions. After a review of some of our material, Griffiths (personal communication, 1974) came to the conclusion that bone islands are no
more common in commercial divers (with at least 4 years experience of diving
to 50 meters or more) than in nondivers of the same age group. The areas
compared were those normally radiographed in the M.R.C. Panel's recommendations for diver bone surveys. The presence of bone islands is something
which in the past radiologists have rightly dismissed as of no significance and
hence no mention has usually been made of them in routine radiological
reports.

Advice

What advice should the doctor give to a diver found to have a bone lesion? This is a difficult question to answer because factual evidence on which
to base the advice is at present scanty. Certainly juxta-articular and shaft lesions should be considered separately.

At the moment, it seems reasonable (certainly in Great Britain where the

Table 8-3
Conditions Reported to be Associated
with Aseptic Necrosis of Bone

Hyperbaric exposure	Trauma
Steroid therapy	Rheumatoid arthritis
Sickle cell anaemia	Gout
Diabetes	Ionizing radiation
Chronic alcoholism	Syphilis
Cirrhosis of the liver	Alcaptonuria
Hepatitis	Arteriosclerosis
Pancreatitis	Hyperlipidaemia
Gaucher's disease	

basis of successful litigation is different from the U.S.A.) to take the view that although a shaft lesion represents a failure to protect the diver from the consequences of diving, shaft lesions almost never result in disability, so the man may continue to dive. Some caution is necessary because Mirra et al.[16] have recently suggested that neoplastic changes may have occurred in shaft lesions in compressed air workers. Men with such lesions should therefore be advised to report to their doctors if any symptom should ever arise in the affected leg. This possibility will have to be watched very carefully over the next few years.

If the lesion is near a joint, the situation is quite different. Each and every juxta-articular lesion is potentially disabling as the articular surface is liable to collapse. Even if the potential disability of one major joint was acceptable, the fact that a continuation of diving might result in a second major joint becoming affected cannot be excluded. For these reasons, it seems sensible to recommend that the presence of a juxta-articular lesion should be taken as a contraindication to further diving. Although the possibility of developing further lesions might be reduced by limiting the diving to say 50 meters, it would still be present. In any case, in the author's view, such a limitation, in Great Britain at the moment, would be impracticable because of the great pressures on men to dive to any depth when required in the North Sea.

The Cause of Aseptic Bone Necrosis in Divers

It is not difficult for those who accept the bubble hypothesis of decompression sickness to believe that aseptic bone necrosis results from the blockage of some critical nutrient blood vessels to bone by gas bubbles liberated at decompression. However, because the bubble hypothesis is not universally accepted and because in any case there is no clear correlation between reported attacks of decompression sickness and subsequent development of bone lesions,[13] several other mechanisms have been suggested for the etiology of bone necrosis in divers. Jones and Sakovich[17] suggest that fat embolism may be an important factor, and Philp, Inwood, and Warren[18] suggest that the blood vessels to bone may be obstructed by platelet thrombi. Puleo and Sobel[19] suggest that modification of the collagen of the bone may occur as a result of its exposure to higher than normal exygen tensions; and Hills[20] points out the osmotic effect of dissolved gases, which would mean that the damage occurs at compression as opposed to the generally accepted idea that the decompression is responsible.

There can be little doubt that much more would be known about the cause of boné lesions if it were not so difficult to induce the condition in laboratory animals by simulated diving. This is probably related to the short circulation time in animals smaller than man, and possibly also to their better regenerative capacity. In recent years, there have been reports of bone changes in mice,[21] rats,[22] and miniature pigs[23] following hyperbaric exposure; but, so far, none of the lesions described appears to be identical to those seen in man. Certainly, the extent of the initiating insult (rapid decompression) has in all these reports been so severe that the mechanism involved in producing the experimental lesion in animals may not be the same as that occurring in man.

An interesting approach to this problem has been the intra-arterial injection into rabbits of spherical glass particles to simulate bubble emboli. By using this technique, lesions of the femoral heads similar to those seen in man have been produced.[24] Thus the difficulty in producing bone lesions in small animals may lie in the short persistence time of bubble emboli.

Treatment

As shaft lesions are not expected to give symptoms or disability, no treatment is indicated. The treatment of aseptic bone necrosis at the juxta-articular site is not yet entirely satisfactory. It would be gratifying if those lesions which are going to break down could be identified early, that is, before disruption of the articular surface and therefore before the onset of pain or limitation of movement. Ideally, this could then lead to successful treatment and return of the damaged bone to normal. Unfortunately, such is not the case at present. A general principle of treatment applied by orthopedic surgeons to damaged joints is to relieve the affected joint of weight bearing in order to give the bone a chance to heal. In the cases of aseptic necrosis of bone in divers, this would mean a period of rest lasting for several months. The difficulty is to select those divers whose lesions are going to break down. This will only be a small minority of the lesions; but, at the moment, there is no way of determining which ones. In general, conservative treatment is unsatisfactory.[25]

Attempts to treat advanced lesions in which the articular surface has already become disrupted have included (1) inserting a bone graft into a drill hole through the underlying living bone into the area of dead bone in order to provide a pathway for revascularization[26]; (2) gouging out the necrotic bone from beneath the cartilage and packing the cavity with fresh cancellous bone chips[27]; or (3) realigning the shaft of the bone to change the line of weight bearing as in a McMurray's osteotomy. None of these methods has met with great success.

The most satisfactory method of treating the seriously affected joint may be to arthrodese the joint or to replace the damaged head of the bone by a prothesis. Although the use of protheses is well established for middle-aged and older patients, questions about the durability of the prothesis become of great importance when it is to be used to treat active young men such as divers.

REFERENCES

1. Jones JP: Alcoholism, hypercortisonism, fat embolism and osseous avascular necrosis, in Zinn WM (ed): Idiopathic Ischaemic Necrosis of the Femoral Head in Adults. Stuttgart, Thieme, 1971, 112-132
2. MRC Decompression Sickness Central Registry. Radiographic appearances of bone lesions in Compressed Air Workers. Newcastle upon Tyne, 1968
3. Davidson JK, Griffiths PD: Caisson disease of bone. X-ray Focus 10:2-11, 1970
4. McCallum RI, Walder DN: Bone lesions in compressed air workers. J Bone Joint Surg 48B:207-235, 1966
5. Citrin DL, Greig WR, Calder JF, et al: Preliminary experience of bone scanning with 99m Tc-labelled polyphosphate in malignant disease. Br J Surg 61:73-75, 1974
6. Cox PT, Walder DN: Strontium scanning in Caisson disease of bone, in Proceedings of the 5th Symposium on Underwater Physiology (in press)
7. Zinn WM: Conclusions, in Zinn WM (ed): Idiopathic Ischaemic Necrosis of the Femoral Head in Adults. Stuttgart, Thieme, 1971, pp 213-214
8. MRC Decompression Sickness Panel. Decompression sickness and aseptic necrosis of bone. Br J Ind Med 28:1-21, 1971
9. Ohta Y, Matsunaga H: Bone lesions in divers. J Bone Joint Surg 56B:3-16, 1974
10. Harrison JAB: Aseptic bone necrosis in naval clearance divers. Proc R Soc Med 64:1276-1278, 1971
11. Elliott DH: The role of decompression inadequacy in aseptic bone necrosis of naval divers. Proc R Soc Med 64:1278-1280, 1971
12. Adams GM, Parker GW: Dysbaric osteonecrosis in US Navy divers. A survey of non-random selected divers. Undersea Biomed Res 1:A20, 1974
13. Walder DN; Caisson disease of bone in Great Britain, in Wada J and Iwa T (eds): Proceedings of the Fourth International Congress on Hyperbaric Medicine. London, Bailliere, Tindall, 1970, pp 83-87
14. Kawashima M, Torisu T, Hayashi K, et al: Avascular necrosis in Japanese Diving Fishermen, in Trapp WG, Banister EW, Davison AJ, Trapp PA (eds): Proceedings of the 5th International Hyperbaric Congress. Burnaby, Simon Fraser University, 1974, pp 855-862

15. Conti V, Sciarli R: Bone lesions in the autonomous diver. Forsvarsmedicin 9:525-527, 1973
16. Mirra JM, Bullough PG, Marcove RC, et al: Malignant fibrous histiocytoma and osteosarcoma in association with bone infarcts. J Bone Joint Surg 56A:932-940, 1974
17. Jones JP, Sakovich L: Fat embolism of bone. J Bone Joint Surg 48A:149-164, 1966
18. Philp RB, Inwood MJ, Warren BA: Interactions between gas bubbles and components of the blood: implications in decompression sickness. Aerosp Med 43:946-953, 1972
19. Puleo LE, Sobel HH: Oxygen-modified collagen and its possible pathological significance. Aerosp Med 43:429-431, 1972
20. Hills BA; Clinical implications of gas-induced osmosis. Arch Intern Med 129:356-362, 1972
21. Chryssanthou C, Kalberer J, Kooperstein S, et al: Studies on Dysbarism. II. Influence of bradykinin and "bradykinin-antagonists" on decompression sickness in mice. Aerosp Med 35:741-746, 1964
22. Wunsche O, Scheele G: Bone cysts in albino rats following decompression from high pressure. Arch Orthop Unfallchir 77:7-16, 1973
23. Stegall PJ, Smith KH, Hildebrandt J: Aseptic bone necrosis and hematologic changes in miniature pigs as the result of compression/decompression exposures. Fed Proc 31:653, 1972
24. Cox PT: Simulated Caisson disease of bone. Forsvarsmedicin 9:520-524, 1973
25. Romer U, Wettstein P: Results of treatment of 81 Swiss patients with II NFH; in Zinn WM (ed): Idiopathic Ischaemic Necrosis of the Femoral Head in Adults. Stuttgart, Thieme, 1971, pp 205-212
26. Phemister DB: Treatment of the necrotic head of the femur in adults. J Bone Joint Surg 31A:55-66, 1949
27. Wagner H: Treatment of idiopathic necrosis of the femoral head, in Zinn WM (ed): Idiopathic ischaemic Necrosis of the Femoral Head in Adults. Stuttgart, Thieme, 1971, pp 202-204

STUDY QUESTIONS

1. Suggest three reasons why the radiological examination of bones in the study of aseptic necrosis is unsatisfactory.
2. What is the commonest site for juxta-articular lesion to appear in a diver?
3. What is the minimum interval advised between routine radiographic surveys in order to avoid exceeding the allowable yearly body dose of irradiation?
4. Name five of the conditions that must be considered in the differential diagnosis of aseptic necrosis of bone.
5. Is there any evidence to justify the continued follow-up of shaft lesions over a number of years?

Joseph C. Farmer, Jr. and
William G. Thomas

9

Ear and Sinus Problems in Diving

When man encounters extreme changes in ambient pressure during diving, significant injuries can develop in the ears and sinuses if adequate pressure equalization does not occur between these air-containing cavities and the ambient atmosphere. Much of the previous literature concerning E.N.T. problems in diving has discussed barotitis media, resulting from inadequate pressure equalization between the middle ear and the ambient atmosphere. This is largely felt to be a reversible and relatively insignificant problem. Lesser mention has been made of barosinusitis, resulting from inadequate pressure equalization between the paranasal sinuses and the ambient atmosphere. This emphasis is very understandable. Barotitis media is a fairly common problem among divers, and though occasionally disabling, is usually reversible with no long-lasting sequelae. Barosinusitis has been rarely encountered and also has not been significantly disabling. However, in recent years, with increased frequency of all diving, particularly deep exposures, more serious and definitely disabling otologic problems involving the inner ear have been encountered. Therefore, the predominance of this chapter will be concerned with otologic problems.

The evolution of an air-containing external and middle ear has presented humans with a device which efficiently transforms air-borne sound energy into a fluid-filled inner ear where this energy is transduced into electrical signals. Proper function of this mechanism requires that the external ear canal and middle ear be air-containing and that pressure differentials between these structures and the ambient atmosphere or inner ear be avoided. With the pressure changes encountered in diving, the existence of a pressure-sensitive middle ear becomes a liability.

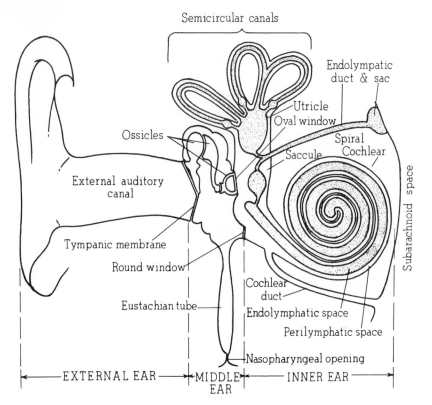

Fig. 9-1. Simplified diagramatic drawing of the external, middle, and inner ear showing air within the external auditory canal, middle ear, and eustachain tube. The fluid-filled inner ear is subdivided into the perilymphatic and endolymphatic spaces which connect with the subarachnoid space via the cochlear duct and endolymphatic duct, respectively.

In terrestrial environments, balance and spatial orientation are dependent upon input to the central nervous system of information from the visual, proprioceptive, and vestibular systems. When man goes beneath the sea, visual and proprioceptive inputs frequently become distorted; thus, spatial orientation under these conditions becomes more dependent upon information received from the vestibular system. As will be noted later in this chapter, vestibular system dysfunction can occur in multiple phases of diving and the subsequent vertigo with nausea and possible vomiting can present significant and life-threatening dangers.

The middle ear cleft (Fig. 9-1) is an irregularly shaped space that connects with air cell systems in the mastoid, petrous, and zygomatic portions of the temporal bone. The total gas volume of this complex varies between individuals depending upon the pneumatization of these areas. With an intact tympanic membrane, the only communication for pressure equalization between this complex and the ambient atmosphere is through the eustachian tube. This tube is approximately 35 to 38 mm in length in the adult and is directed downward, forward, and medially from the middle ear to the nasopharynx. The nasopharyngeal ostium is normally closed except when opened by a positive middle ear pressure or when opened by muscular action of the pharyngeal and palatine muscles upon the surrounding tubal cartilage during swallowing.

The eustachian tube is lined by respiratory epithelium which is similar to that lining the nose, sinuses, and nasopharynx. Abnormal nasal function can result from acute or chronic inflammatory diseases; allergy; chronic irritation from excessive smoking or prolonged use of nose drops; or from chronic obstruction from internal and/or external nasal deformities or mass lesions. This contributes to inadequate eustachian tubal function which, in divers can cause middle ear or even inner ear barotrauma. Also, inadequate ventilation of and barotrauma to the paranasal sinuses can occur.

The inner ear (Fig. 9-1) consists of a system of perilymph-filled bony channels within the temporal bone. In these channels are located membranous structures which contain endolymph. The membranous inner ear is divided into two parts: the vestibular system containing the semicircular canals, utricle, and saccule; and the cochlear system containing the spiral cochlear or auditory system. These two systems are interconnected and similar anatomically. The blood supply to both systems is through the internal auditory artery which originates from the basilar or inferior cerebellar artery. This is an end artery which supplies only the inner ear and has no collaterals with other vessels. Changes in cerebrospinal fluid (CSF) pressure can be directly transmitted to the inner ear compartments. Therefore, any maneuver that increases cerebrospinal fluid pressure, such as a Valsalva maneuver, can cause an increased pressure in the inner ear fluid compartments with bulging of the round window membrane into the middle ear. With marked pressure changes, possible round window rupture can occur and, as will be described later, can be seen in diving, even in shallow exposures.

Use of Systemic and Topical Drugs to Improve Nasal Function

While the use of systemic and topical vasoconstrictor agents can improve nasal function with the subsequent improvement in paranasal sinus and middle ear ventilation, such agents should be employed cautiously in divers. Rebound phenomena when the effect of the drug wears off, especially after topical nose drops, can lead to even greater nasal congestion with greater problems of pressure equalization in the ears and sinuses. Prolonged use of topical nasal medications can result in chronic nasal irritation and mucosal inflammation with similar pressure equalization problems during diving.

In general, any individual who has difficulty with middle ear ventilation at the surface or a past history of significant tympanomastoid disease such as cholesteatoma, recent draining ear, or chronic mastoiditis should probably not dive. Such individuals and those who have chronic nasal obstruction, history of frequent upper respiratory infections, or history of nasal allergies should have a complete otolaryngological evaluation before diving.

SYMPTOMS OF OTOLOGIC DYSFUNCTION

The common symptoms of otologic dysfunction are ear fullness or pain, tinnitus, hearing loss, and vertigo. It is not within the scope of this chapter to present a complete discussion of each of these symptoms. However, a brief review is in order.

Ear Fullness and Pain

Ear fullness or the sensation of a blocked ear commonly occurs as a result of a high or low middle ear pressure relative to ambient pressure. The resultant tensing of the eardrum and increased ossicular chain impedance causes a decrease in sound transmission to the inner ear. The patient feels that the ear has become occluded. With marked pressure differentials, pain occurs from sensory pain receptors in the eardrum and middle ear mucosa. Increased pain will be felt with eardrum rupture.

Hearing Loss

Hearing loss is classified into three types:

1. Conductive hearing loss resulting from dysfunction of any component of the sound conduction system, i.e., the external auditory canal, the eardrum, or the ossicular chain.

   Complete, airtight occlusion of the external auditory canal, such as from a cerumen plug, will cause a conductive hearing loss. Partial occlusion, or nonairtight seal of the canal, will not result in hearing loss unless the occluding material lies against the eardrum and thus impedes vibration. Conductive hearing loss can also occur from any process which interferes with the transmission of sound energy into the inner ear or impedes the movement of the eardrum and the ossicles. Such processes can include inflammation and swelling of the eardrum or middle ear mucosa, middle ear effusion or exudates, changes in middle ear gas density such as seen during hyperbaric exposures, pressure differentials across the eardrum, fixation of the ossicles, loss of elasticity of the eardrum from scarring, large eardrum perforations, interruption of the ossicular chain, etc.

2. Neurosensory or nerve hearing loss resulting from dysfunction in the inner ear, the auditory nerve, or the brain stem cochlear nuclei.

Such dysfunction can result from occlusion of the cochlear blood supply with ischemia, mechanical disruption of inner ear or brain stem structures from trauma or bubbles, leakage of perilymph from a round window rupture, idiopathic hydrops or excess fluid pressure in the endolymphatic space (Meniere's disease), inflammatory disease in the inner ear (Labyrinthitis), idiopathic degenerative processes such as presbycusis, degeneration of cochlear structures from excessive noise exposure, etc.

3. Mixed or combined conductive and neurosensory hearing losses resulting from simultaneous dysfunction in the middle and inner ear.

This can be seen in coexisting middle and inner ear barotrauma, middle and inner ear otosclerosis, or the development of acute middle or inner ear dysfunction with preexisting disease in the other area.

Tinnitus

Tinnitus or spontaneous noise in the ear is difficult to quantitate and is poorly understood. It can occur with middle ear disease which results in a conductive hearing loss, but it is usually seen with inner ear or central auditory disease. With the former, tinnitus is thought to represent the sounds of cochlear and cranial blood flow which are perceived because the conductive hearing loss results in a loss or decrease of the masking effect of usual, background noise. With inner ear disease, tinnitus is thought to be due to the spontaneous firing of injured, but viable, auditory neurons or cochlear hair cells. However, this is not well understood, for destructive labyrinthectomies in patients with recurrent vertigo, tinnitus, and nonfunctional hearing have frequently not resulted in relief of the tinnitus.

Evaluation of Hearing Loss

The determination of the type of hearing loss is essential in the evaluation and management of any patient with suspected otologic dysfunction. This is best done with soundproof booth audiometry by a trained audiologist. However, in some instances, such testing is not available or practical, and some preliminary information can be gained by testing with a 512 Hz or 1024 Hz tuning fork in quiet surroundings. A 256 Hz fork can be used, but the examiner has to be careful that the patient does not respond to vibratory sensation which will be more predominently perceived at the lower frequencies.

Weber Test. The struck tuning fork is placed on the forehead or the upper incisor teeth and the patient is asked if the sound is louder in either ear or is the same intensity in both ears. With a conductive hearing loss, a sound source placed on either of these midline skull locations will be heard louder in the affected ear; with a neurosensory hearing loss, such sounds will be heard louder in the unaffected ear. With equal hearing in both ears, i.e., normal hearing or with bilaterally equal hearing losses, the sound will not lateralize.

Rinne Test. A vibrating tuning fork is alternately placed against the patient's mastoid tip and then held about 2 inches from the ear canal. The patient is asked to ascertain in which position the sound is louder or heard longer. In a normal hearing ear, or in an ear with a pure neurosensory hearing loss, bone-conducted sound will be heard less loud and heard for a shorter time than air-conducted sound. This phenomenon is due to the enhancement affects upon airborne sound by the middle ear transformer, i.e., the eardrum and the ossicular chain. With a moderate or severe conductive hearing loss, bone-conducted sound will become equal to or louder than air-conducted sound, depending on the degree of the loss. With mild conductive hearing losses, normal results can be obtained.

Schwabach Test. The examiner who knows he has normal hearing first places a vibrating tuning fork on the patient's mastoid tip. At the precise moment the patient no longer hears the sound, the fork is placed on the examiner's mastoid tip. If the sound is then heard by the examiner, decreased bone conduction or a nerve hearing loss in the patient's tested ear is indicated.

In general, fork tests are difficult to adequately perform, particularly by untrained examiners. Patient suggestibility, decreased alertness or discomfort, plus excessive background noise can adversely affect the results. Also, the presence of mixed hearing losses, either unilateral or bilateral, can make interpretation of the results difficult. Adequate audiometry by trained personnel should be obtained as soon as possible to supplement and confirm the results of fork testing. Individuals who dive regularly should have routine, periodic audiometry to detect unnoticed hearing losses and to provide baseline data for future references.

Vertigo

True vertigo often is not differentiated from other vague symptoms of balance disturbances such as dizziness, lightheadedness, unsteadiness, faintness, swaying, etc. Even when vertigo is specifically described, adequate evaluations are frequently not done to differentiate end organ from central vestibular dysfunction or to properly determine whether such affected individuals are suited for further diving after apparent recovery. These deficiences are very understandable, for dizzy patients often present complex and perplexing diagnostic problems even to otologic physicians. A systematic approach to the evaluation and management of dizzy patients must be undertaken. To develop this type of approach, several points should be emphasized:[1]

1. The first distinction that should be made is whether a dizzy individual is experiencing nonvestibular dizziness or true vestibular vertigo, defined as a specific alteration of spatial orientation involving the sensation of rotary motion of either the subject or his environment. Dysfunction in many body systems can produce dizziness. However, if a dizzy individual does not have rotary vertigo, his dizziness is unlikely to be related to primary or secondary vestibular system dysfunction.

2. Vestibular dysfunction of any severity will always be accompanied by classical labyrinthine nystagmus with a defined quick and slow component. If, by visual observation and electronystagmography, an acutely dizzy patient does not have such accompanying nystagmus, the dizziness is not due to vestibular system dysfunction.

3. Nystagmus resulting from nonacute end organ (inner ear) vestibular dysfunction is frequently suppressed by visual fixation and, therefore, not observable. Thus, electrical recordings of ocular motion in the dark or with eyes closed, i.e., electronystagmography, is important in the evaluation of a dizzy patient.

4. Vestibular system pathology does not usually produce continuous and nonepisodic symptoms for more than 3 weeks. If dizziness lasts continually for a longer period of time, the cause is probably not due to vestibular system dysfunction.

5. Vestibular dysfunction is frequently accompanied by nausea, vomiting, visual disturbances, presyncope, and other symptoms. Thus, the presence of these symptoms does not necessarily mean a more extensive central nervous system injury.

6. Once it has been established that dizziness is due to primary vestibular dysfunction, the next distinction that should be made is whether the pathology is located in the end organ or in the central vestibular system. In some cases, this determination is not difficult, for there are other accompanying neurological signs that point to a centrally located lesion. However, in many cases, such accompanying signs are lacking and this determination is more difficult. The presence of accompanying auditory symptoms or signs of injury to the tympanic membrane or middle ear as seen by otoscopic examination is more frequently, but not always, associated with end organ injury. The presence of vertical nystagmus almost always means central pathology.

7. Further evaluation such as electronystagmography, pure tone and speech audiometry, temporal bone and skull radiography, and complete otological and neurological examinations should be done as soon as feasible.

8. Vertigo after an acute, unilateral, vestibular end organ injury characteristically subsides over a varying time period of several days to 3 to 4 weeks. This improvement in symptoms results either from a functional recovery of the injured structure and/or from central nervous system compensation. Thus, a disappearance of symptoms does not necessarily mean that the injured part of the vestibular system has been restored to its previous healthy state. Individuals who have compensated from a permanent end organ vestibular injury can be generally asymptomatic. Many do experience transient vertigo and/or loss of spatial orientation with certain positions or motions. These symptoms can be intensified with loss of some proprioception and vision during underwater conditions. Therefore, all divers who experience vestibular injuries should be evaluated by specialists in vestibular problems after their symptoms have disappeared. Only in this way can rational judgments be made regarding an individual's suitability for exposure to future situations in which vertigo or spatial disorientation might endanger his life or the lives of others.

Vertigo is the most hazardous otologic symptom to occur during diving. It is frequently accompanied by otalgia, hearing loss, and tinnitus. It is described in multiple phases of diving.[2] However, many of the reports are not well documented or have discussed vertigo only as an incidental observation. Possible causes suggested for vertigo in divers include decompression sickness, hypoxia, hypercarbia, nitrogen narcosis, seasickness, alcoholic hangovers, sensory deprivation, hyperventilation, impure breathing gas, unequal caloric stimulation, and difficulties with middle ear pressure equilibration. One can readily appreciate that these causes can encompass a wide variety of pathological mechanisms, the management of which will be vastly different depending upon which mechanism is involved.

Edmonds[3, 4] has undertaken a complete review of the various causes of vertigo in diving. His classification of this problem is basically broken down into those causes due to unequal vestibular stimulation, including caloric stimulations, barotrauma, and decompression sickness; and those causes due to unequal vestibular responses to equal stimuli. This latter group includes subjects who, when exposed to conditions in which multiple vestibular stimuli are encountered, develop vertigo as a result of one vestibular apparatus being more sensitive than the other. Such individuals might have vertigo with caloric stimulation resulting from equal amounts of cold water entering the external ear canal. This would be particularly noted when the diver is swimming in a position in which the lateral semicircular canal is vertical in orientation such as a prone or supine position with the head flexed 30°. Edmonds further includes in this classification vertigo resulting from a unilateral hypofunctioning vestibular end organ in situations in which equal and symmetrical pressure changes occur in the middle ear cavities during ascent and descent. Also included are cases of vertigo and dizziness seen in nitrogen narcosis, although there is doubt as to whether this dizziness includes vertigo and results from true vestibular system dysfunction; the dizziness, nausea, and tremor that has been described in the high pressure nervous syndrome; the dizziness seen during oxygen toxicity; and sensory deprivation.

A modification of this classification is offered which separates those diving situations causing true vertigo and other otologic symptoms into those in which transient otologic dysfunction has been described and those in which permanent otologic injury has been seen.

TRANSIENT OTOLOGIC DYSFUNCTION IN DIVING

Middle Ear Barotrauma (Aerotitis Media, Aural Barotrauma, Ear Squeeze)

The most common transient otologic problem seen with diving is middle ear barotrauma resulting from inadequate pressure equalization between the middle ear and the external environment. During compression, the nasopharyngeal ostium of the eustachian tube, which is normally closed, can fail to open if the diver does not make active attempts to clear the ears by swallowing or if local inflammation and swelling prevents opening. Thus, middle ear pressure will become negative relative to the increasing ambient pressure (Fig. 9-2). With increasingly negative middle ear pressure, opening of the eustachian tube becomes more difficult because of the nasopharyngeal valve effect (Fig. 9-2B). At a pressure differential of approximately 90 mm Hg, it is impossible to open the tube voluntarily[5] (Fig. 9-2C). Fullness and pain usually occur at a pressure differential of approximately 60 mm Hg and the tympanic membrane has been found to rupture at pressure differentials ranging from 100 to 500 mm Hg[5] (Fig. 9-2E). With a forceful Valsalva maneuver under these conditions, the existing pressure differential between inner ear and middle ear can become greater and round window rupture with leakage of perilymph and inner ear injury (inner ear barotrauma, see the following section) can occur (Fig. 9-2D). Animal studies have demonstrated such ruptures when CSF pressure has been increased 120 to 300 mm Hg.[20]

Clinical presentation. Symptoms consist initially of a sensation of ear blockage. With further descent and greater pressure differentials, frank otalgia occurs. A conductive hearing loss is always present, but may not be a primary complaint because of ear pain. Mild tinnitus and vertigo may occur. With eardrum rupture, pain is usually severe and vertigo can be seen from a

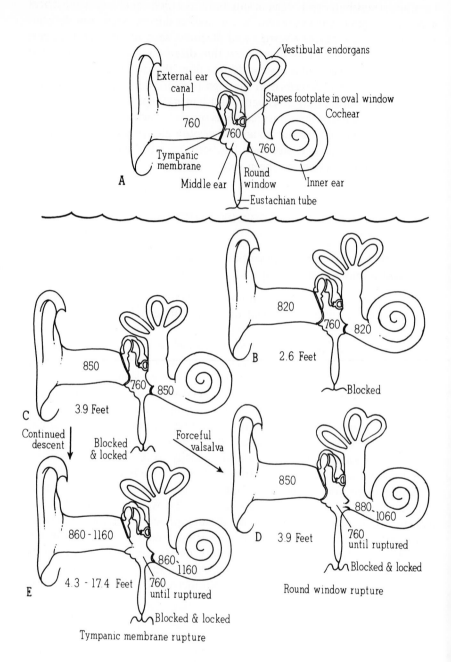

A

External ear canal

Vestibular endorgans

Stapes footplate in oval window

Cochear

760

760

760

Tympanic membrane

Round window

Inner ear

Middle ear

Eustachian tube

B   2.6 Feet

820

760   820

Blocked

C   3.9 Feet

850

760   850

Continued descent

Blocked & locked

Forceful valsalva

D   3.9 Feet

850

880   1060

760 until ruptured

Blocked & locked

Round window rupture

E   4.3 - 17.4 Feet

860 - 1160

860   1160

760 until ruptured

Blocked & locked

Tympanic membrane rupture

caloric effect if water enters the middle ear. If hearing loss, tinnitus, and vertigo are severe in association with a no-decompression dive, possible inner ear barotrauma with round window rupture and inner ear damage should be suspected. These individuals should immediately be referred to an otolaryngologist. Recompression therapy should not be attempted with suspected inner ear barotrauma, since this exposes the diver to the same pressure differentials which resulted in the initial injury and thus can cause further round window and inner ear damage.

The presence of predive nasal dysfunction such as congestion and discharge makes the occurrence of poor eustachain tubal function and subsequent middle ear barotrauma more likely. However, the lack of predive nasal symptoms should not suggest that a diver with these ear symptoms has not had middle ear barotrauma.

Physical signs. The obvious physical signs of middle ear barotrauma are seen with otoscopic examination. One should note that pathological changes occur in the entire middle ear and are not confined to the eardrum. These changes include edema and hemorrhages in the middle ear mucosa as well as inflammation and collections of serous fluid and/or blood in the middle ear.

Six grades of middle ear barotrauma are described:[6]

Grade 0. Symptoms without otoscopic signs.
Grade 1. Diffuse redness and retraction of the tympanic membrane.
Grade 2. Grade 1 changes plus slight hemorrhage within the tympanic membrane.
Grade 3. Grade 1 changes plus gross hemorrhage within the tympanic membrane.

Fig. 9-2. Otologic barotrauma of descent. Theoretical sequence of events in the right ear of a diver who does not equilibrate middle-ear pressure during descent. Pressures are shown in mm Hg. (A) Surface condition with equal pressures (760 mm Hg) throughout and patent eustachian tube with normally closed nasopharyngeal ostium. (B) Depth of approximately 2.6 feet after diver failed to open the eustachian tube upon entering the water. Pressure differential of 60 mm Hg exists. Tympanic membrane and round window are bulging into the middle ear. Diver notices pain and pressure in the ear with a conductive hearing loss and possible vertigo. (C) Depth of approximately 3.9 feet with 90 mm Hg pressure differential and blocked and locked eustachian tube. (D) Forceful Valsalva can lead to rupture of the round window with resulting leak of perilymph into the middle ear. The exact pressure differentials at which rupture occurs in humans are unknown. Studies in cats[19] have indicated that round window ruptures occur when a pressure of 120 to 300 mm Hg is added to the cerebrospinal fluid space of a cat at 1 ata. (E) Continued descent can lead to tympanic membrane rupture at pressure differentials of 100 to 400 mm Hg or depths of 4.3 to 17.4 feet. The actual rupture point is quite variable.

Grade 4. Dark and slightly bulging tympanic membrane from free blood in the middle ear; a fluid level might be present.

Grade 5. Free hemorrhage into the middle ear with tympanic membrane perforation. Blood can be seen outside or within the ear canal.

This classification has limited practical value, for the otoscopic findings in middle ear barotrauma frequently include combinations of changes in different grades. Eardrum scarring from previous perforations or nondiving related middle ear disease can obscure the middle ear findings. Occasionally, no or minimal signs will be seen initially, only to have obvious signs of negative middle ear pressure, with eardrum injection and retraction or middle ear inflammation and effusion, develop 2 to 24 hours later. Also, treatment is not completely dependent upon which of these five grades are present.

Treatment: Cases with postdive symptoms, but with no otoscopic signs either immediately or 24 hours postdive.

1. Avoid any further diving until (a) any preexisting nasal symptoms have cleared; (b) the individual can easily auto-inflate both ears at surface; and (c) all ear symptoms have cleared.
2. Systemic decongestants such as Sudafed, 30 to 60 mg orally, three times daily, and long-acting topical nasal decongestants such as Afrin nose drops, 2 to 3 drops into each nostril twice daily with the head extended, can be used. Nose drops should not be used longer than 5 days. Nasal sprays are not as effective. Systemic antihistamines are not indicated unless preexisting nasal allergy is suspected or exists.

Treatment: Cases with symptoms plus otoscopic findings and no eardrum perforation.

1. Rest and the avoidance of further diving until complete resolution as seen by otoscopic exam has occurred and the diver can easily auto-inflate both ears at surface. This usually requires 3 to 10 days depending upon the severity of the injury.
2. Use of systemic and topical nasal decongestants as just described.
3. Systemic antibiotics should be used prophylactically. This is controversial; however, eustachian tube function is usually poor because of middle ear and tubal mucosal inflammation and swelling. Under these conditions, secondary middle ear bacterial infection is more likely.
4. With an intact eardrum, topical eardrops containing antibiotics, steroids, or anesthetic agents are of no benefit, for these substances do not readily cross the outer, squamous epithelial layer of the tympanic membrane. An inert, oily preparation such as Auralgan, warmed to body temperature and instilled into the ear, may provide partial relief of pain.

5. Pain relief is best achieved with systemic analgesics.

Treatment: Cases with symptoms and otoscopic findings which include eardrum perforations. These divers should be referred to an otolaryngologist as soon as practical. Until such referral can be obtained, the following should be done:

1. Avoid further diving until compelte otologic evaluation has been performed and the middle ear process has resolved with healing or surgical repair to the eardrum. Many of these perforations will heal spontaneously and surgical repair will not be necessary. Persistence of poor eustachian tubal function and/or middle ear inflammation from secondary infection will delay eardrum healing.
2. Ear cleansing with 1.5 percent hydrogen peroxide warmed to body temperature should be done if significant amounts of blood and other debris are in the ear. Such a solution can be prepared by mixing commercially available 3 percent hydrogen peroxide with equal amounts of water, which has been warmed so that the temperature of the resulting solution approaches body temperature. This solution is then instilled into the ear three to four times daily with a small, rubber bulb ear syringe. If the solution temperature is too warm or too cool, vertigo and nausea might result from a caloric effect. Solutions containing alcohol or strong acids should not be used when a tympanic membrane perforation exists, for these substances will further irritate the middle ear. Once blood and purulent material or other debris have cleared, the peroxide irrigations can be discontinued.
3. Topical eardrops containing antibiotics and steroids, i.e., Cortisporin Otic solution, should be used to prevent infection and decrease inflammation. If peroxide irrigations are used, these drops should be instilled after each irrigation. Once these irrigations have been discontinued, the drops should be used three to four times daily until the ear is clean and dry or the eardrum is completely healed. If inner ear barotrauma with a round window fistula is suspected, preparations containing Neomycin or other ototoxic chemicals should be avoided and antibiotic solutions such as chloromycetin otic solution should be used instead.
4. Systemic and topical nasal decongestants should be employed as just described.
5. The use of systemic antibiotics prophylactically is controversial. The author favors such use of a broad spectrum antibiotic, given orally for a 7- to 10-day period, because of the increased possibility of secondary middle ear or mastoid infection either from the entry of contaminated water into these areas or secondary infection related to persistent eustachian tubal inflammation and obstruction. One can decide not to use prophylactic systemic antibiotics. However, if purulent otorrhea or

rhinorrhea develops, these drainages should be cultured and systemic antibiotics should then be administered.

6. Analgesia, if needed, should be given systemically. Topical otic solutions containing topical anesthetics are usually unsatisfactory for analgesia.

External Ear Canal Barotrauma (External Ear Squeeze, Reverse Ear Squeeze)

This problem is related to blockage of the external ear canal during descent or ascent. With such blockage, ear canal pressure becomes negative (descent) or positive (ascent) relative to ambient and middle ear pressure. The resulting tissue damage consists of congestion, hemorrhage, outward or inward bulging, and possible rupture of the tympanic membrane. The common causes of external auditory canal obstruction are cerumen or other foreign bodies, the use of mechanical ear plugs, and the use of tight-fitting diving hoods.

Cases of external ear canal barotrauma with no eardrum perforations should be treated in a similar fashion as the treatment just described for cases of middle ear barotrauma with otoscopic findings and no eardrum perforation. If an eardrum perforation has occurred, treatment is similar to those cases of middle ear barotrauma with eardrum perforation.

The best treatment of external ear squeeze is prevention. External ear canal patency during pressure changes must be assured. Accumulated masses of cerumen which can potentially obstruct the ear canal should be removed by washing the ear with a lukewarm water solution using a rubber bulb syringe. Care should be taken before such washing to ensure that a tympanic membrane perforation does not exist. The use of tight-fitting hoods, solid ear plugs, or headphones which can completely seal the external ear canal should be avoided.

Transient Vertigo Due to Caloric Stimulation

Under most diving conditions, vestibular end organs are stimulated equally and vertigo does not occur. In certain situations, unequal stimulation with subsequent vertigo occurs especially when there are preexisting pathological changes. Unequal entry of cold water into the external auditory canal secondary to obstruction of one canal by cerumen, otitis externa, ear plugs, bony exostosis, etc., can produce a caloric response particularly when the diver is oriented in a position in which the lateral semicircular canal is in a vertical plane, i.e., prone or supine with the head flexed 30°. Tympanic membrane perforations, such as seen with otic barotrauma during descent or preexisting trauma or middle ear disease, can result in unequal stimulation of one semicircular canal by the entry of cold water into the middle ear.

Transient Vertigo Resulting From Unequal Middle Ear Pressure Equilibration during Ascent (Alternobaric Vertigo)

Transient vestibular dysfunction secondary to asymmetrical middle ear pressure equilibration has been described primarily during ascent by Lundgren[7], who coined the term alternobaric vertigo; Vorosmarti and Bradley[8]; and by Terry and Dennison[9]. Lundgren attributes such vertigo to increased middle ear pressure on one side during ascent with resulting unequal vestibular end organ stimulation. Indeed, some individuals who have experienced alternobaric vertigo at depth can produce vertigo and vestibular nystagmus by performing the Valsalva maneuver and unequally inflating the middle ears at 1 ata. Many of these individuals have encountered difficulty during diving with middle ear pressure equalization, usually unilaterally. Disappearance of the vertigo has been noted with stopping the ascent or descending again or shortly after a sudden hissing of air into one ear. Further work by Tjernstron,[10] using a special technique for measuring middle ear pressure changes with simultaneous electronystagmographic recordings, has shown true vestibular nystagmus during conditions of asymmetrical equilibration of middle ear pressure during ascent from shallow depths.

The exact frequency of alternobaric vertigo is not known. A more recent work by Lundgren et al[11] involving a questionnaire answered by 2053 Swedish divers indicates that of 453 divers who have experienced vertigo during diving, 343 were likely to have had alternobaric vertigo. Of these divers 97 percent indicated that vertigo lasted from a few seconds up to 10 minutes. Divers who had experienced vertigo had logged more dives than those without vertigo experience and reported middle ear pressure equilibration difficulties more frequently. Such divers also noted that these pressure equilibration difficulties were more dominant in one ear.

The occurrence of vertigo during shallow underwater exposures can be quite hazardous. The resulting spatial disorientation with possible nausea and vomiting may explain some of the previously unexplained deaths of experienced scuba divers. The best treatment is that of prevention. First, individuals should not dive if difficulties with ear clearing exist or if a Valsalva maneuver at 1 ata produces vertigo. Second, if a diver notices any ear fullness or blockage, or vertigo during compression, further descent should be stopped and the diver should ascend until the ears can be cleared. Third, if such symptoms are noted during ascent, the ascent should be stopped abruptly and the diver should descend until the symptoms disappear if gas supplies and other conditions permit. Fourth, diving with a companion is always a safe precaution.

Transient Dizziness and "Vertigo" Associated with the High Pressure Nervous Syndrome

Transient symptoms suggestive of vestibular system dysfunction, vertigo, dizziness, and tinnitus with nausea have been reported in association with the high pressure nervous syndrome.[12, 13] More recent investigations[14] have indicated that these symptoms are not accompanied by demonstrable electronystagmographic nystagmus. Such symptoms during the high pressure nervous syndrome are felt to be related to dysfunction in more centrally located structures and not to unilateral end organ and/or primary vestibular neuron dysfunction.

PERMANENT OTOLOGIC INJURY IN DIVING

In recent years, reports of permanent cochlear and/or vestibular injury in multiple phases of diving have occurred with increased frequency. The mechanisms of injury and proper treatment appear to differ depending upon which phase of diving the injury occurred. Thus, these injuries are organized as follows:

1. Injuries occurring during descent or compression
2. Injuries occurring at stable deep depths
3. Injuries occurring during ascent, decompression, or shortly after decompression from deep depths
4. Injuries related to high background noise during diving conditions.

Injuries Occurring during Descent or Compression (Inner Ear Barotrauma)

Australian investigators[15, 20] have collected a series of cases of cochlear injury with and without vestibular damage occurring after shallow air dives. In each case, there was apparent difficulty with ear clearing during descent and/or evidence on otoscopic examination of middle ear barotrauma. The depth and duration of these dives makes decompression sickness very unlikely. The neurosensory deafness can be total or partial, occurs with varying degrees of vestibular dysfunction, and can be noted concurrently with the middle ear barotrauma, or can follow it by several days.

Goodhill[16] postulated that with a forceful Valsalva maneuver or straining, intracochlear pressure rises significantly from the transmission of the accompanying increased cerebrospinal fluid pressure. With inadequate middle ear pressure equalization during compression in diving, this increased intracochlear pressure results in an increase in an already existing pressure differential between the cochlea and the middle ear with resulting rupture of round window membrane into the middle ear and subsequent perilymph fistula[17, 18] (see Fig. 9-2D). Recent studies by Harker et al.[19] have shown that increased CSF pressure results in bulging and rupture of the round window membrane in cats. Later investigations by Edmonds et al.[20] have actually demonstrated round window ruptures in divers who develop cochlea and/or vestibular symptoms during shallow, no-decompression dives, in which there were difficulties with middle ear clearning during compression. Subsequent surgery to repair these round window fistulae has resulted in improvement of hearing and/or disappearance of vestibular dysfunction.

Any diver who experiences persistent vertigo and/or neurosensory hearing loss and tinnitus following dives in which decompression sickness is unlikely should be considered as a possible case of inner ear barotrauma and labyrinthine fistula. Such divers should be immediately placed on bed rest with head elevation. Care should be taken that CSF and middle ear pressure are not increased. Valsalva maneuver, coughing, nose blowing, and straining at defecation must be avoided.[20] If no improvement in hearing loss and/or dizziness occurs within 48 hours, an exploratory tympanotomy for closure of a possible perilymph fistula should be considered.[16] Hyperbaric oxygen therapy exposes the diver to the same pressure changes which initially caused the injury. Thus, it is potentially harmful and should not be used. Drugs that supposedly increase intracranial and inner ear blood flow are generally not effective, or are potentially harmful because of possible hemorrhage from traumatized tissue. Thus, these agents plus anticoagulants should be avoided.

Otologic Problems Occurring at Stable Deep Depths

Inner ear problems occurring while at a stable, deep depth have been described by Sundmaker[21] and Lambertsen.[22] These episodes were noted in one dive at the University of Pennsylvania in late summer of 1971. Three divers experienced a sudden onset of vertigo, nausea, and nystagmus shortly after starting to breathe by mask a gas mixture which contained a second inert gas, neon or nitrogen, in addition to the background helium-oxygen atmosphere. Follow-up evaluation after the dive revealed a total unilateral loss of labyrinthine function in one subject, a partial unilateral loss in another subject, and a recovery of function after an initial partial unilateral loss in the third subject. No losses of auditory function were noted and no evidence of central nervous system lesions were found.

Further work has suggested that the etiology of these injuries is related to gas counterdiffusion problems between inner ear compartments. When divers change from one breathing mixture to another, the diffusion of the new dissolved inert gas into body tissues and fluid spaces with the reversed diffusion of the previous dissolved inert gas results in bubbles at various interfaces, such as the partitions in the inner· ear between the perilymphatic and endolymphatic spaces. This bubble formation produces displacement and/or disruption of the inner ear structures and occurs without changes in total ambient pressure. Blenkarn et al.[23] and Graves et al.[24] have noted gas-filled blister formations in skin following the sequential exposure to various inert gases at constant ambient pressures. This eruption is felt to represent gas bubble formation in the deep layers of the skin resulting from the counterdiffusion of different inert gases across tissue interfaces.

Until the exact mechanisms of these injuries at stable deep depths have been established, changes between inert gases at deep depths should be avoided.

Permanent Otologic Injuries Occurring during Ascent, Decompression, or Shortly after Decompression from Deep Depths.

Classical descriptions of decompression sickness have mentioned otologic manifestations only in association with massive central nervous system bends where the inner ear symptoms were of secondary importance and, in many cases, were probably related to centrally located lesions. Otologic symptoms have not been felt to occur during decompression without other manifestations of decompression sickness. Such symptoms have been occasionally ignored. However, with more frequent helium-oxygen exposures to deeper depths, reports of vertigo and/or hearing loss during or following decompression without other signs of decompression sickness have become more frequent.[25, 26, 27] In a series of 20 such cases, Farmer and Thomas[28] noted a significant correlation between prompt recompression treatment, relief of symptoms, and a lack of residual deficits. This, plus the fact that in each case the symptoms began either during or shortly after decompression strongly suggests that these injuries are a form of decompression sickness and are related to bubble formation either in the perilymphatic or in the endolymphatic spaces, or in the internal auditory artery system. In this series, inner ear barotrauma with round window rupture was an unlikely contributing factor in that no divers noted difficulties with ear clearing during compression. In trying to implicate other possible mechanisms of injury, such as hemorrhage into the inner ear or vascular spasm or thrombosis with subsequent ischemia, one would not expect to obtain prompt relief with recompression.

In the author's experience, the following measures should be taken in regards to otologic symptoms appearing during or shortly after decompression from dives in which decompression sickness is possible and in which middle ear barotrauma is unlikely:

1. Isolated cochlear and/or vestibular symptoms during such dives should be considered forms of decompression sickness and should be recompressed promptly.

2. Divers who experience such symptoms during or shortly after a switch to an air environment during decompression from a deep helium oxygen exposure should be recompressed promptly and switched back to the presymptom helium-oxygen atmosphere.

3. The exact treatment depth, or depth of recompression to be followed, is at present controversial. Obviously, the depth at which relief of symptoms occurs would be a good end point. However, in some cases bubble formations in the inner ear will have caused structural deformities, such as membrane breaks, and relief will not be seen even though an adequate depth of recompression to drive the bubbles back into solution has been achieved. Thus, the optimum depth of recompression for otologic decompression sickness is best defined as the lesser of the depth of relief or the bottom depth. However, in some instances, returning to the bottom depth in the open sea is hazardous or impractical. Thus, the authors recommend that the optimum treatment depth in these situations should be at least 3 atm above the depth at which symptoms occurred.

4. The use of other measures in the treatment of otologic decompression sickness, such as anticoagulants, low molecular weight dextran, and intermittent oxygen breathing, has not been adequately evaluated. In the authors' view, anticoagulation can cause additional harm, particularly if the inner ear bubble formation has caused structural destruction and subsequent hemorrhages. Therefore, anticoagulation is specifically not recommended. Conversely, the breathing of oxygen treatment gases during the treatment of otologic decompression sickness is unlikely to cause additional harm and might be beneficial.

5. The use of Valium, 5 to 15 mg intramuscularly, has been associated with significant symptomatic relief of vertigo during otologic decompression sickness. Other agents, such as Antivert, Dramamine, Bonine, have not been found to be as useful in this regard.

Otologic Injuries Related to High Background Noises during Diving Conditions

Coles and Knight[29] in a survey of Royal Navy divers concluded that high-frequency neurosensory deafness seen in the usual diving population could be explained on the basis of previous nondiving noise exposures. Divers with no history of previous excessive noise exposure had high frequency losses similar to the overall nondiving population when allowances were made for age. However, recent investigations by Summitt and Reimers[30] and Murray[31] have demonstrated excessive noise levels in various diving conditions. By using existing damage-risk criteria,[32] the allowable exposure time in such noise levels may be as short as 15 or 20 minutes before one runs the risk of permanent noise-induced hearing loss. It is not known whether the previously noted reversible and depth-related conductive hearing losses, secondary to decreased sound transmission by the eardrum and ossicles in compressed gas,[33, 34, 35] are sufficient to provide attentuation from excessive noise during diving. Temporary threshold shifts have been seen in air helmet dives.[30] This would suggest that these conductive hearing losses do not provide sufficient attentuation to protect divers from the excessive noise frequently encountered in multiple phases of diving.

Until more data are available regarding the actual damage risks from excessive noise in diving, chambers and helmets should be made as quiet as possible. If excessive noise during these conditions is likely, some types of protective attentuation such as ventilated earplugs or earmuffs should be provided.

OTITIS EXTERNA

Alterations in the continuity of the squamous epithelium lining the ear canal or in its slightly acid pH can result in infection and inflammation of the external auditory canal wall skin, otitis externa. This is not uncommon in diving. Excessive exposure to water or humid atmospheres can produce maceration of the epithelium and cause pH shifts toward the alkaline side. Also, divers are occasionally exposed to water with a high bacterial count. Other factors such as collections of cerumenous debris, local trauma, seborrheic dermatitis, bony auditory canal exostoses, and poorly fitting or improperly cleaned earplugs can contribute to otitis externa.

In divers, the bacterial flora found in otitis externa is frequently mixed with *Pseudomonas* and *Proteus* predominating with *Staphyloccus aureus*.[36] Symptoms include irritation with itching or burning, thin and serous discharge, and pain. Examination shows an acutely inflamed, swollen, and extremely tender external auditory canal. With progression, erythema of the surrounding pinnae and skin, anterior cervical lymphadenitis, and complete obstruction of the ear canal with subsequent abscess formation and possible involvement of bone and cartilage can occur.

Treatment consists of relief of pain, cleansing the auditory canal, and specific therapy to provide topical antibiotics and a more normal pH to the canal. One should not hesitate to prescribe narcotics for relief of pain, which is often severe. The method of choice for cleansing is by ear irrigation using lukewarm tap water, with care being taken to dry the ear canal afterward. A gentle stream of compressed air blown into the canal can aid in such drying. If an eardrum perforation exists, the ear tip suction and cotton wipes should be used instead. Specific therapy should consist of an agent which is on the neutral or acid pH side and contains topical antibiotics. One should keep in mind that the predominating organism can be killed, only to be replaced by another organism that is resistant to the antibiotics being used. Thus, if no response to treatment occurs within 24 to 36 hours, cultures should be obtained to more precisely identify the causative organisms. Adequate amounts of the specific agents should be used three to four times daily. If ear canal swelling is sufficient to prevent the agent from getting into the entire auditory canal, a cotton wick impregnated with the agent should be inserted and the agent instilled on the wick several times daily. All swimming and diving should cease until the infection has cleared.

Attempts can be made to prevent otitis externa by ensuring that adequate cleansing of the ear canal is present and none of the previously described predisposing factors exist. A useful prophylactic topical ear solution in humid and aqueous environments is Otic Domeboro solution, which should be applied several times daily. Alcohol instilled into the ears has been used as a prophylactic measure with variable success. However, alcohol will dissolve and remove the longer chain fatty acids in cerumen which are felt to be protective. Thus, alcohol used in this manner probably should be avoided.

PARANASAL SINUS BAROTRAUMA

This entity has been described mainly in fliers.[37, 38, 39] It is rarely described in divers.[40] As just noted, adequate ventilation and pressure equalization in both the middle ear and paranasal sinuses are dependent to a large degree upon nasal function. Inflammation and congestion of the nasal mucosa, nasal structural deformities, or nasal mass lesions can result in blockage of the paranasal sinus ostia. This blockage leads to a series of changes within the paranasal sinuses consisting of absorption of preexisting air and vacuum formation; swelling, engorgement, and inflammation of the sinus mucosa; and the collection of a transudate in the sinus cavity. When such blockage occurs during descent while diving or flying, the intrasinus vacuum becomes greater and the resulting pathological changes are more severe with actual hemorrhage into the sinus in some instances.

Paranasal sinus barotrauma has also been noted during ascents. Here, the pathological mechanism is felt to be related to a one-way valve blockage of the sinus ostium by inflamed mucosa or cysts or polyps located within the sinus. Thus, pressure equilibration can occur during descent, but is impaired during ascent.

Symptoms of paranasal sinus barotrauma include fullness and pain over the involved sinus or in the upper teeth. Paresthesias over the infraorbital nerve distribution have been seen. Also, epistaxis has been noted particularly in cases occurring during ascent. Purulent nasal discharge is seen with secondary infection.

Treatment consists of the use of topical and systemic vasoconstrictor agents to promote nasal mucosal shrinkage and opening of the sinus ostia. In cases occurring during descent and in which severe pain is present, ascent or decompression has been used with some success in relief of pain. If purulent nasal discharge exists, cultures should be obtained and antibiotic therapy administered.

Most cases of paranasal sinus barotrauma will recover in 5 to 10 days without serious sequelae. Individuals who have symptoms for longer periods should be referred for complete otolaryngologic and paranasal sinus x-ray evaluation.

REFERENCES

1. McCabe B: Vestibular physiology: Its clinical application in understanding the dizzy patient, in Paparella M, Schumrick D (eds): Otolaryngology, vol 1. Philadelphia, Saunders, 1973, p 318-328
2. Kennedy R: A bibliography of the role of the vestibular apparatus under water and at high pressure. US Naval Medical Research Institute Report M4306.03.5000 BAK 9. No 3, 1973
3. Edmonds C: Vertigo and disorientation in diving, in Edmonds C, Freeman P, Thomas R, et al (eds): Otological Aspects of Diving. Sidney, Australian Medical Publishing Co, 1973, p 55
4. Edmonds C: Vertigo in diving, in Guedry F (ed): The Use of Nystagmography in Aviation Medicine, AGARD Conference Proceedings No 128. Naval Aerospace Medical Research Institute, Pensacola, 1973
5. Keller A: A study of the relationship of air pressure to myringorupture. Laryngoscope 68:2015-2029, 1958
6. Edmonds C, Freeman P, Thomas R, et al: Otological Aspects of Diving. Sidney, Australian Medical Publishing Co, 1973, p 32
7. Lundgren C: Alternobaric vertigo—a diver's hazard. Br Med J 2:511-513, 1965
8. Vorosmarti J, Bradley J: Alternobaric vertigo in militarydivers. Milit Med 135:182-185, 1970
9. Terry L, Dennison W: Vertigo amongst divers. US Navy Submarine Medical Center Special Report, No 66-2, 1966
10. Tjernstrom O: On alternobaric vertigo—experimental studies. Forsvarsmedicin (Stockholm) 9:410-415, 1973
11. Lundgren C, Tjernstrom O, Ornhagen H: Alternobaric vertigo and hearing dis-

turbances in connection with diving: An epidemiologic study. Undersea Biomed Res 1:251-258, 1974

12. Buhlmann A, Matthys H, Overrath H, et al: Saturation exposures at 31 ata. Aerosp Med 41:394-402, 1970

13. Bennett P, Towse E: Performance efficiency of men breathing oxygen-helium at depths between 100 feet and 1500 feet. Aerosp Med 42:147-156, 1971

14. Farmer J, Thomas W, Smith R, Bennett P: Vestibular function during the high pressure nervous syndrome. Undersea Biomed Res 1:A11, 1974 (abstract)

15. Freeman P, Edmonds C: Inner ear barotrauma. Arch Otolaryngol 95:556-563, 1972

16. Goodhill V: Sudden deafness and round window rupture. Laryngoscope 81:1462-1474, 1971

17. Goodhill V: Inner ear barotrauma. Arch Otolaryngol 95:588, 1972

18. Pullen F: Round window membrane rupture: A cause of sudden deafness. Trans Am Acad Ophthalmol Otolaryngol 76:1444-1450, 1972

19. Harker L, Norante J, Rzu J: Experimental rupture of the round window membrane. Trans Am Acad Ophthalmol Otolaryngol 78:448-452, 1974

20. Edmonds C, Freeman P, Tonkin J: Fistula of the round window in diving. Trans Am Acad Ophthalmol Otolaryngol 78:444-447, 1974

21. Sundmaker W: Vestibular function, in Lambertsen C (ed): Special Summary Program, Productive Studies III, University of Penn, 1973 (in press)

22. Lambertsen C: Collaborative investigation of limits of human tolerance to pressurization with helium, neon, and nitrogen. Simulation of density equivalent to helium-oxygen respiration at depths to 2000, 3000, 4000 and 5000 feet of sea water, in Lambertsen C (ed): Proceedings of the Fifth Symposium on Underwater Physiology. Washington, FASEB (in press)

23. Blenkarn G, Aquadro C, Hills B, Saltzman H: Urticaria following the sequential breathing of various inert gases at a constant pressure of 7 ATA: A possible manifestation of gas induced osmosis. Aerosp Med 42:141-146, 1971

24. Graves D, Idicula J, Lambertsen C, Quinn J: Bubble formation in physical and biological systems: a manifestation of counterdiffusion in composite media. Science 179:582-584, 1973

25. Buhlmann A, Waldvogen W: The treatment of decompression sickness. Helv Med Acta 33:487-491, 1967

26. Gehring H, Buhlmann A: So-called vertigo bends after oxygen-helium dives, in Lambertsen C (ed): Proceedings of the Fifth Symposium on Underwater Physiology. Washington, FASEB (in press)

27. Rubenstein C, Summitt J: Vestibular derangement in decompression, in Lambertsen C (ed): Proceedings of the Fourth Symposium on Underwater Physiology. New York and London, Academic Press, 1971, pp 287-292

28. Farmer, J, Thomas W: Vestibular injury during diving. Forsvarsmedicin (Stockholm) 9:396-403, 1973

29. Coles R, Knight J: Aural and audiometric survey of qualified divers and submarine escape training instructors. Med Res Counc Ser (Lond) Report RNPL 61/1011, 1961

30. Summitt J, Reimers J: Noise: A hazard to divers and hyperbaric chamber personnel. Aerosp Med 42:1173-1177, 1971

31. Murray T: Noise levels inside Navy diving chambers during compression and decompression. Naval Submarine Medical Center, Report No 643, 1970

32. Eldredge D., Miller J: Acceptable noise exposures—damage risk criteria, in Ward D, Fricke J (eds): Noise As a Public Health Hazard, ASHA Report 4, pp 110-120, 1969

33. Fluur E. Adolfson J: Hearing in hyperbaric air. Aerosp Med 57:783-785, 1966

34. Farmer J, Thomas W, Preslar M: Human auditory response during hyperbaric helium-oxygen exposures. Surg Forum 22:456-458, 1971

35. Thomas W, Summit J, Farmer J: Human auditory thresholds during deep saturation helium-oxygen dives. J Acoust Soc Am 55:810-813, 1974

36. Edmonds C, Freeman P, Thomas R, et al: Otological Aspects of Diving. Sidney, Australian Medical Publishing Co, 1973, p 20

37. Wright B, Boyd H: Aerosinusitis. Arch Otolaryngol 41:193-203, 1945

38. Campbell P: Aerosinusitis—a resume. Ann Otol Rhinol Laryngol 54:69-83, 1945

39. Campbell P: Aerosinusitis—its cause, course and treatment. Ann Otol 53:291-301, 1944

40. Idicula J: Perplexing case of maxillary sinus barotrauma. Aerosp Med 43:891-892, 1972

STUDY QUESTIONS

1. An experienced diver surfaces from a 10-minute 30-foot scuba dive complaining of roaring tinnitus in the left ear and vertigo. Preliminary evaluation shows a retracted and injected left tympanic membrane with right-beating horizontal nystagmus. Further evaluation shows a severe neurosensory hearing loss in the left ear.
   a.   The most likely diagnosis is _____ .
   b.   The recommended treatment is _____ .

2. During decompression from a 450-foot, 35-minute bottom time, helium oxygen dive, a diver complains of severe vertigo, nausea, and vomiting shortly after a switch to an air environment at 120 feet. No other symptoms are present and no prior ear symptoms have occurred during this dive.
   a.   The most likely diagnosis is _____ .
   b.   Treatment steps should be _____ .

3. _____ in diving has been described as transient vertigo resulting from unequal middle ear pressure equilibration most often during
   a.   ascent
   b.   descent

4. Otologic dysfunction occurring while at stable, deep depths has been seen shortly after switching to a different inert gas mixture. It is thought to be due to
   (a) _____ formation at tissue interfaces from the counter diffusion of different
   (b) _____ .

5. Temporary auditory threshold shifts from excessive noise levels that can permanently damage the cochlear have been found after diving in
   a.   Diving helmets

b. Scuba gear
c. None of these
d. Both of these

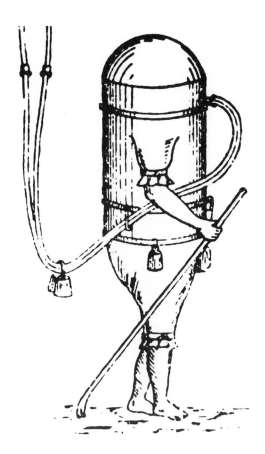

Successful enclosed diving dress. From *History of Diving,* U.S. Navy Diving Manual, 1973.

Robert B. Cook

10
Eyes, Vision, and Diving

Evolution has lifted man from floundering within the dark primeval ooze of the bottom of prehistoric seas to a life where vistas range in light years. Yet despite the fact that man's retinas record patterns of distant planets, diving is still practiced in bodies of water where visual phenomena rapidly dissipate to flashes of perceived light from the pull of one's own vitreous body. If anyone has ever had the dubious experience of diving in the Anacostia River in Washington, D.C., or in any equivalently polluted mixture of half water and half matter, the consistency of a chocolate frappe, then one would not have to be convinced of the importance of vision underwater. Save for a few souls vainly searching for a true second uterine experience, all diving is carried out with at least the desire, if not definite need, to see. Although many underwater jobs must be done in utter darkness in harbors where the bottom is defined by relative silt consistency, most people agree that efficiency, enjoyment, and safety soar with the added benefit of visual capability.

Transmission of Light by Water

The spectrum of vision underwater varies from utter blackness to visibility at distances of approximately 200 feet. Natural light coursing down in shimmering beams in clear water can support photosynthesis to a depth of approximately 650 feet. Occupants of bathyscaphes have described the sensation of light from the sunny surface as deep as 1500 feet.

Once light pierces the surface of the water, changes begin. The difference in the index of refraction between air ($n = 1.000$) and water ($n = 1.333$)

135

causes refraction of incident light beams striking the water surface at oblique angles. This phenomenon results in visual distortion of objects when viewed through the phase change.

Perhaps more important in relation to diving, however, is the fact that more energy is sapped from the light as it traverses water than when it traverses air. Indeed, the logarithmic attenuation coefficient of the decay curve is 1000 times greater in water than in air. As an example, in clear water and at a depth of 15 feet, approximately one-fourth of the incident energy is still progressing on course, while at 50 feet only one-eighth of the incident energy is heading for the depths.

In very simple terms, the rapid attenuation of light energy is due to two components. First, there is the effect of scattering of the harmonic waves by collision with particles in the water. The visual effect of this phenomenon is to reduce contrast between objects and the general background. Obviously, such an effect reduces the opportunity for resolution acuity as well as stereoacuity (sense of the relative distance of objects).

The second cause of attenuation and perhaps the more interesting is the absorption of light energy by the water and its contained materials. This phenomenon is very variable depending on the particular body of water (its turbidity, dissolved and particulate matter, the amount of plankton, etc.) and the wavelength of the incident light. This causes a varying degree of penetrability by light in different bodies of water. Even within the same body of water there is a differential absorption of various wavelengths. The net result, of course, is certain distortions of color. In general terms, one can say that the longer wavelengths, such as red and orange, begin to fade first. This effect becomes noticeable below approximately 40 feet in clear water. Yellow and green begin to fade in clear water around 120 feet. Blue is visible for the greatest distance in clear water.[1, 2]

An example of this phenomenon occured when a diver was warned not to handle a particularly mischievous red starfish. However, the dive was carried out to 80 or 90 feet, and the diver found that even the green starfish he found bit him. A lesson in differential wavelength absorption was learned as green blood issued forth from his newly acquired wound.

For the purpose of color coding and camouflaging, quite a bit of work has been carried out in relation to color visibility underwater. For a comprehensive review of this the reader is referred to the bibliography.[1, 3] Some generalizations, however, are appropriate. The first concerns the fact that there is a great difference in color appreciation between clear and turbid waters. In clear water, short wavelengths (the blue end of the spectrum) are favored. In turbid waters, the longer wavelengths are treated with more respect.[1] For visibility, fluorescent paints are better in general than non-fluorescent paints, although this benefit diminishes as the turbidity increases.[2] When one switches from natural light to artificial light, (e.g., to mercury or tungsten), further changes in color appreciation are noted because of the differences in the emitted wavelengths must be available in the source. This fact is particularly true for fluorescent paints that rely heavily on a good source of short wavelength energy to fluoresce. Thus mercury light is superior to tungsten light for fluorescent paints. For color coding, not necessarily visibility, Luria and Kinney have suggested that green, orange, and black cause the least confusion.

Refraction

Whenever one puts his head beneath the surface and opens his eyes, he is immediately impressed by the tremendous ground glass appearance of his surroundings. It is difficult even to count fingers at 2 or 3 feet. The reason for this is that the air cornea interface is responsible for approximately two-thirds of the refraction carried out by the eye. When water with an index of refraction of $n = 1.333$ replaces the air in front of the cornea ($n = 1.376$), the corneal refraction is lost. Duane found that a plus lens ($+ 64.5$ diopters in air), when placed in front of the submerged eye, restored visual acuity.[4] This means that the unaided submerged eye is tremendously hyperopic, with the light rays focusing well behind the retina.

Correcting the hyperopia by using a high plus lens leaves a lot to be desired. First of all, it does not provide any protection for the eye. In saltwater, this is a very important factor. In addition, looking through such a high plus lens results in a visual field of approximately 20°, and a 20° visual field is a tremendous visual handicap. A 10° visual field qualifies one for legal blindness, despite the acuity.

Better methods of attacking the problem were devised. Goggles, helmets, masks, and contact lenses were tried. Goggles protect the eyes from the water, restore the cornea-air interface, but generally limit ability of the diver to equalize the pressure, which can lead to eye squeeze. Goggles also offer very narrow visual fields. Helmets cause field defects and decrease mobility. At the other end of the spectrum, contact lenses are superb in relation to maintaining mobility and the visual field. Indeed, tests have shown that scleral contact lenses designed for diving resulted in a visual field loss of only 10 to 14 percent.[5] However, swimmers' contact lenses are frightfully expensive. The usual hard lens cannot be used because the lens tends to float off of the cornea. Soft lenses have the same drawback, as well as the difficulty of incorporating an air space. Hence, scleral contact lenses must be used. Even with scleral contact lenses, decentering occurs with the optical portion of the lens occassionally riding away from the visual axis and causing some mild diplopia (double vision). The biggest problem with scleral contact lenses for swimmers, other than the expense, is the unsolved problem of conjunctival irritation and corneal clouding.[5]

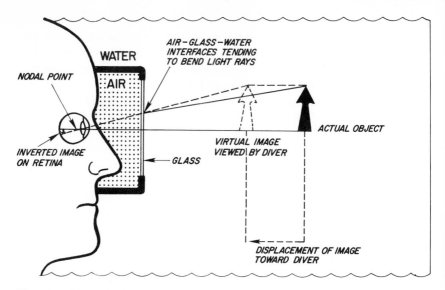

Fig. 10-1. When the diver wears a facemask, vision is clear, but an object appears to be closer than it actually is.

Hence, the typical diving mask seems to be the best compromise. The eye is protected, the cornea-air interface is retained, and the cost is small.

However, placing a glass in front of the face underwater creates another minor difficulty. The water-air interface acts as a refraction surface and light rays are bent. A virtual image is formed, which then becomes the image the swimmer perceives. This virtual image appears to be approximately 3/4 of the distance to the actual object, and it appears to 4/3 the size of the original object (see Fig. 10-1).

This phenomenon of the object appearing closer and larger results in a spurious increase of visual acuity underwater as compared with air. This apparent increase is only at very short distances before attenuation at longer distances causes a rapid drop off of acuity. The reason the increased acuity compared with vision in air is spurious is because of the magnification. In other words, the virtual image is actually subtending a larger arc on the retina. An equivalent situation would be for someone to view a visual acuity chart in air with a device to magnify the 20/10 line so he could read it. Obviously one would not say that that person had better visual acuity than usual. The magnification of objects underwater has a practical effect in distance estimation. It has been found empirically that, within 1.2 meters in clear water, distances tend to be underestimated. Beyond 1.2 meters, the distances are progressively overestimated, especially as turbidity increases.[6]

The use of a mask also affords the opportunity to correct refractive errors in the diver. Regular glasses within the mask are impractical, although they probably work reasonably well within a diving helmet. The most efficient method of including one's own correction in a mask has been to grind a lens with the corrective surface on the inside and a plano surface on the outside. These lenses can then be bonded to the inner aspect of the diving mask with an optically clear glue. In this fashion, customizing for anisometropia (difference in the power between the two eyes), astigmatism, vertex distance, and varying interpupillary distances can be easily accomplished at modest cost.[4]

Visual Fields

The problems of curtailed field of vision can be best illustrated by watching a diving physician trying to view consecutively all his gauges while looking for potential denizens of the deep. Because of the relative tunnel-like vision and small field, the head is incessantly gyrating and swiveling with dizzying rapidity within the confines of 4° of freedom. Even the lack of hydrodynamic design of the mask does not keep the anxious doctor from attempting to visualize continuously the sphere of space about himself. The result is a comical constant motion machine.

Indeed, the problem of reduced field of vision has not been solved. Attempts to construct wraparound masks have resulted in peripheral distortion as annoying as the lack of field. Side-view ports have resulted in large disquieting image jumps.

The reduction of the visual field comes from two components. One is the simple blinder effect caused by the sides of the mask infringing on vision. The other component is the critical angle of reflection as light rays coming from the water impinge on the glass surface of the mask. Any rays hitting the mask at an angle greater than 48.5° from the perpendicular are totally reflected, and do not pass through the glass. Therefore, the peripheral field of vision is limited to 97° in both vertical and horizontal meridians. The normal visual field is approximately 130° in the vertical and 200° in the horizontal.

As was mentioned earlier, stereoacuity is less in water than in air. At first, this effect was presumed to be due to loss of contrast by scatter and absorption. Later it was found that the reduction in the stereoacuity was greater than that which could be accounted for by mere loss of contrast. Some further work has suggested that the decrease in stereoacuity underwater is due to the decrease in field as well as the decrease in peripheral clues (Ganzfeld).[7, 8] The condition labled *instrument myopia* has also been implicated.[9]

Adaptation

Despite the psychological effects on vision and the actual physical distortions, human beings are able to visually adapt quite well to an underwater environment. Testing has suggested that there is a rather rapid adjustment in terms of hand-eye coordination. This adjustment seems to be facilitated by multiple exposures rather than a mass trial, even if the duration of time is the same. There seems to be a definite correlation between diving experience and visual adjustment, although with specific tasks, there is some dependence on the specific optic condition of the particular body of water.[10-13]

Visual Standards

There is no agreement on visual standards for diving. The U.S. Navy insists upon 20/30, correctable to 20/20 in the worst eye. Alley suggests that those individuals with vision ranging from 20/40 to 20/200 should have optical corrections within their face masks and that those whose best eye is 20/200 or worse, uncorrected, should not dive.[14] Williams feels that vision correctable to at least 20/40 should be acceptable despite the uncorrected vision.[4] Strauss and Kupfer (personal communication) suggested that divers with vision 20/100 or worse should be advised to wear corrected masks. They also pointed out that a person with poor but correctable vision can obtain approximately 20/40 vision on the surface without a corrected face mask by squinting.

Eye Squeeze

Conjunctival or eye squeeze is obviously not related to vision underwater, although it does involve the eyes. This problem is caused by a relative negative pressure gradient between ambient pressure and the pressure to which the eyes are exposed. The topic of squeeze is dealt with at length in Chapter 5.

Oxygen Toxicity

Any discussion concerning vision underwater would be incomplete if the effect of oxygen were not included. Indeed, Behnke et al. noted in 1935 that breathing pure oxygen for 4 hours at 3 atm caused a progressive contraction of the visual fields, dilation of the pupils, and impairment of central vision.[15] They went on to show that the effect was reversible within their experimental time frame, after 1 hour of breathing air at atmospheric pressure.

Subsequent work has suggested that the toxic effects of hyperbaric oxygen on the eye are not always reversible. Indeed one of the most exciting investigative sagas in medicine involves the implications of oxygen as the nasty culprit in producing retrolental fibroplasia in the immature retinas.[16] Admittedly, this fact has little significance in relation to diving medicine other than suggesting that premature infants should not dive deeply on air. Yet other work has shown that prolonged hyperbaric oxygen can have deleterious effects on the mature retina as well. This fact may have significance in saturation diving and during oxygen treatment. Hyperbaric oxygen has been implicated in retinal detachment in dogs,[17] as well as degeneration of the visual receptors in rabbits.[18]

For sometime it has been known that oxygen decreases the caliber of retinal vessels. In normal subjects, the small arterioles were noted to contract their diameter by 30.2 percent, while breathing oxygen at 1 atm.[19] While breathing oxygen at 2 atm the small arteriols contracted by a mean of 42.3 percent.[20] (For more information on this subject, see Chapter 11 and the bibliography at the end of this chapter).

One possible benefit of hyperbaric oxygen in relation to the eye concerns the difficult treatment of central retinal artery occlusion. By utilizing hyperbaric oxygen, the choroidal circulation is theoretically able to supply oxygen to the entire retina.[21] This theory was upheld by the experiments with animals,[16, 22] but failed to effect a change in human patients under the experimental protocol of Anderson et al.[23] and Haddad and Leopold.[16]

Increased partial pressures of carbon dioxide at normal oxygen levels do not seem to effect the retinal circulation in terms of vessel size or retinal circulation time, although blood flow increases. At higher oxygen tensions, increased carbon dioxide, however, tends to inhibit the oxygen induced vasoconstriction.[24]

Summary

Immersion in water and breathing compressed gas causes alterations in the function of the eyes. The distortions result from psychological and physical factors. Even with the protection of a mask, there are alterations in contrast, visual acuity, stereoacuity, distance estimation, color appreciation, and field of vision. Light rays falling on the retina have undergone differential attenuation, refraction, and reflection. The retinal vessels and the choroidal sinusoids respond to fluctuation of the partial pressure of the respiratory gas causing alterations of the pattern of blood flow. Yet, despite these cummulative effects and with adequate protection, the submerged human shows effective adaption.

And the future? What could one hypothesize as the ultimate optical solution. Taking clues from the aquatic creatures, one could imagine, as suggested by Williamson,[5] phacoprosthesis (lens prosthesis) of the appropriate diopter power (roughly equivalent to a fish lens) to offset the loss of the air-cornea interface; and a protective substance similar to the secretion of the Harderian glands in seacows and manatees.[4] The result would be an individual perfectly adapted optically to the underwater environment without the need of a mask.

His vision would be good; he would have little if any optical distortion; and his visual field would be normal. The only problem would be that out of the water his phacoprosthesis would make him horribly myopic.

REFERENCES

1. Kinney JA, et al: Visibility of colors underwater. J Opt Soc Am 57 (6) 802-809, 1967.
2. Luria SM, Kinney JS: Underwater vision. Science 167: 1454-1461, 1970
3. Kinney JA, et al: Visibility of colors underwater using artificial illumination. J Opt Soc Am 59 (5) 624-628, 1969
4. Williamson DE: Correction of ametropia in skin and scuba divers. J Fl Med Assoc 56 (2) 98-103, Feb. 1969
5. Faust KJ, Beckman EL: Evaluation of a swimmer's contact air-water lens system. Milit Med 779-788, Sept 1966
6. Ferris SH: Magnitude estimation of absolute distance underwater. Percep Mot Skills 35: 963-971, 1972
7. Luria SM, et al: Stereoscopic acuity underwater. Am J Psychol 81 (3) 359-366, 1968
8. Luria SM: Stereoscopic and resolution acuity with various fields of view. Science 164: 452-453, 1969
9. Luria SM, Kinney JS: Peripheral stimuli and stereo-acuity underwater. Percept Psychophys 11: 437-440, 1972
10. Kinney JA, et al: Responses to the underwater distortions of visual stimuli. US Naval Submarine Medical Center, Report 541, 1968
11. Kinney JS, et al: Effects of diving experience on visual perception underwater. US Naval Submarine Medical Center, Report 612, 1970
12. Kinney JS, et al: The improvement of divers' compensation for underwater distortions. US Naval Submarine Medical Center, Report 633, 1970
13. McKay CL, Kinney JS, Luria SM: Further tests of training techniques to improve visual-motor coordination of navy divers underwater. US Naval Submarine Medical Center, Report 684, Oct 1971
14. Alley RH: Scuba examinations: A guideline for the physician. J Am Coll Health Assoc 15: 194-196, 1966
15. Behnke ARK, Forbes H, Motley EP: Circulatory and visual effects of oxygen at three atmospheres. Am J Physiol 114: 436, 1935
16. Haddad HM, Leopold IH: Effect of hyperbaric oxygenation on microcirculation. Invest Ophthalmol 4: 1141, 1965
17. Beehler CC, et al: Retinal detachment in adult dogs resulting from oxygen toxicity. Arch Ophthalmol 71: 665, 1964
18. Noel WK: Metabolic injuries of the visual cell. Am J Ophthalmol 39: 589, 1955
19. Dollery CT et al: Oxygen supply to the retina from the retinal and choroidal circulation at normal and increased arterial oxygen tension. Invest Ophthalmol 8: 588, 1969
20. Dollery CT, et al: High oxygen pressure and retinal blood vessels. Lancet 1: 291, 1964

21. Flower RW et al: The effect of hyperbaric oxygenation on retinal ischemia. Invest Ophthalmol 10: 605-616, 1971
22. Carlisle R, Lanphier EH, Rahn H: Hyperbaric oxygen and persistance of vision in retinal ischemia. J Appl Physiol 19: 914, 1964
23. Anderson B Jr, Saltzman HS, Heyman A: The effects of hyperbaric oxygenation on retinal arterial occlusion. Arch Ophthamol 73: 315, 1965
24. Frayser R, Hickam JB: Retinalvascular response to breathing increased carbon dioxide and oxygen concentrations. Invest Ophthalmol 8: 427, 1964

ADDITIONAL BIBLIOGRAPHY

Ashton N and Pedler C: Studies on developing retinal vessels-reaction of endothelial cells to oxygen. Br J Ophthalmol 46: 257, 1962
Ferris SH: Improvement of absolute distance estimations underwater. Percept Mot Skills 35: 299-305, 1972
Kent PR: Vision underwater. Am J Optom and Arch Am Acad Optom 43 (9) 553-565, 1966
Kinney JA, et al: Effect of turbidity on judgments of distance underwater. Percept Mot Skills 28: 331-333, 1969
Luria SM, et al: Estimates of size and distance underwater. Am J Psychol 180: 282-286, 1967
Luria SM: Acuity-luminance function for extreme refractive error. Am J Optom and Arch Am Acad Optom 47 (3) 205-211, 1970
Luria SM et al: Judgments of distance under partially reduced cues. Percept Mot Skills 26: 1019-1028, 1968
Miles S: Vision, hearing and special senses, Underwater Med 160-165, 1962
US Navy Diving Manual
Wise GN, Dollery CT, Henkind P: The retinal circulation in The Pharmacology of Retinal Circulation. New York, Harper & Row, 1971, pp 120-129

STUDY QUESTIONS

1. When submerged, is the human eye myopic or hyperopic? Why is this so?
2. No matter how large the faceplate of a diving mask is, the visual field is limited to 97° vertically and horizontally. Why is this so?
3. Hyperbaric oxygen causes visual effects. What is the major part of the eye affected by hyperbaric oxygen?
4. Vision is limited underwater because of rapid attenuation. What are the two major sources of this attenuation?
5. How does one explain the fact that color appreciation varies from one body of water to another?

David A. Youngblood and
Walter G. Wolfe

11

Unearthly Atmospheres: Some Dangerous Aspects of Diving Gases

AIR

Almost all sport divers and many commercial divers breathe air underwater; it is abundant, cheap, and relatively constant in composition. In fact, air is such a standard substance that there are, as yet, no federal specifications; we are forced to accept what nature has provided and make every effort not to contaminate it during compression, transport, or storage.

Air Purity for Diving Purposes

The U.S. Navy has provided purity standards for compressed air to be used as a diver's breathing gas[1]:

Oxygen concentration-20 to 22 *percent* by volume
Carbon dioxide—not more than 0.05 *percent* (500 ppm)
Carbon monoxide—not more than 0.002 *percent* (20 ppm)
Oil vapor—not more than 5 mg/m^3
Gross moisture, dust, and other foreign matter—must be free of these contaminants

Common Sources of Air Contamination

An occasional cause of serious contamination is the vapor of those halogenated hydrocarbons used to clean the air hoses. These solvents are highly soluble in synthetic rubber compounds. However, a more common source of contamination is the compression of impure air. For instance, methane or hydrogen sulfide fumes may be present in air pumped near polluted harbors or putrefying fish products—and at 5 ata pressure, as little as 0.002 percent hydrogen sulfide could be lethal. Furthermore, many air compressors in common use are lubricated by petroleum base products; improper maintenance or ordinary wear can allow excessive amounts of oil vapor contamination.

The most common contaminant, however, is carbon monoxide from the compressor's engine, although other carbon monoxide sources, such as high ambient levels during peak traffic hours at urban-based compressor installations, should not be overlooked.

CARBON MONOXIDE

Pathophysiology of Carbon Monoxide Toxicity

Although carbon monoxide is a normal waste product of human metabolism, its rate of production is inconsequential in most diving operations.[2] The primary toxic effect of contaminant carbon monoxide is its efficiency in competing with oxygen for the Fe^{2+} binding sites in the hemoglobin molecule. The carbon monoxide affinity for hemoglobin is more than 200 times greater than the oxygen affinity for hemoglobin, which implies that breathing air with a carbon monoxide concentration of only 0.1 percent could at 1 atm produce equal concentrations of blood carboxyhemoglobin and oxyhemoglobin at the time of equilibrium.[3] This decrease in arterial oxygen content causes tissue hypoxia, even in the presence of a relatively normal P_{O_2}.

Furthermore, carbon monoxide appears to react with hemoglobin forms which normally enter into the most labile combination with oxygen. The remaining hemoglobin molecules that combine with oxygen seem to be more stable forms which release oxygen only at a considerably lowered P_{O_2}. This relative increase in the affinity of hemoglobin for oxygen is an important secondary factor in the hypoxia of carbon monoxide poisoning. A diver surfacing with 60 percent carboxyhemoglobin would probably lose consciousness and perish, whereas an anemic patient with a hemoglobin content of only 40 percent of normal is in no immediate danger. The tension at which oxygen is unloaded in the tissue capillary in the absence of carboxyhemoglobin provides an adequate pressure differential for diffusion into the cells.

Chronic Toxicity

Chronic carbon monoxide poisoning is relatively common. It occurs chiefly among cigarette smokers, who may have carboxyhemoglobin concentrations as high as 7 percent, but poorly ventilated charcoal or petroleum

Table 11-1
Carbon Monoxide Poisoning

% Blood Saturation with COHb	Symptoms and signs
0-10	No prominent symptoms; insidious decreases in judgment and psychomotor performance
10-20	Mild frontal headache; dilation of cutaneous blood vessels
20-30	Headache, throbbing in temples; nausea
30-50	Severe headache, weakness, dizziness, dimness of vision, nausea and vomiting, collapse and syncope, increased pulse and respiration
50-80	Syncope, increased pulse and respiration, coma and convulsions with progression to Cheyne-Stokes respiration, weak pulse, respiratory failure, and death

stoves can be an unsuspected cause as well as faulty exhaust systems aboard boats, aircraft, or automobiles. Aside from any cumulative or residual effects of chronic carbon monoxide poisoning, there are two real and immediate dangers to divers. The first is decreased psychomotor performance[4] and the second is the obvious compromise in the time available before onset of symptoms in the event of a subsequent acute exposure.

Acute Toxicity

The onset of acute carbon monoxide toxicity is related to two factors: the baseline level of carboxyhemoglobin acquired during any prior exposure, and the rate of uptake during the acute exposure phase. The latter is a function of *time, inspired concentration,* and *alveolar ventilation.*[3] During diving operations, exposure time is directly related to the total dive time, whereas the inspired concentration must be calculated as partial pressure of carbon monoxide. Alveolar ventilation varies with exercise, and during a hard-working dive, the onset of acute carbon monoxide toxicity can be greatly accelerated.

Symptoms and Signs

The symptoms and signs of carbon monoxide poisoning are principally those that one would associate with tissue hypoxia, as shown in Table 11-1.

Some of the signs of carbon monoxide poisoning, on the other hand, contrast significantly with the cyanosis usually associated with hypoxia. The carbon monoxide victim often presents with pink cheeks, characteristic "cherry red" lips, and reddish blotches on the skin, although these findings are by no means constant.

Treatment of Carbon Monoxide Poisoning

Carbon monoxide is eliminated most rapidly by ensuring a maximum partial pressure gradient between the carboxyhemoglobin and any gas in the alveoli. The half-time for CO elimination breathing pure air at atmospheric pressure, with the patient at rest, is between 4 and 5 hours.[5] If oxygen can be administered by mask at atmospheric pressure, the half-time can be reduced to approximately 1 hour.[6]

If a recompression chamber equipped for hyperbaric administration of oxygen is available, the half-time for CO elimination can be reduced to less than half an hour, while greatly improving tissue oxygenation during the recovery period. A standard 135-minute U.S. Navy Treatment Table 5 would be adequate in most diving situations. If respiration is depressed, artificial ventilation may be necessary.

Theoretically, an increase in alveolar ventilation would also enhance elimination of carbon monoxide, and effective experiments have been performed using 5 to 7 percent CO_2 added to oxygen at atmospheric pressure.[7] Such mixtures are rarely available in diving situations, and would be contraindicated in the hyperbaric treatment of CO poisoning because of the possibility of accelerating the onset of oxygen convulsions.[8]

Residual Effects of Carbon Monoxide Poisoning

Although recovery is apparently complete following mild CO poisoning, the hypoxic injury associated with acute, chronic, or recurrent exposures may cause transient or even permanent damage to the heart, central nervous system, or other organs having a high oxygen demand.[9] Careful postrecovery evaluation of such patients is essential, with special attention toward the assessment of cardiac, renal, and neurological function.

Except for contaminants, the dangerous aspects of all diving gas mixtures, including air, are a result of the hyperbaric properties of their ordinary components. The pressure effects of "inert" compounds such as nitrogen and helium will be considered in another chapter. In what follows, we will consider the toxic effects of carbon dioxide and oxygen during diving situations.

CARBON DIOXIDE

The Normal Role of Carbon Dioxide

Carbon dioxide is a normal metabolic product of oxidative metabolism. In this context, it is not a toxin, but an essential component of the body's internal environment—a chemical messenger influencing the regulation of respiration and circulation. Carbon dioxide is the primary stimulant in respiratory control through changes produced in the hydrogen ion concentration of the blood, brain, and cerebrospinal fluid.[10] This carbon dioxide respiratory control involves a direct relationship between arterial P CO_2 and ventilation, in which metabolically produced CO_2 actually maintains ventilation at a natural "set point" at rest and increases ventilation proportionately as metabolism produces more CO_2. The normal "set point" of the CO_2 sensitive respiratory neurons seems to be about 50 mm Hg. Evidence accrued from studies performed upon experienced breath-hold divers indicates that this CO_2 "set point" may become elevated through conditioning and training. With such a change, there is an increased possibility of hypoxia and unconsciousness during prolonged breath-holding.

Carbon Dioxide Intoxication

Carbon dioxide poisoning results from its accumulation through inadequate respiratory exchange or through the inhalation of elevated concentrations of it. The toxic effects are a consequence of the severe cellular acidosis produced.

Acute Toxicity.   Carbon dioxide intoxication during diving operations is most commonly caused by an accumulation of endogenously produced CO_2 in hose-supplied diving helmets or masks secondary to inadequate gas flow. Closed or semiclosed-circuit scuba, with its requirement for chemical removal of CO_2, ranks high among the causes of carbon dioxide fatalities and closed space contamination of recompression chambers, diving bells, underwater habitats, and submersibles, is a constant threat.[11-15] The adverse effects of acute carbon dioxide poisoning in normal persons at rest are shown in Table 11-2.

With acute exposure to carbon dioxide, exercise tolerance is decreased due to interference with elimination of mataboically produced CO_2. Short-term exposure to these simultaneous stresses of high inspired CO_2 and heavy exercise do not produce apparent adverse effects.[16]

Chronic Toxicity.   Chronic carbon dioxide toxicity is not a serious problem in diving medicine; only during exceptionally prolonged saturation

Table 11-2
Effects of Acute Carbon Dioxide Poisoning

Percent CO_2 (sea level equivalent*)	Adverse Effects
0-3	No detectable respiratory or other discomfort
4-6	Increasing respiratory stimulation and general arousal
7-10	Dyspnea and mental deterioration
10-20	Progressive dyspnea, violent respiratory distress, unconsciousness, spasmodic neuromuscular twitching, and convulsions

*As depth increases, the biological effect of an inspired gas becomes greater because its partial pressure increases, although its percentage remains constant.

dives with woefully inadequate CO_2 removal systems would one expect to encounter it at all. The body is capable of acclimatizing to chronically high levels of inspired CO_2 through alterations in the acid-base characteristics of blood and cerebrospinal fluid, the respiration and respiratory responsiveness, the deposition of calcium and carbonate in the skeleton, and in the tolerance to exercise. All of the physiological changes associated with acclimatization to chronic CO_2 exposure appear to be completely reversible with the resumption of normal air breathing.[16]

Acceptable CO_2 Concentrations for Diving Operations

Commercial saturation operations employing submersible decompression chamber-deck decompression chamber complexes with a chemical CO_2 removal capability often attempt to maintain a CO_2 partial pressure of 2 mm Hg or less in accordance with recommendations in the *U.S. Navy Diving Operations Handbook*[17] and are frustrated by their inability to achieve such efficient CO_2 "scrubbing." Since normal men can tolerate with impunity long-term exposure to CO_2 partial pressures of 21 mm Hg, or 3 percent surface equivalent,[18] it would seem reasonable to establish more realistic guidelines. For saturation diving, CO_2 exposures of 10.5 mm Hg, or 1½ percent surface equivalent, seem a reasonable recommendation. Although this level can cause a decrease in respiratory frequency, it is accompanied by a concomitant increase in tidal volume. Total pulmonary ventilation remains relatively constant, and this change in breathing pattern might even be considered desirable in helping to prevent mild atelectasis secondary to the inactivity often associated with saturation diving.

OXYGEN

Experimentation with the biological role of oxygen began immediately following its isolation in 1772. Lavoisier, the first to describe the true nature of the interchange of pulmonary gases in the lung, referred to the "incendiary action" upon the lungs of animals exposed to this gas. In the nineteenth century, Paul Bert recorded the first formal account of oxygen toxicity restricted exclusively to hyperbaric pressures.[19] J. Lorrain Smith is credited with first describing the pathology of pulmonary oxygen toxicity.[20] As early as 1897, he recognized that the inherent toxicity of oxygen might limit its clinical application. The importance of this toxic effect of oxygen on the lung has not been appreciated by physicians engaged in patient care until the last 15 to 20 years. The toxic effect of high partial pressures of inspired oxygen upon the eyes of newborn infants was the first clinical evidence of the dangerous effect of oxygen administered at atmospheric pressure.[21, 22]

Pulmonary oxygen toxicity is essentially the only major manifestation of oxygen overdosage which is observed in clinical practice, with the exception of retrolental fibroplasia in neonates. Central nervous system toxicity, which consists mainly of grand mal seizures, is a matter of concern only in unusual environments in which oxygen is inspired at pressures greater than 2.5 atm. Complete reviews on the subject of oxygen toxicity have been published by Wood,[23] Clark,[24] and Wolfe.[25]

Oxygen toxicity which occurs at oxygen tensions greater than one atmosphere differs from that seen in patients exposed to high oxygen tensions at atmospheric pressure for prolonged periods. Bean[26] reviewed the effect of oxygen at hyperbaric pressure in 1945. Early signs of oxygen poisoning at hyperbaric pressures are muscular twitching, nausea, vomiting, dizziness, tunnel vision, hearing difficulty, and difficulty with breathing described as "air hunger." These symptoms are accompanied by anxiety, fatigue, and poor coordination. Grand mal convulsions of short duration are brought on by exposure to high pressure oxygen. Toxicity of this type is seen during inhalation of 100 percent oxygen in the treatment of decompression sickness.

It was formerly believed that central nervous system effects of oxygen would herald pulmonary toxicity. Bean[26] felt that the pulmonary effects of high oxygen tension were related to the CNS effect and convulsions, thus postulating a noxious extrapulmonary agent. Reich[27] pointed out that pulmonary oxygen toxicity could result rapidly with systemic hyperoxia and that convulsions (CNS toxicity) were not necessary for significant pulmonary injury.

The mechanism by which high systemic oxygen tension produces pulmonary injury is not clear. Perhaps systemic hyperoxia causes formation of an extrapulmonary agent toxic to the lung. However, it is possible that higher than normal oxygen tension in mixed venous blood may act directly upon the lung.

An extrapulmonary noxious agent was postulated by Kistler.[28] Because of the chronological finding of endothelial injury before alveolar epithelial injury, he felt that a bloodborne agent might be necessary for oxygen poisoning of the lung. However, the major body of evidence still points to the importance of the local toxic effect of high concentration of oxygen on the airway and lung tissue.

Many of the physiologic responses seen in the cardiovascular system after introduction of 100 percent oxygen are well documented.[29] There is an increase in systemic vascular resistance that occurs in response to hyperoxia with decline in cardiac output. Hyperoxia has been shown to produce an increase in pulmonary arterial pressure. However, the changes in pulmonary artery pressure in dogs appear to be relatively insignificant.

A decline in dynamic pulmonary compliance in man in the absence of chest film changes has been reported.[30] Atelectasis and edema have been ruled out by the absence of radiologic evidence or alteration of the alveolar-arterial oxygen gradient. Exposure of human volunteers to high oxygen pressures has permitted measurement of altered respiratory function many hours before development of anatomical changes of irreversible toxicity.[31] The rate of development of severe symptoms is variable. One of the earliest signs of pulmonary oxygen toxicity in man is chest pain. One of the major changes occurring in lung function is a change in vital capacity.[32] In several studies, vital capacity continued to fall after chest pain had disappeared, suggesting that the subject's discomfort was not the primary cause of such a change. Caldwell's study[32] showed that the vital capacity of one subject decreased 35 percent after 74 hours of exposure and that several weeks elapsed before the preexposure value was restored. Also, in Caldwell's subjects, the cause of impairment of vital capacity was not established, but on the basis of associated decrease in carbon monoxide diffusing capacity, beginning at 48 hours, it was proposed that early alveolar edema formation had occurred. However, the absence of either radiologic changes or a low alveolar-arterial oxygen gradient make this explanation unlikely. Clark and Lambertsen[33] suggested that the diminution of vital capacity is the best index of the development of oxygen toxicity in man.

Absorptive atelectasis has been implicated as the mechanism whereby the decrease in vital capacity is induced in human toxicity.[34] However, this cannot be verified on the basis of chest films. Another possible mechanism could be muscle weakness, due to fatigue, and discomfort, which is described as retrosternal soreness induced by deep inspiration. This appears to be substantiated by the observation that reduction of vital capacity seems to occur mainly at the expense of the inspiratory reserve volume.

Other changes observed in man include abnormalities of compliance, diffusion capacity, pulmonary blood volume, and airway resistance. All of these studies have inherent difficulties when obtained from patients breathing 100 percent oxygen. Technical difficulties arise in measuring pulmonary diffusion capacity or changes in compliance that might be observed, but are reversed by deep breathing. This difficulty in measurement of pulmonary capillary volumes makes the significance of measured changes unclear. Studies in humans breathing 95 percent oxygen show a drop in diffusing capacity to 81 percent of control after 48 hours and to 73 percent after 74 hours. Total lung capacity fell to 73 percent of control value after 74 hours. These results might be explained on the basis of increase in blood tissue barrier, decrease in pulmonary capillary surface area, or alveolar edema formation as observed in animal studies.[30, 32] Morphological changes in man are similar to those seen in monkeys exposed to prolonged hyperoxia. Also, in these studies, there was a progressive fall in the diffusing capacity in patients breathing 60 to 100 percent oxygen for periods longer than 3 days.[35]

Currently, it appears that pulmonary oxygen toxicity will not develop in humans if the inspired tensions are below one-half atmosphere, and it is doubtful that significant oxygen toxicity develops in patients breathing pure oxygen at one atmosphere for less than 24 hours.[36] There is no known contraindication to the use of pure oxygen for brief periods in emergency situations. One must remember that the development of oxygen toxicity is a function of inspired tension, atmosphere pressure, and duration of exposure. There is *no indication* for breathing oxygen (that is, O_2 at concentrations greater than 20 to 22 percent by volume) in sport scuba diving.

REFERENCES

1. US Navy Diving Manual, 1973, Appendix IIA
2. Coburn RF, Blakemore WS, Torster RE: Endogenous carbon monoxide production in man. J Clin Invest 42:1172, 1963
3. Lambertsen CJ: Effects of excessive pressures of oxygen, nitrogen, carbon dioxide, and carbon monoxide: Implications in aerospace and undersea environments, in: Mountcastle VC (ed): *Medical Physiology.* St. Louis, Mosby, 1968, p 836
4. Beard RR, Westheim GA: Behavioral impairment associated with small doses of carbon monoxide. Am J Public Health 57:2112, 1967
5. Roughton FJW: The average time spent by the blood in the human being capillary and its relation to the rates of CO uptake and elimination in man. Am J Physiol 143:621, 1945
6. Pace N, Strajman E, Walker EL: Acceleration of carbon monoxide elimination in man by high pressure oxygen. Science 111:652, 1950
7. Henderson Y, Haggard HW: Noxious Gases and the Principles of Respiration Influencing their Action. New York, Chemical Catalog Co, 1927
8. Lambertsen CJ: Effects of oxygen at high partial pressure, in Tenn WO, Rahn H

(eds, respir sect): Handbook of Physiology, vol. 2 Baltimore, Williams & Wilkins Co, 1965

9. Beck HG, Suter GM: Role of carbon monoxide in the causation of myocardial disease. JAMA 110:1982, 1938

10. Lambertsen CJ: Chemical control of respiration at rest, in DePalma JR (ed): Drill's Pharmacology in Medicine, (ed 4) New York, McGraw-Hill, 1971

11. Lambertsen CJ: Therapeutic gases: Oxygen, carbon dioxide and helium, in DePalma JR (ed): Drill's Pharmacology in Medicine, (ed 4). New York, McGraw-Hill, 1971

12. Lambertsen CJ: Carbon dioxide and respiration in acid-base homeostasis. Anesthesiology 21:642, 1960.

13. Dripps RD, Comroe JG Jr: The respiratory and circulatory response of normal man to inhalation of 7.6 and 10.4 percent CO_2 with a comparison of the maximal ventilation produced by severe muscular exercise, inhalation of CO_2 and maximal voluntary hyperventilation. Am J Physiol 149:43, 1947

14. Lambertsen CJ: Effects of excessive pressures of oxygen, nitrogen, carbon monoxide: Implications in aerospace and undersea environments, in Mountcastle VB (ed): St. Louis, Medical Physiology. Mosby, 1968, p 836

15. Sinclair RD, Clark JM, Welch BE: Comparison of physiological responses of normal man to exercise in air and in acute and chronic hypercapnea, in Lambertsen CJ (ed): Underwater Physiology. New York, Academic Press, 1971

16. Lambertsen CJ: Carbon dioxide tolerance and toxicity. Philadelphia, Pennsylvania, Institute for Environmental Medicine, University of Pennsylvania Medical Center, 1971

17. US Navy Diving Operations Handbook, NAVSHIPS, 0994-009-6010, p 171

18. Clark JM, Sinclair RD, Welch BE: Rate of acclimatization to chronic hypercapnia in man, in Lambertsen CJ (ed): Underwater Physiology. New York, Academic Press, 1971

19. Bert P: Barometric Pressure: Researches in Experimental Physiology. (transl Hitchcock MA, Hitchcock FA) Columbus, Ohio, Longs College Book Co, 1943, p 5

20. Smith JL: The influence of pathological conditions on active absorption of oxygen by the lungs. J Physiol 22:307, 1897-1898

21. Cusick PL, Benson OO Jr, Boothby WM: Effect of anoxia and of high concentrations of oxygen on the retinal vessels. Proc Mayo Clinic 15:500, 1940

22. Gerschman R, Nadig PW, Snell AC Jr, Nye SW: Effect of high oxygen concentrations on eyes of newborn mice. Am J Physiol 179:115, 1954

23. Wood JD: Oxygen toxicity, in Bennett PB, Elliot DH (eds): *The Physiology and Medicine of Diving* (ed 2). London, Bailliere and Tindall, 1975

24. Clark JM: The toxicity of oxygen. Am Rev Respir Dis 110:40, 1974; Clark JM, Lambertsen CJ: Pulmonary oxygen toxicity: A review, Pharmacol Rev 23:37-133, 1971

25. Wolfe WG, DeVries WC: Oxygen toxicity. Ann Rev Med 26:203, 1975

26. Bean JW: Effects of oxygen at increased pressure. Physiol Rev 23:1, 1945

27. Reich T, Tait J, Suga T, Naftchi NE, Demeny M: Pathogenesis of pulmonary oxygen toxicity: Rose of systemic hyperoxia and convulsions. J Appl Physiol 32:374, 1972

28. Kistler GS, Caldwell PRB, Weibel ER: Development of fine structural damage to alveolar and capillary lining cells in oxygen poisoned rat lungs. J Cell Biol 33:605, 1967
29. Eggers GW, Paley HW, Leonard JJ, et al: Hemodynamic responses to oxygen breathing in man. J Appl Physiol 17:75, 1962
30. Fisher AB, Hyde RW, Puy RJM, et al: Effect of O_2 at 2 atmospheres and the pulmonary mechanics of normal man. J Appl Physiol 24:529, 1968
31. Burger EJ Jr, Mead J: Static properties of lungs after oxygen exposure. J Appl Physiol 27:191, 1969
32. Caldwell PRB, Lee WL Jr, Schildkraut HS, et al: Changes in lung volume, diffusing capacity, and blood gases in men breathing oxygen. J Appl Physiol 21:1477, 1966
33. Clark JM, Lambertsen CJ: Rate of development of pulmonary O_2 toxicity in man during O breathing at 2 atmospheres. J Appl Physiol 30:739, 1971
34. Michel EL, Langevin RW, Gell CF: Effect of continuous human exposure to oxygen tension of 418 mm Hg for 168 hours. Aerosp Med 31:138, 1960
35. Kapanci Y, Tosco R, Eggermann J, et al: Oxygen pneumonitis in man: Light- and electron-microscopic morphometric studies. Chest 62:162, 1972
36. Van DeWater JM, Kagey KS, Miller IT, et al: Response of the lung to 6 to 12 hours of 100 percent oxygen inhalation in normal man. N Engl J Med 283:621, 1970

STUDY QUESTIONS

1. According to U.S. Navy standards, what is the maximum allowable concentration of carbon monoxide in compressed air?
2. List several possible contaminants of compressed air, with their sources.
3. What is the primary principle of treatment in carbon monoxide poisoning?
4. In closed-circuit scuba, accumulation of CO_2 can lead to convulsions.
   a. True
   b. False
5. Breathing oxygen underwater may cause convulsions which in turn may lead to death by drowning or air embolism.
   a. True
   b. False
6. Pulmonary oxygen toxicity is not a significant problem among sport divers.
   a. True
   b. False

Peter B. Bennett

12

The Physiology of
Nitrogen Narcosis and
The High Pressure Nervous Syndrome

This text discusses the majority of the medical and physiological problems of diving summarized in Figure 12-1. It is apparent that two problems, nitrogen narcosis and the high pressure nervous syndrome (HPNS), appear as major hazards. The former is likely to occur in scuba or other divers breathing compressed air deeper than 100 feet (4 atmospheres absolute or ata). The latter is found only in very deep diving to depths greater than 500 feet (16 ata) in divers breathing oxygen-helium and, therefore, commonly today in divers used in support of the offshore oil drilling industry.

At first glance, there would seem to be little relationship between these two conditions, since they have very different signs and symptoms. However, it will become clear that there is, in fact, a very close relationship between them, although they are in a sense opposites. It will not be possible to consider these subjects in detail here. Further information may be obtained from more extensive reviews elsewhere.[1-5] The relevance of these problems to our knowledge of the mechanism of anesthesia also is described in another volume.[6]

NITROGEN NARCOSIS

The condition known as "nitrogen narcosis" or compressed air intoxication was first observed as long ago as 1835 when a Frenchman, Junod, noted that when breathing compressed air "the functions of the brain are activated,

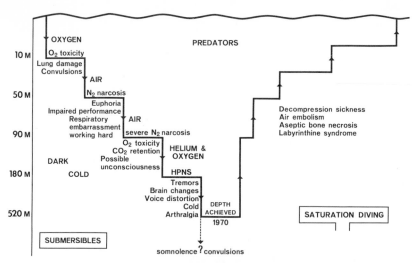

Fig. 12-1. Physiological problems of diving.

imagination is lively, thoughts have a peculiar charm and in some persons, symptoms of intoxication are present." Green[7] seems to have been the first American to have noted narcosis. At 160 feet (5.8 ata), he reported sleepiness, hallucinations, and impaired judgment, which he considered required an immediate return to atmospheric pressure.

The Royal Navy carried out a thorough investigation[8] when it was found that during 17 of 58 dives between 200 to 350 feet (7-11.6 ata) a condition resulting in "semi-loss of consciousness" occurred. The condition was regarded as serious, since the diver would continue to give all the normal hand signals at depth, but after decompression could not remember any of the events that took place underwater.

Much speculation about the possible cause resulted, but it was not until 1935 that Behnke and co-workers[9] correctly attributed the narcosis as due to the raised partial pressure of nitrogen in the compressed air. They characterized the narcosis as "euphoria, retardment of the higher mental processes and impaired neuromuscular coordination."

The signs and symptoms start to be noticed at about 100 feet (4 ata) and become increasingly more severe the greater the depth. Laughter, loquacity, and a light-headed sensation may be apparent with feelings of stimulation and excitement. With increased effort at self-control, it may be possible to overcome such behavior to some extent. There is a slowing of mental activity with delays in auditory and olfactory stimuli and a tendency to word idea fixation, as often seen in hypoxia. The resulting limitation of the power of association and perception is made especially dangerous due to the presence of overconfidence.

Memory will be impaired, especially short-term memory. Errors may be

Table 12-1
Effect of Pressure on Psychometric Tests[73]

Pressure (feet)	0	90	100	125	150	175	200	225	250	275	300
Mean additional time to solve problems (seconds)	0.35	11.09	6.89	7.65	9.74	11.95	13.98	17.17	26.07	26.53	31.42
Mean additional errors in solving problems	0.18	0.86	0.49	0.42	0.72	0.84	1.22	0.88	2.18	2.66	3.02
Mean decrease in numbers crossed out	—	− 0.59	− 0.09	− 2.26	− 2.30	− 2.49	− 2.55	− 4.24	− 5.85	− 6.43	− 8.74
Average reaction time (seconds)	0.214	—	—	—	0.237	—	0.242	—	0.248	—	0.257
Mean additional time to solve problems (acclimatized subjects)	1.64	2.55	3.42	3.91	4.66	8.00	11.75	15.73	16.33	17.09	24.36

Table 12-2
Mean Percentage Impairment in Ability of 14 Subject to
do an Arithmetical Test during Rest and Work on a
Bicycle Ergometer (300 kg/minute[74])

Absolute air pressures	4 atm	7 atm	10 atm	13 atm
At rest	− 3.2	− 6.9	− 24.6	− 61.6
During exercise	− 2.1	− 11.6	− 39.8	—

made in recording arithmetic data (Table 12-1.) For example, 43 minutes may be confused with 48 minutes and 12:15 written as 15:15. Handwriting becomes increasingly larger with the severity of the narcosis. There may be a change in the sense of time. Intellectual capacities are affected more severely than psychomotor or manual abilities. However, the ability to carry out fine movements will be impaired, usually due to overexaggeration of movements. If the movements are carried out more slowly than usual, the impairment of efficiency is likely to be less severe.

There may be some numbness and tingling of the lips, legs, and feet and a characteristic "dead pan" look to the face.

At depths greater than 180 feet (6.5 ata), no trust should be placed in human performance or efficiency in men breathing compressed air.

At depths greater than 300 feet (10 ata), the signs and symptoms are severe with the possibility of the diver becoming unconscious. Orders may be ignored. Intensity of vision and hearing, voice reverberation, stupor, and a sense of impending blackout and disorientation occur. Manic or depressive states can also occur, with changes in personality and a sense of levitation.[10]

These signs and symptoms are very similar to those seen in alcoholic intoxication and the early stages of hypoxia and anesthesia, with an equally wide variation in susceptibility. Nitrogen narcosis is an especially important danger to the compressed air diver. The perceptual narrowing that results may permit the diver to carry out a specific task with varying degrees of competency; but, in the event of something unusual occurring, he or she will be unable to function effectively in an emergency. Many divers who chose to ignore the narcosis problem or believed, as with alcohol, that it is more "manly" to be able to imply you are unaffected by the condition have perished as a result.

The narcosis is usually more severe immediately on arrival at depth, and there may be some improvement shortly afterward followed by a relatively stable level of narcosis.

Recovery is rapid upon decompression, although some amnesia may occur about events that occurred while narcotic. For example, a diver may have specific instructions to perform a certain task underwater; he will make the dive, become narcotic, and either not perform the task or perform it badly.

On return to the surface, he will report that the task has been completed satisfactorily!

Many factors potentiate the severity of the narcosis for a given depth, in addition to individual susceptibility. In particular, any increase in exogenous or endogenous carbon dioxide will synergistically potentiate the narcosis. For this reason, the narcosis is likely to be more severe in the swimming or working diver wearing breathing apparatus than in a pressure chamber (Table 12-2.) Similarly, hard work will facilitate narcosis as will very rapid compression, alcoholic excess or hangover, and apprehension.

Interestingly, variations in the oxygen percentage of the breathing mixture also will affect the degree of narcosis. Thus, at a constant nitrogen pressure, an increase in oxygen partial pressure will cause a greater narcosis.[11] Although a reduction of the oxygen partial pressure may reduce the narcosis if the nitrogen partial pressure is constant, this is not the case if the reduction means a concomitant increase in the nitrogen partial pressure. Albano and associates[12] noted, for example, that at 300 feet (10 ata) seven divers were more narcotic breathing 96 percent nitrogen/4 percent oxygen than breathing air (Table 12-3), a finding confirmed by Barnard and co-workers.[13]

The novice diver may expect to be relatively seriously affected by nitrogen narcosis, but subjectively, at least, there will be some improvement with experience. Frequency of exposure does seem to result in some adaptation. However, adaptation to narcosis is an area about which little is known and more research is required before any definite statements may be made.

Causes and Mechanisms of Inert Gas Narcosis

Although this chapter refers to nitrogen narcosis, the more general term inert gas narcosis is more correct. Inert, in this case, is in reference to the inability of the respired nitrogen to interact biochemically in the body. Any mechanism of narcosis must therefore be biophyiscal in nature. Further, nitrogen is not alone in its ability to cause signs and symptoms of narcosis or indeed anesthesia. Behnke and associates[9] related their inference of nitrogen as the causative agent in compressed air to an old, but still very valid, hypothesis that narcotic potency is related to the affinity of an anesthetic for lipid or fat. This Meyer-Overton hypothesis[14] affirms that "all gaseous or volatile substances induce narcosis if they penetrate the cell lipids in a definite molar concentration which is characteristic for each type of animal (or better, type of cell) and is approximately the same for all narcotics." This concentration, for example, Meyer calculated as 0.07 moles/liter for mice.

In fact, the narcotic potency of inert gases may be related to many physical constants including molecular weight,[15] adsorption coefficients,[16] thermodynamic "activity," [17-19] Van der Waal's constants,[20] and the formation of clathrates.[21, 22] Of these many constants, lipid solubility gives the best correla-

Table 12-3
Arithmetic Test Results at 10 Atmospheres Absolute[12].

Subject	Figures multiplied			Percentage of errors			Difference	
	(1) Ambient pressure	(2) 10 atm air	(3) 10 atm 96% N_2-4% O_2	(4) Ambient pressure	(5) 10 atm air	(6) 10 atm 96% N_2-4% O_2	(5)-(4)	(6)-(5)
A.G.	23	18	12	4.35	22.2	41.6	17.85	19.4
P.V.	24	19	15	4.25	79	86.6	74.75	7.6
R.S.	50	43	33	–	23	21.8	23.00	– 1.2
M.E.	40	20	14	10	30	42.8	20.00	12.8
S.V.	36	32	28	28	53.6	71.4	25.60	17.8
C.B.	27	24	20	7.4	50	60	42.60	10.0
C.U.	45	34	30	–	26.4	30	26.40	3.6
						M =	32.88	10.0
						t =	4.30	4.20
						P =	<0.01	<0.01

162

Table 12-4
Correlation of Narcotic Potency of the Inert Gases Hydrogen,
Oxygen, and Carbon Dioxide with Lipid Solubility and Other
Physical Characteristics

Gas	Molecular weight	Solubility in lipid	Molar Vol. (cm³)	Polarizability	Relative narcotic potency*
He	4	0.015	32.00	0.20	4.26
Ne	20	0.019	16.72	0.39	3.58
H_2	2	0.036	28.3		1.83
N_2	28	0.067	35.4	1.74	1
A	40	0.14	28.6	1.63	0.43
Kr	83.7	0.43	34.7	2.48	0.14
Xe	131.3	1.7	43.0	4.00	0.039 (surgical anesthesia)
O_2	32	0.11	27.9	1.58	
CO_2	44	1.34	38.0	2.86	

*In order from least narcotic to most narcotic.

tion, although polarizability and molar volume also are important in relation to the mechanism of the narcosis (Table 12-4), which involves interaction of the molecule with neuronal membranes. Thus, the size of the molecule and the degree of electrical charge upon it are important considerations.

Although nitrogen is widely recognized as the cause of compressed air intoxication, mention must be made of an alternative, but erroneous, theory that has been promoted from time to time.[23-27] This theory infers that due to the increased density of the breathing gas there is a respiratory insufficiency leading to carbon dioxide retention, and this increased carbon dioxide tension is the cause of the narcosis.

In fact, measurements of arterial carbon dioxide (Table 12-5) in men breathing either compressed air or oxygen-helium (helium being only a very weak narcotic at the most) showed that there is no increase in arterial carbon dioxide at 286 feet (9.6 ata) and 190 feet (6.7 ata). However, nitrogen narcosis occurred when nitrogen was present, but not helium.[28] Similarily measurements of alveolar carbon dioxide by Rashbass[29] and Cabarrou[30, 31] do not support the carbon dioxide theory. More recently Hesser et al.[32] have shown also that the effects of raised pressures of nitrogen and carbon dioxide merely are additive and that carbon dioxide is not the cause of compressed air intoxication.

There can be no doubt that the site of action of the narcosis in the brain is

Table 12-5
Mean Results of Human Mental Performance and Arterial Carbon
Dioxide in Air and 20/80 Oxygen-Helium

	Control	20/80 He/O_2	Air 20/80 N_2/O_2
At 286 Feet			
Arithmetic Correct	16.8 ± 1.78	15.67 ± 2.08	11.00 ± 1.73
Visual Analogy Test	50.5 ± 5.61	51.50 ± 5.80	44.50 ± 1.21
P_{aCO_2}	−	35.38 ± 4.36	34.73 ± 3.84
At 190 Feet			
Arithmetic Correct	16.8 ± 1.78	18.67 ± 1.53	15.67 ± 2.08
Visual Analogy Test	50.5 ± 5.61	50.00 ± 5.42	51.70 ± 4.19
P_{aCO_2}	−	35.05 ± 2.56	32.68 ± 1.60

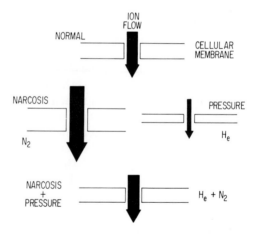

Fig. 12-2. Diagram of the action of nitrogen or
similar anesthetic agents on a nerve membrane. In the
normal membrane there is a normal ion (sodium,
chloride) flow. Under increased nitrogen pressures
the membrane expands 0.4-5 percent and a larger
flow of electroloyes occurs. As helium does not ad-
sorp to the membrane, pressure contracts the
membrane and the electrolyte flow is less than normal. The correct balance of nitrogen narcosis and
helium applied pressure, as with trimix, results in a
normal membrane and electrolyte flow.

Table 12-6
Comparative Percentage Impairment in Psychometric Performance of
Subjects Compressed to 600 feet and 800 feet While Breathing 5/95
Oxygen-Helium[43,44]

	600 ft (6) (%)	800 ft (4) (%)
Sums correct	− 18	− 42
Sums attempted	− 4	− 6
No. of ball bearings	− 25	− 53

at synapses or nerve junctions where there is a very small gap of 200 Å between the presynaptic terminal of one nerve and the postsynaptic terminal of another.[33-40] The mechanism therefore involves interferences with the electricochemical mechanisms necessary for the transfer of the electrical potential across the synaptic gap of central synapses. Polysynaptic regions of the brain, such as the ascending reticular activating system and the cortical mantle, are likely to be the regions of the brain most affected.

Contemporary theory as to the mechanism of anesthesia is relevant in explaining how synaptic transmission is impaired. It is believed that anesthesia occurs when the synaptic membrane is modified by adsorption of the anesthetic molecule of the lipid constituent. Such adsorption causes the membrane to expand, and when it expands beyond a critical volume, transmission fails and narcosis or anesthesia results, depending upon the number of synapses affected.[6, 41]

Expansion of the membrane permits its interior to be more fluid and free so that passage of ions such as sodium and chloride occurs more readily and increased permeability results (Fig. 12-2). As narcosis proceeds to loss of consciousness and anesthesia, this increased permeability may turn into a block.[42]

THE HIGH PRESSURE NERVOUS SYNDROME

On the basis of the lipid solubilities shown in Table 12-4, it might be expected that helium narcosis would not occur comparable to that due to compressed air at 300 feet (10 ata) until about 1400 feet (43 ata), and this resulted in the selection of helium as an alternative to compressed air for deep diving.

However, in 1965 during simulated dives with rapid compressions of 20 to 100 feet/minute to 600 feet and 800 feet for 1 to 4 hours, a marked decrement in performance was noted during the first hour of exposure (Tables 12-6 and 12-7) which, unlike nitrogen narcosis, was followed by a slow improve-

Table 12-7

Mean Percentage Change in Performance in Subjects Breathing 95/5 Helium/Oxygen at 600 feet for 4 hours Compared with Performance at Atmospheric Pressure[43,44]

Test	Surface (air)	600 ft 20 min (%)	600 ft 1½ hr (%)	600 ft 2 hr (%)	600 ft 2½ hr (%)	600 ft 3 hr (%)	600 ft 3½ hr (%)	300 ft (decomp) (%)
Arithmetic (no. correct)	15.67	− 18	+ 1.02	− 9.6	+ 9.6	+ 10.06	+ 7.4	+ 21.25
Arithmetic (no. attempted)	19.67	− 4.2	− 2.61	− 7.0	+ 4.33	+ 6.95	− 0.88	+ 6.6
Ball-bearing (no. of balls)	10.67	− 25	+ 9.37	+ 17.15	+ 26.53	+ 9.37	± 15.5	+ 17.15

ment. Further, in an opposite manner to narcosis, there was a more marked decrement in psychomotor tests, such as the ball bearing test (which required the subject to pick up ball bearings one at a time with forceps and place each in a tube of the same diameter), than intellectual tasks such as arithmetical efficiency.[43, 44] This was due to the associated presence of a marked tremor (6-10 Hz) of the hands, arms, or even whole body, together with dizziness, nausea, and sometimes vomiting. This was the first report at such depths of a condition now recognized as the high pressure nervous syndrome (HPNS), which appears to reflect a general excitation of the brain compared to the decreased excitation of inert gas narcosis.

Similar changes were reported in animals by Brauer and associates[45] in mice and monkeys. In such animals, the HPNS appears during compression with tremors and ratchety movements. As the pressure increases, localized myoclonic jerks occur, which progress to clonic seizures. If the animal is maintained at this pressure, intermittent seizure activity will occur for as long as 12 hours. Compression beyond this point results in tonic seizures, coma, and death. Such convulsions have yet to be reported in man.

Susceptibility to HPNS increases with increasing complexity and development of the nervous system.[46] Brauer and co-workers[47]—based on the fact that during 10 man dives at a compression rate of 24 atm/hour and, with an oxygen partial pressure of 0.5 atm and temperature of 30°-33°C, the mean threshold pressure for the onset of tremors was 26.4 atm (22-27 atm)—calculated that convulsions should occur in man under similar conditions at 66.3 ± 7.8 atm or 2300 feet. The onset of HPNS, however, is markedly affected by the rate of compression and slowing the rate of compression will result in the tremors and convulsions occurring at greater pressures and vice versa.

Thus, in 1968, a dive was performed at Duke University Medical Center to 1000 feet (31 ata) with a compression rate of 40 feet/hour without any tremors or other of the signs of HPNS reported during the earlier British dives in 1964-1965 to 600 and 800 feet at 100 feet/minute.[48]

However, during a further series of experiments by the French, known as Physalie[49] with compression rates averaging about 500 feet/hour, four of the dives exceeded 1000 feet (31 ata).

Tremors appeared at 21 ata (660 feet), and changes were seen in the electroencephalogram (EEG) at about 31 ata (1000 feet), with a marked increase in theta activity (4-6 Hz) accompanied by a depression of alpha (8-13 Hz) (see Fig. 12-3). As the pressure increased, the EEG changes became worse and were accompanied by intermittent bouts of somnolence with sleep stages 1 and 2 in the EEG. If the subjects had work to do, they were able to function; but if they stopped, they lapsed into what has been termed microsleep. Due to the severity of the microsleep and EEG changes at that time, the deepest dive was aborted after only 4 minutes at 1190 feet (37 ata).

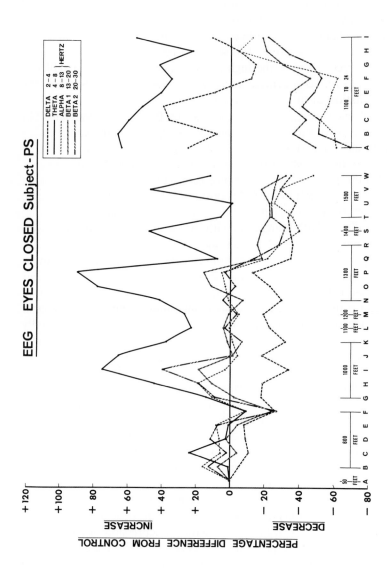

Fig. 12-3. Spontaneous cortical electrical activity of the brain (EEG) in a subject compressed in stages to 1500 feet (46 ata) with on-line frequency analysis shows a rise in theta (4-8 Hz) activity with a fall in overall activity from 1300 feet (40 ata).[51]

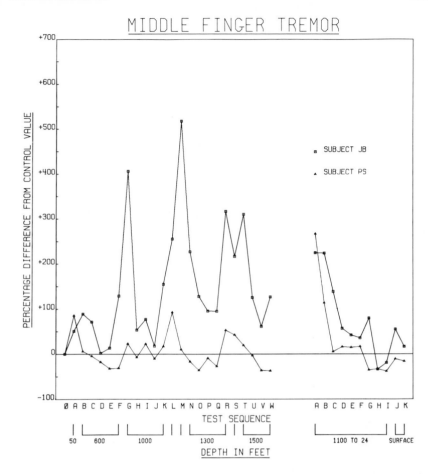

Fig. 12-4. Percentage change in tremor of the hand measured by a transducer on the finger of men compressed to 1500 feet (46 ata) oxygen-helium. Each compression phase causes a marked increase in tremor in one subject, but little affect on the other. The tremor sensitive subject also shows an increase in base tremor.[50]

Subsequently, further depth has been achieved by the use of slower rates of compression, with or without stages.

Thus, in 1970, two men were compressed for the first time to 1500 ft (46 ata), where they stayed for 10 hours. The compression rate was fast at 16-17 feet/minute (i.e., 100 feet/hour), but some 24 hours were spent at 600 feet, 1000 feet and 1300 feet (19, 31, and 40 ata). During this dive, the divers were extensively monitored.[50-53]

All of the characteristics of the HPNS were seen, but the divers were able to function reasonably well. A number of points were clarified by this dive.

First, in regard to the EEG, the rise in theta activity was initiated on

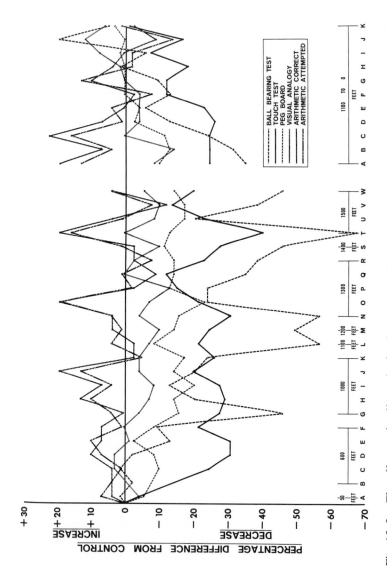

Fig. 12-5. The effect on intellectual (visual analogy, arithmetic) and psychomotor performance (ball bearing, peg board) of compression to 1500 feet (46 ata) oxygen-helium. Intellectual tasks are unaffected, indicating that helium does not cause narcosis; but, due to the pressure induced tremors, psychomotor tasks are impaired.[50]

compression, especially at pressures greater than 31 ata (1000 feet). The theta continued to rise for 6 hours, even though compression had ceased and then fell over 12 hours to lower levels (Fig. 12-3). On compression again, the cycle repeated. The rise in theta did not seem to correlate with any of the other signs of HPNS. There was an interindividual susceptibility that also was apparent in the tremors. One diver showed a considerable increase in tremor, whereas the other had little response (Fig. 12-4). The occurrence of tremor in diving has been reviewed in more detail elsewhere,[4] but it should be pointed out that the tremor is in the frequency range of 8-12 Hz, which is normal resting tremor and not that of Parkinson's or cerebellar disease which is 3-8 Hz. Cold, alcoholism, and thyrotoxicosis also cause tremor in the 8-12 Hz range.

For the first time, too, it could be clearly seen that helium did not cause signs and symptoms of narcosis. Arithmetic performance was unaffected, but psychomotor tests, such as the ball bearing and peg board tests (Fig. 12-5), showed a decrement mostly due to the tremors and muscular jerks.

On June 2, 1972, the French, using the system of such exponential type compression, with stages, reached a depth of 2001 feet (60.5 ata), which remains the deepest dive at present and which is close to the predicted depth for convulsions.

Nevertheless, at this remarkable depth, the diver efficiency was rather better than that seen in the 1500-foot British dive which used faster compression rates. Thus, manual dexterity was impaired by only 16-20 percent.[54] However, HPNS was certainly present and much further research is required and with some caution, due to the wide variation in individual susceptibility, if we are to avoid seeing the first HPNS convulsions in man at depths in excess of 2000 ft.

The Cause of HPNS

Clearly HPNS is a complex syndrome composed of more than one factor. Hunter and Bennett,[3] in a more extensive review than is possible here, point out that it is in reality composed of two phenomena, a "compression" syndrome and a "hydrostatic pressure" syndrome, for helium is but the carrier of pressure. Thus, liquid-breathing rodents show the same tremors and convulsions when only the hydrostatic pressure is increased.[55]

There have been many causes suggested as producing the HPNS, and these are discussed in some detail elsewhere.[3] Of these, the two most significant will be mentioned here:

The first mechanism infers that gas-induced osmosis is the cause due to fluid shifts in tissues as a consequence of differential saturation by the inert gases.[56, 57] As equilibrium in the tissues occurs with time, this also would account for the amelioration of the HPNS with time.

French workers[58-60] have developed mathematical relationships for calculation of compression rates which have been successful in amelioration of the HPNS. However, care must be utilized in relating this success to prevention of gas induced osmosis; for whichever method of calculation is used, the profiles developed are exponential in nature and, sometimes, with stages, and, as such, must be expected to be considerably better than the early linear over-rapid compressions.

Further, as already stated, HPNS is seen in liquid-breathing mice where inert gas osmosis cannot be a component.[61, 62] Again, in the experiments of Kylstra, et al[56] the osmotic shifts stabilized in 20 minutes, but HPNS can require 18 hours for EEG changes to stabilize, and the initial HPNS signs and symptoms often require over 60 minutes.

The second mechanism appears more logical and is related to the "critical volume" hypothesis, described earlier in this chapter in association with the cause of inert gas narcosis and as illustrated in Fig. 12-2.

However, the cell membrane in this case is not expanded by helium, or at least to such an extent as to be neglible, and the important parameter is the pressure itself.

This causes compression of the membrane making its interior tighter and the passage of ions more difficult. In fact, pressure can reverse anesthesia,[63-65] and it does so, theory directs, by restoring the expanded membrane to normal size. Thus, tadpoles given sufficient ethyl alcohol to cause them to fall to the bottom of a tank will wake up and resume swimming upon application of 100 atm pressure.

Conversely, it is reasonable to assume that membranes already compressed by the pressure in a helium dive may be re-expanded by the addition of a narcotic, anesthetic, or indeed nitrogen, and so prevent HPNS. That this is the case will be described in the final section of this chapter.

Prevention of HPNS

If the HPNS is to be avoided as much as possible, yet still permit realistic operational procedures, it is clearly of significant importance for the rate of compression to be optimally slow at depths greater than 500 feet (16 ata). But just how much slower than the conventional rate of 60 feet/minute is not clear, since there is insufficient systematic data upon which to make a judgment. However, it is advantageous to employ an exponential slow rate and stages.

Fructus et al.[54] have exposed men to 2001 feet (61 ata) using the formula for compression speed below, and although HPNS was present the divers were functional.

$$\frac{dP}{dt} = \frac{\text{Log } 2 \times G}{T\,(1 - G')}$$

where

P = depth
T = half-time of the tissue
$G(P)$ = the proposed gradient function
G' = $\dfrac{dG}{dP}$

Whatever rate is utilized, if a saturation mode of diving is chosen and sufficient time is available, it will be profitable to let the divers rest for the first 2-3 hours before starting work.

Another method, which also utilizes saturation diving is to use a saturation depth considerably less than the work depth and make excursions to the work site. Recent research at Duke University Medical Center[4] suggests, for example, that it is possible to saturate at a depth of 870 feet (27 ata) by slow compression without the occurrence of HPNS and then to make excursions at 100 feet/minute without the onset of HPNS. This is an area that merits much further investigation, especially at depths in excess of 1000 feet (31 ata).

Finally, there is the use of anesthetic or narcotic agents as alluded to earlier. Brauer and co-workers[66] found the addition of various concentrations of hydrogen, nitrogen, or nitrous oxide of significant value in alleviating HPNS. For example, 0.3 percent nitrous oxide added to heliox permitted 30 percent greater depths to be attained in mice and monkeys before HPNS occurred. Other agents, such as nongaseous barbiturates, were able to raise the HPNS convulsion threshold by over 50 percent.[67]

The use of nitrogen as the narcotic additive was investigated by Zaltsman and his colleagues[68 69] as early as 1961 and resulted in some very successful deep diving to 527 feet (17 ata), or so, by using trimix. Vigreux[70] also reported that a mixture of helium, nitrogen, and oxygen effectively prevented HPNS in dives to 394 feet (13 ata). However, these are relatively shallow depths and only minor HPNS would have been expected even without trimix.

More recently, studies have been made at Duke University with various nitrogen percentages and at depths to 1000 feet (31 ata).[71] These experiments involved comparison of the effects of the same procedures when diving on heliox alone, or trimix, or air containing the same partial pressure of nitrogen (5.6 ata).

The effect of the presence of 18 percent nitrogen (5.6 ata) at 1000 ft on the tremor of HPNS is illustrated in Fig. 12-6. Without the nitrogen, there is a marked increase in tremor as shown by the transducer. On addition of nitrogen at 600 feet (19 ata), there is a progressive reduction of tremor. At 850 feet (26.6 ata), on return to helium and oxygen for the decompression,

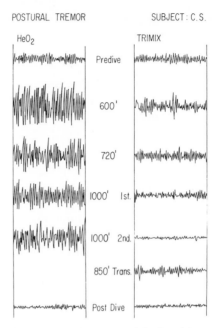

POSTURAL TREMOR   SUBJECT : C.S.

HeO₂   TRIMIX

Predive

600'

720'

I000'   I st.

I000'   2nd.

850' Trans.

Post Dive

Fig. 12-6.   Postural tremor of the hand in a subject
exposed either to 1000 feet (31 ata) oxygen-helium
alone or Trimix (He/O₂ with 18 percent nitrogen)
with the same compression time of 33 minutes. Without the nitrogen present, the classic tremor may be
seen. With nitrogen added at 600 feet (19 ata) in the
trimix, the tremors are suppressed. On changing back
to oxygen-helium during the decompression at 850
feet (26.6 ata), the tremor returns.[71]

the tremor again increases. Presumably, as the nitrogen now comes out of the
cell membranes, they contract and HPNS occurs.

However, although the 18 percent nitrogen was very effective in preventing HPNS, it was found that the percentage of nitrogen was too high and narcosis occurred in some subjects.

Accordingly, a mathematical method was developed for calculating the
correct balance of nitrogen and hydrostatic pressure to produce neither narcosis nor HPNS, which was based on the Gibbs adsorption equation.[6] The
model developed assumed

1. Anesthetics act at specific membrane sites with the same oil-water
   partition coefficients as olive oil.
2. At all pressures, the gases obey Henry's Law.
3. Helium compresses membrane, whereas nitrogen and oxygen expand it.

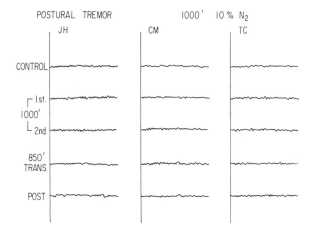

Fig. 12-7. Tremor transducer measurements in three subjects compressed in 33 minutes to 1000 feet (31 ata) in trimix (He/O$_2$ with 10 percent nitrogen). No HPNS tremors are seen.[72]

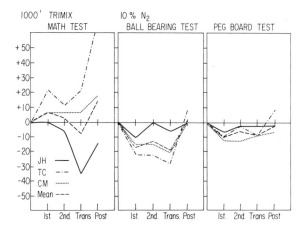

Fig. 12-8. Percentage change in performance tests in three men exposed to 1000 feet (31 ata) in 33 minutes breathing trimix (He/O$_2$ with 10 percent nitrogen). Measurements on arrival at depth (first) and before leaving 1 hour 40 minutes later (second) indicate no nitrogen narcosis and little psychomotor decrement.[72]

4. Conditions for elimination of HPNS and narcosis are that the membrane volume is constant at the pressure desired.

Calculations showed that the correct proportion of nitrogen to helium is 1 to 10. Men compressed to 1000 feet (31 ata) in 33 minutes, when breathing 3.2 ata nitrogen (10 percent), 0.5 ata oxygen, and the remainder helium,[72] were in fine condition with no tremors (Fig. 12-7) narcosis, nausea, dizziness, or other signs of HPNS (Fig. 12-8).

This appears to be a promising avenue for extension of the limits to which man may be exposed beneath the sea.

REFERENCES

1. Bennett PB: Inert gas narcosis, in Bennett PB, Elliott DH (ed): The Physiology and Medicine of Diving and Compressed Air Work (ed 2). London, Bailliere Tyndall, 1975
2. Bennett PB: The high pressure nervous syndrome: In Man, in Bennett PB, Elliott DH (ed): The Physiology and Medicine of Diving and Compressed Air Work (ed 2). London, Bailliere Tyndall, 1975
3. Hunter WL, Bennett PB: The causes, mechanisms and prevention of the high pressure nervous syndrome. Undersea Biomed Res 1:1-28, 1974
4. Bachrach A, Bennett PB: Tremor in diving. Aerosp Med 44:613-623, 1973
5. Bennett PB: Pharmacology of inert gases and hydrogen, in Lambertsen CJ (ed): Proceedings 5th Symposium on Underwater Physiology, Aug 1972. Washington, FASEB (in press)
6. Bennett PB, Simon S, Katz Y: High pressures of inert gases and anesthetic mechanisms, in Fink R (ed): Molecular Mechanisms of Anesthesia. Baltimore, Williams & Wilkins, 1974
7. Green JB: Diving with and without Armour. Buffalo, Leavitt, 1861
8. Hill L, Davis RH, Selby RP, et al: Deep Diving and Ordinary Diving. London, British Admiralty Report, 1933
9. Behnke AR, Thomson RM, Motley EP: The psychologic effects from breathing air at 4 atmospheres pressure. Am J Physiol 112:554-558, 1935
10. Adolfson J, Muren A: Air breathing at 13 atmospheres. Psychological and physiological observations. Sartryck ur Forsvars Medicin 1:31-37, 1965
11. Frankenhaeusser M, Graff-Lonnevig V, Hesser CM: Effects on psychomotor functions of different nitrogen-oxygen gas mixtures at increased ambient pressures. Acta Physiol Scand 59:400-409, 1963
12. Albano G, Criscuoli PM, Ciulla C: La sindrome neuropsichica di profondita. Lav Um 14:351-358, 1962
13. Barnard EEP, Hempleman HVH, Trotter C: Mixture Breathing and Nitrogen Narcosis. Report UPS 208, London, Medical Research Council, RN Personnel Research Committee, 1962
14. Meyer HH: Theoris der alkoholnarkose. Arch Exp Pathol Pharmacol 42:109, 1899

15. Behnke AR, Yarbrough OD: Respiratory resistance, oil-water solubility and mental effects of argon compared with helium and nitrogen. Am J Physiol 126:409-415, 1939
16. Case EM, Haldane JBS: Human physiology under high pressure. J Hyg (Lond) 41:225-249, 1941
17. Ferguson J: The use of chemical potentials as indices of toxicity. Proc Roy Soc B 197:387-404, 1939
18. Ferguson J, Hawkins SW: Toxic action of some simple gases at high pressure. Nature 164:963-964, 1949
19. Brink R, Posternak J: Thermodynamic analysis of relative effectiveness of narcotics. J Cell Physiol 32:211-233, 1948
20. Wulf RJ, Featherstone RM: A correlation of Van der Waal's constants with anesthetic potency. Anesthesiology 18:97-105, 1957
21. Miller SL: A theory of gaseous anesthesia. Proc Natl Acad Sci 47:1515-1524, 1961
22. Pauling L: A molecular theory of anesthesia. Science 134:15-21, 1961
23. Bean JW: Changes in arterial pH induced by compression and decompression. Fed Proc 6:76, 1947
24. Bean JW: Tensional changes of alveolar gas in reactions to rapid compression and decompression and question of nitrogen narcosis. Am J Physiol 161:417-425, 1950
25. Seusing J, Drube H: The importance of hypercapnia in depth intoxication. Klin Wochenschr, 38:1088-1090, 1960
26. Buhlmann A: Deep diving, in Eaton B (ed): The Undersea Challenge. London, The British Sub-Aqua Club, 1963
27. Vail EG: Hyperbaric respiratory mechanics. Aerosp Med 42:536-546, 1971
28. Bennett PB, Blenkarn GD: Arterial blood gases in man during inert gas narcosis. J Appl Physiol 36:45-48, 1974
29. Rashbass C: The unimportance of carbon dioxide in nitrogen narcosis. Report UPS 153, London Medical Research Council, RN Personnel Research Committee, 1955
30. Cabarrou P: L'invresse des grandes profondeurs. Presse Med 72:793-797, 1964
31. Cabarrou P: Introduction a la physiologie de 'Homo Aquaticus.' Presse Med, 74:2771-2773, 1966
32. Hesser CM, Adolfson J, Fagraeus L: Role of CO_2 in compressed air narcosis. Aerosp Med 42:163-168, 1971
33. Carpenter FG: Depressant action of inert gases on the central nervous system in mice. Am J Physiol 172:471-474, 1953
34. Carpenter FG: Anesthetic action of inert and unreactive gases on intact animals and isolated tissues. Am J Physiol 178:505-509, 1954
35. Carpenter FG: Inert gas narcosis, in Goff LG (ed): Proc 1st Underwater Physiology Symposium. Washington, National Research Council, National Academy Sciences, 1955
36. Larrabee MG, Posternak JM: Selective action of anesthetics on synapses and axons in mammalian sympathetic ganglia. J Neurophysiol 15:91-114, 1952
37. French JD, Verzeano M, Magoun HW: A neural basis of the anesthetic state. Arch Neurol Psychiat 69:519-529, 1953

38. Arduini A, Arduini MG: Effect of drugs and metabolic alterations on brain stem arousal mechanism. J Pharmacol 110:76-85, 1954
39. Bennett PB: Neurophysiologic and neuropharmacologic investigations in inert gas narcosis, in Lambertsen CJ, Greenbaum LJ (eds): Proceedings 2nd Underwater Physiology Symposium. Washington, National Research Council, National Academy of Sciences, 1963
40. Bennett PB: The effects of high pressures of inert gases on auditory evoked potentials in cat cortex and reticular formation. Electroencephalogr Clin Neurophysiol 17:388-397, 1964
41. Miller KW, Paton WDM, Smith RA, Smith EB: The pressure reversal of general anesthesia and the critical volume hypothesis. Mol Pharmacol 9:131-143, 1973
42. Anderson NB: Dual effects of general anesthetics on active and passive sodium fluxes and on sympathetic response in toad, in Fink RB (ed): Cellular Biology and Toxicity of Anesthetics. Baltimore, Williams & Wilkins, 1972
43. Bennett PB: Psychometric impairment in men breathing oxygen-helium at increased pressures. Report No 251, London, Medical Research Council, RN Personnel Research Committee, Underwater Physiology Sub-Committee, 1965
44. Bennett PB, Dossett AN: Undersirable effects of oxygen-helium breathing at great depths. Report No. 260, London, Medical Research Council, RN Personnel Research Committee, Underwater Physiology Sub-Committee, 1967
45. Brauer RW, Johnson DO, Pessotti RL, Redding RW: Effects of hydrogen and helium at pressures to 67 atmospheres on mice and monkeys. Fed Proc 25, 1966
46. Brauer RW, Way RO, Perry RA: Narcotic effects of helium and hydrogen in mice and hyperexcitability phenomena at simulated depths of 1500 to 4000 ft of sea water, in Fink BR (ed): Toxicity of Anesthetics. Baltimore, Williams & Wilkins, 1968
47. Brauer RW, Dimov S, Fructus X, Fructus P, Gosset A, Naquet R: Syndrome neurologique et electrographique des hautes pressions. Rev Neurol, 121:264-265, 1969
48. Summit JK, Kelly JS, Herron JM, Saltzman HA: Joint US Navy-Duke University 1000 ft saturation dive. Report 3-69, Washington D.C., U.S. Navy Experimental Diving Unit, 1969
49. Fructus X, Brauer RW, Naquet R: Physiological effects observed in the course of simulated deep chamber dives to a maximum of 36.5 atm in a helium-oxygen atmosphere, in Lambertsen CJ (ed): Proceedings 4th Symposium on Underwater Physiology. New York, Academic Press, 1971
50. Bennett PB, Towse EJ: Performance efficiency of men breathing oxygen-helium at depths between 100 ft and 1500 ft. Aerosp Med 42:1147-1156, 1971
51. Bennett PB, Towse EJ: The high pressure nervous syndrome during a simulated oxygen-helium dive to 1500 ft. Electroencephalogr Clin Neurophysiol 31:383-393, 1971
52. Bennett PB, Gray SP: Changes in human urine and blood chemistry during a simulated oxygen-helium dive to 1500 ft. Aerosp Med 42:868-874, 1971
53. Morrison JB, Florio JT: Respiratory function during a simulated dive to 1500 ft. J Appl Physiol 30:724-732, 1971
54. Fructus X, Charpy JP: Etude psychometrique de 2 subjets lors d'une plongee fictive jusqu'a 52.42 ata. Report No 7, Bulletin Medsubhyp, Service d'Hyperbare,

Hospital Salvator Marseille, 1972

55. Kylstra JA: Hydraulic compression of mice to 166 ATM. Science 158:793-794, 1967

56. Kylstra JA, Longmuir IS, Grace M: Dysbarism; Osmosis caused by dissolved gas. Science 161:289, 1968

57. Hills BA: Gas-induced osmosis as a factor influencing the distribution of body water. Clin Sci 40:175-191, 1971

58. Fructus X, Conti V: Le syndrome nerveau des hautes pressions. Medecine de Plongee Gas Hop 35:1031-1036, 1971

59. Fructus X, Agarate C, Sicardi F: Postponing the high pressure nervous syndrome down to 500 meters and deeper. Study of compression rates for very deep dives, in Lambertsen CJ (ed): Proceedings 5th Symposium on Underwater Physiology. Washington, FASEB, 1972, (in press)

60. Chouteau J, Ocana de Sentuary JM, Pironti L: Theoretical, experimental and comparative study of compression as applied to intervention dives and saturation dives at great depths. Report 1-71, Centre d Etudes Marines Avancees Marseille, 1971

61. Kylstra JA, Nantz R, Crowe J, et al: Hydraulic compression of mice to 166 atmospheres. Science 158:793-794, 1967

62. Ornhagen HC, Lundgren CEG: Hydrostatic pressure tolerance in liquid breathing mice, in Lambertsen CJ (ed): Proceedings 5th Symposium on Underwater Physiology. Washington, FASEB 1972. (in press)

63. Johnson, FH, Flagler EA: Hydrostatic pressure reversal of narcosis in tadpoles. Science 112:91-92, 1950

64. Lever MJ, Miller KW, Paton WDM, Smith EB: Pressure reversal of anesthesia. Nature 231:368-371, 1971

65. Johnson SM, Miller KW: Antagonism of pressure and anesthesia. Nature 228:75-76, 1970

66. Brauer RW, Goldman SM, Sheehan ME: N_2, H_2 and N_2O antagonism of high pressure neurological syndrome in mice. Undersea Biomed Res 1:59-72, 1974

67. Brauer RW: Studies concerning the high pressure hyperexcitability in the squirrel monkey. Final Report Office of Naval Research Contract N00014-69-C-0341, 1972

68. Zaltsman GL: Physiological principles of a sojurn of a human in conditions of raised pressure of the gaseous medium (engl transl) Foreign Technology Div, Ohio Wright Patterson AFT AD 655360, 1967

69. Zaltsman GL (ed): Hyperbaric Epilepsy and Narcosis. Leningrad, Sechenov Institute Evolutionary Physiol Biochem. USSR Academy of Sciences, 1968

70. Vigreux J: Contribution to the Study of the Neurological and Mental Reactions of the Organism of the Higher Mammal to Gaseous Mixtures Under Pressure. Toulouse University, M.D. Thesis, 1970

71. Bennett PB, Blenkarn GD, Roby J, Youngblood D: Suppression of the high pressure nervous syndrome in human deep dives by $He/N_2/O_2$. Undersea Biomed Res 1:221-237, 1974

72. Bennett PB, Roby J, Simon S, Youngblood D: Optimal use of nitrogen to suppress the high pressure nervous syndrome. Aviat Space Eviron Med 46:37-40, 1975

73. Shilling CW, Willgrube WW: Quantitative study of mental and neuromuscular reactions as influenced by increased air pressure. US Navy Med Bull, 35:373-380, 1937
74. Adolfson J: Deterioration of mental and motor functions in hyperbaric air. Scand J Psychol 6:26-31, 1965

STUDY QUESTIONS

1. Compressed air narcosis is first apparent at
   a   60 feet
   b. 100 feet
   c. 180 feet
   d. 300 feet
   e. 400 feet
2. Signs and symptoms of compressed air intoxication are similar to those of
   a. The bends
   b. Oxygen toxicity
   c. Alcoholic excess
   d. Carbon dioxide poisoning
3. The action of an increased carbon dioxide tension on nitrogen narcosis is to
   a. Potentiate
   b. Ameliorate
   c. Have no effect
4. At a constant nitrogen pressure, the action of an increase in oxygen partial pressure on nitrogen narcosis is to
   a. Potentiate
   b. Ameliorate
   c. Have no effect
5. Which one of the physical constants listed gives the best correlation with narcotic potency of the inert gases?
   a. Molecular weight
   b. Thermodynamic activity
   c. Clathrate formation
   d. Lipid solubility
   e. Polarizability
   f. Molar volume
6. Name three of the signs and symptoms of the high pressure nervous syndrome.
   a. _____
   b. _____
   c. _____

7. The mechanism of inert gas narcosis and the high pressure nervous syndrome is due to
   a. Meyer-Overton hypothesis
   b. Carbon dioxide
   c. Critical volume hypothesis
   d. Gas-induced osmosis
8. Name three methods for helping to lessen the signs and symptoms of high pressure nervous syndrome
   a. _____
   b. _____
   c. _____
9. Under HPNS, cell membranes are believed to
   a. Expand
   b. Contract
   c. Show no change
   d. Disrupt
10. What is believed to be the correct percentage of nitrogen to add to helium to prevent HPNS without causing narcosis?
   a. 18 percent
   b. 25 percent
   c. 5 percent
   d. 10 percent
   e. 15 percent

Arthur J. Bachrach* and
Glen H. Egstrom

13

Human Performance Underwater

Human performance underwater occurs when a commercial diver inspects a pipeline, a sport diver engages in underwater photography, or a Navy diver repairs a propeller. The performance of the underwater worker is affected by a number of variables; the principal ones are *the environment, breathing mixture, equipment, training, diver condition,* and *type of work.* Some of these variables may be objectively measured, such as the environmental factors of current, water temperature, depth, and breathing mix; others, particularly those involving diver condition, may not be as easily measured: for example, states of anxiety or the level of motivation. Nonetheless, these six rubrics may be useful in discussing the important factors in underwater performance. A fuller consideration of methodological perspective in measuring underwater performance appears in Bachrach.[1]

ENVIRONMENTAL FACTORS

To begin, let us consider aspects of the environment and their impact on the diver. The water environment itself necessarily alters performance. Movements in a viscous medium are obviously different from those accomplished

*From the Naval Medical Research and Development Command, Navy Department, Research Task No. MPN10.03.2040DAC9. The opinions and statements contained herein are the private ones of the writers and are not to be construed as official or reflecting the views of the Navy Department or the naval service at large. The excellent editorial work by Mrs. M. M. Matzen and manuscript preparation by Mrs. Phyllis Shapiro are warmly acknowledged.

in air. For example, subjects trained in water on the U.C.L.A. Pipe Puzzle learned the task in a manner clearly superior (25 percent faster) to a group who were trained on dry land and then performed the task underwater.[2]

The water environment degrades performance in a number of ways; its tractionless environment particularly affects the use of tools. Current that is strong enough can markedly interfere with work and can make entering the water with the necessary equipment and gear difficult for the diver. Temperature effects, particularly cold stress, markedly affect performance when the required protective clothing impedes manual performance and movement. Frequent conditions of low visibility occasioned by turbidity or other obscuring elements in the water make the diver's task more difficult.

Dangerous marine animals, such as sharks, can pose hazards both real and perceived beyond their actual threat. In a recent shark-research panel report, Zahuranec[3] noted that a number of Navy diving missions, as well as a training mission for the recovery of the Apollo-15 astronauts, had been canceled when sharks were sighted in the vicinity. He states:

> The shark hazard to Navy Divers has been a continual threat over the years, both in the sense of producing actual casualties and in the psychological effect of degrading effectiveness of divers who must work in waters in which sharks have recently made an attack.

The understandable diver concern about such predators is not mitigated by the very favorable ratio of shark sightings to actual shark attacks.

The feeling of anxiety itself can interfere with the diver's performance. In some cases, however, performance for experienced divers improves under stressful conditions. Evidence tends to support the idea that danger increases the diver's anxiety level, which influences performance by producing a narrowing of attention. An experienced diver's attention will be narrowed to the task at hand, whereas the novice will be overly involved with the danger.

Cold

As diving technology and life-support systems have improved, there has been a corresponding increase in the diver's ability to work deeper and longer. These greater exposures to the effects of cold have resulted in reduced performance levels, early termination of dives, and other similar problems. The state of the art in diver heating is progressing, but cold still remains as a prime cause of impaired diver performance.

Studies of heat loss from the body reveal that conductive and convective losses were modified by factors such as the thickness of the insulating materials, the temperature gradient, respiratory rate, heart rate, metabolic rate, adaptation, and the conformation of the diving dress to the body, to name a few. Thus, it is obvious that the effect of a dive in cold water cannot be

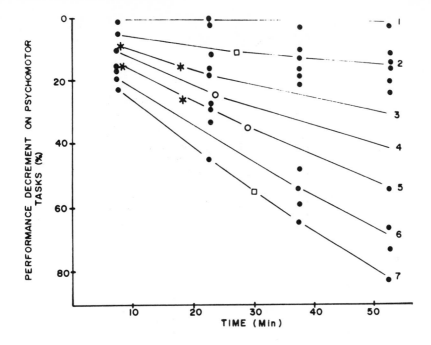

Fig. 13-1.   Effect of exposure length on psychomotor task performance in cold water while insulated with wet suits. (From Egstrom and Weltman.[39])

adequately assessed until the thermal protection variables are considered. A diver without thermal protection in 65°F water may suffer markedly more degradation than a diver in a well-fitted wet suit at 45°F in the same time span.

The problems associated with cold exposure and underwater perfor-mance are demonstrated in Fig. 13-1, which synthesizes the results of several

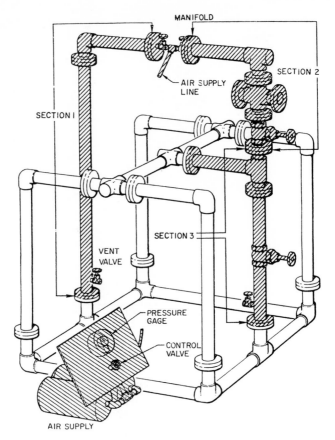

Fig. 13-2.   Schematic of the U.C.L.A. pipe puzzle.

investigations on cold effects on psychomotor tasks. The studies[1, 4-6] were
made on divers wearing wet suits, boots, gloves, and hoods while performing
moderate work. The diver's performance was primarily affected by three
variables: temperature gradient between the diver and his environment; exposure time; and task complexity. In the series of studies with the U.C.L.A.
pipe puzzle, (Fig. 13-2), efforts to measure useful work output and quality of
work revealed that manipulative operations such as assembly and disassembly
were lengthened and simple task portions such as pressurization were
shortened. It must be recognized that the compression of the insulating layer
of neoprene rubber will result in greater heat loss at depth.

Studies of cognitive efficiency in cold water[1, 4, 5, 7, 8] (Fig. 13-3) have
revealed only a slight impairment. An examination of memory, reasoning
ability, and vigilance of 14 subjects wearing wet suits during exposure to 40°F
and 80°F water was conducted in an enclosed tank at U.C.L.A. The tests used
sentence comprehension, vigilance to a peripheral visual stimulus while per-

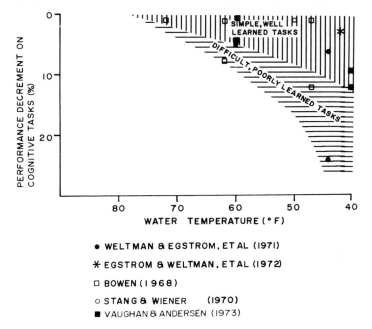

Fig. 13-3. The effect of water temperature on cognitive task performance. (From Egstrom and Weltman.[39])

forming mathematical computations, and a 30-minute postdive recall and recognition of material learned after a 1-hour exposure in the water. The cold exposures resulted in a mean loss of 1.3°F measured with a 3-inch rectal thermistor. This loss did not significantly affect either vigilance or reasoning ability. Memory, however, was significantly impaired as a result of the cold stress. It was of particular interest that tasks for which a diver was poorly trained, and therefore more dependent upon memory for effective performance, were affected to a greater degree than those for which he was well trained.

Fortunately, the diver is able to make some longer-term physiologic adaptation to the effects of cold, which may well result in a less stressful exposure and a consequent improved performance. Nevertheless, regular exposure to the rigorous environment is a necessary price for the adaptive process.

Pressure

A crucial environmental variable is pressure itself. The effects of pressure, according to Workman,[9] can be divided into both direct (or mechanical) and indirect effects resulting from "changes in the partial pressure of respired gases." Pressure directly affects the ears, sinuses, lungs, and other body components. Such problems are discussed in other chapters in this volume.

In discussing the indirect effects of pressure resulting from the changes in partial pressure of respired gases, Workman[9] lists two major effects. The first, nitrogen narcosis, is described as "a state of light anesthesia," probably beginning at around 33 feet of seawater (fsw), or 2 ata, with increasing effects upon the brain as the descent continues; it is perhaps exacerbated by carbon dioxide retention owing to inadequate pulmonary ventilation. The second indirect effect of pressure is oxygen toxicity which can occur when a diver is breathing compressed oxygen at a depth sufficient to increase the partial pressure of the gas to around 1 ata. These problems are also discussed more fully in other chapters.

The problems under hydrostatic pressure become markedly important in deep dives. As Fenn[10] observed "you would not be surprised . . . if pressure *per se* became the limiting factor in deep dives." Aside from the changes in respiration and other physiological events, such as otological effects, pressure can effect certain neurophysiological changes, particularly at high rates of compression and at marked depths. Hunter and Bennett[11] differentiate between the high pressure nervous syndrome as manifested during compression and hydrostatic pressure alone, which suggests that the terms compression syndrome and hydrostatic pressure syndrome may be useful to make such a differentiation. The compression syndrome as part of the high pressure nervous syndrome is characterized by changes in the electroencephalogram (particularly in increased theta activity), the appearance of both intention and postural tremor, and neuromuscular incoordination—for example—a loss of balance.[11-13] These effects have been measured in deep chamber dives up to 49.5 ata.[14, 15] As noted, research has suggested that the depth interferes with different types of functions. The high pressure nervous syndrome that occurs generally at depths below 31.3 ata is consistent with findings that neuromuscular motor performance is most affected by deep dives (where the diver breathes a helium-oxygen mixture), while intellectual or cognitive performance is much less affected. The opposite appears to be true in hyperbaric air where intellectual cognitive functions appear to be more degraded than psychomotor skills.[16] How much of this is a function of pressure, and how much is a function of breathing helium versus breathing hyperbaric air with its aspects of nitrogen narcosis, is not entirely clear.

BREATHING MIX

As just noted, the effects of hyperbaric air and possible effects of helium on performance are very much a matter of concern for the operational diver and the researcher. It is necessary to be cautious in the use of the word "inert," as in "inert gas narcosis." The very term nitrogen narcosis appears to be a contradiction, if indeed nitrogen is considered to be inert. The meaning is clearer if one adheres to the definition provided by Featherstone and Muehlbaecher[17] that inert is used "in a metabolic sense and includes those gases which are generally considered to exert their biological effects without undergoing any change in their own chemical structures while modifying the primary chemical structure of other substances." There have been questions, chemical as well as biological, regarding the physiological effects of such gases as helium and nitrogen. Nitrogen narcosis, more fully discussed in the chapter by Bennett in this volume, has been implicated frequently in performance degradation by divers using scuba and breathing compressed air at depths approaching 130 fsw (4.5 ata). To consider such effects as purely a function of breathing mix is obviously incorrect; for, as a number of investigators have shown in both animal and human research, adaptation to environmental factors over time can be objectively seen and measured.[13,18-22] Such adaptation to pressure and breathing mix has not been sufficiently studied in terms of mechanisms, but is a part of both the anecdotal and research literature. It has long been felt that helium itself has no physiological effects. The search for any subtle effects of helium is presently in progress.

The high pressure nervous syndrome can be suppressed using a trimix breathing gas containing helium, oxygen, and added percentages of nitrogen.[23] Mechanisms of such actions appear to be related to the *critical volume hypothesis,*[11, 24] in which the anesthetic potency of an agent is related to the ability of its molecules to modify the dimensions of lipid phases, possibly those in cell membranes. In one theoretical position, anesthesia is thought to occur when the surface of the hydrophobic portion of the cell membrane is expanded beyond a "critical volume" of 0.4 to 0.5 percent.[25] Increased permeability of the membrane occurs, and anesthesia results, when more nitrogen molecules are absorbed at such a level. This may be implicated in nitrogen narcosis. When pressure of 100 ata is applied to a membrane, there is a return to normal size and permeability while the anesthetic (or nitrogen) is still in the cell membrane. The 30-ata pressure alone without the narcotic (for example, in a helium breathing mix) compresses the membrane, and permeability is inhibited. This is implicated in the occurrence of the high pressure nervous syndrome. The evidence that general anesthesia can be reversed by pressure has been advanced as an explanation for such a phenomenon. In a compressed expanded cell membrane, an appropriate dose of anesthetic (or nitrogen) theoretically would reverse the effects of hydrostatic pressure on cell membranes by reexpanding the membrane to its normal volume. This is the basis of a trimix in which a nitrogen percentage of approximately 10 percent is added to the standard heliox mixture to damp out the symptomatology of the high pressure syndrome. If the critical volume hypothesis is correct and the trimix breathing mixture is successful, diving at greath depths without central nervous system problems might be expected.

In sum: the breathing mix, whether it be hyperbaric compressed air or helium-oxygen, appears implicated in physiological changes that appear to affect performance adversely.

EQUIPMENT

The impact of protective equipment on the diver's performance can be profound. Although the obvious need for breathing gear and clothing to protect the diver from the undersea environment is well recognized, there is nevertheless a marked inadequacy in equipment design and engineering that requires the diver to compensate for shortcomings in the apparatus. This is true in both sport and industrial diving equipment as Egstrom[26] noted:

> Faceplates have remained virtually unchanged since the 30's and few major problems have been resolved. The faceplate still provides tunnel vision, magnification, refraction, and in some cases, distortion. The sport diver adapts to these limitations and generally finds little fault with faceplates. However, the increasing demands on working divers should result in a closer look at the problem.

There is very little systematic human engineering of diving equipment.[27, 28] Certainly one of the problems with equipment has been a lack of standardization which forces divers under certain circumstances to shift operational modes because of differences in equipment intended for similar uses. A biomechanical analysis was made comparing the standard hard hat Mark V diving system with the newer U.S. Navy prototype Mark XII. Fourteen biomechanical measurements believed to be important in work in the hard hat rigs were used to compare flexibility in the Mark V and Mark XII with baselines accomplished in swimsuits. The assumption was that range of movement is limited by internal mechanical stops; therefore, joints were measured to determine the external mechanical limitations of the particular diving suits. In addition, physiological measures were taken[27] showing that heart rate measured by acoustical telemetry[29] can give indication of levels of work and presumably the physiological cost of the particular equipment used. A greater heart rate was measured in one diver (up to 184 beats/minute) in the Mark V system as compared with a lower heart rate in the Mark XII (Fig. 13-4), which suggests, at least in this particular diver under these work conditions, a greater physiological cost of the one system over the other.

Diver tools are another important aspect of the diver's equipment as it affects performance.[30] The diver should be provided with tools that are safe and efficient; however, tools designed without consideration of environmental factors, such as poor visibility, diver buoyancy, and cold, can contribute to diver fatigue, and thus degrade performance.

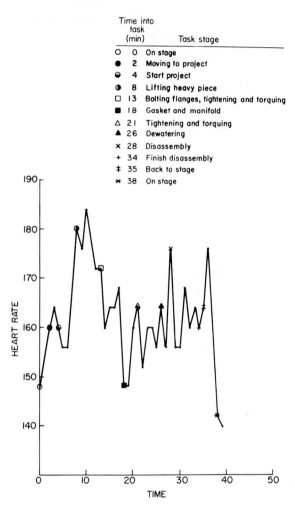

Fig. 13-4. Heart rate recordings for a subject working on the U.C.L.A. pipe puzzle while wearing the Mark V, He-O$_2$ mode, breathing air. (From Bachrach and Egstrom.[27])

DIVER TRAINING

Obviously, the performance of a diver underwater is going to be significantly affected by the type of training he has for the particular work to be accomplished, as well as the use of the underwater equipment that provides the transportation of his work site. There are variations in the type of training both sports and commercial divers receive, and this variation in training often presents problems. Too little application of the principles of learning theory has gone into diver training.[31] Much of what is called training in diving is actually a type of examination, for example, "Can the trainee dive down to the bottom of a 25-foot tank and clear his mask?" The required terminal behavior of clearing the mask should be staged, with phases of steps leading to the goal. All too often, the training of a particular technique becomes a demonstration by example rather than an actual experience for the individual trainee.

Certain kinds of techniques necessary to the working environment have not been incorporated into diver training.[32] For example, escape from entanglement was a highly significant item of performance, yet many divers indicated they had not had training in escape from entanglement in their diving courses. In a similar fashion, the emphasis in sport diver training is frequently on decompression, which is understandable in view of the importance of decompression in diving. Yet most diving accidents have been at relatively shallow depths, where decompression sickness is unlikely.[31] In a survey of diving fatalities in Puget Sound from 1970 to 1974, there were a total of 46 fatalities, of which only 60 percent occurred at or near the surface.[33] Deep diving was not a factor in these fatalities: the average depth of the dives was 40 fsw. So, it is perhaps more appropriate for sport diver training to emphasize hazards of tachypnea or hyperpnea and air embolism, which may well be more crucial to diver performance and difficulty.

DIVER CONDITION

Perhaps the most important factor in underwater human performance is the condition of the diver himself. Given optimal diving conditions and superbly engineered equipment, the physical and psychological state of the diver remains the crucial element. The diver in good physical condition is more likely to be able to perform adequately and to cope readily with problems encountered in the underwater environment. Physically, this means that he should have sufficient stamina and strength to withstand the stresses of the underwater environment plus the ability to handle his equipment effectively. Behaviorally, it means that the diver in good condition has a sense of confidence in his own skills (in large measure a function of adequate training), and thus provide sufficient competence to cope with impending problems. A combination of effective training and good physical condition seems to be a crucial requisite of coping behavior in divers. The level of work involved in sport diving should be kept well within aerobic limits. Divers should be trained to recognize the signs of overexertion and use them as "alarms" to trigger behavior designed to reduce the work load until respiration rate and pulse rate are back at a comfortable level.

THE PROBLEM OF PANIC

The lack of confidence and competence, coupled with less than adequate physical condition, can lead to a loss of control which seems to be implicated in most sport diving accidents. This problem of loss of control or diver panic has been approached in recent years by several authors.[31, 34-38] Bachrach and Egstrom[35] summarize aspects of apprehension and panic and its implications for improved diver training and performance. As they note, a certain amount of apprehension may be expected in a diver experiencing a situation such as kelp or cave diving for the first time. The diver who is performing adequately obtains as much information as possible about the particular dive: the conditions, the equipment needed, and the possible problems—thus reducing apprehension by information gathering. While apprehension may be brought under control by proper planning and adequate knowledge (among other variables), panic is a loss of control state wherein an individual perceives that he is losing control, but cannot extricate himself from the dangerous situation.

In virtually all of the accidents that have been studied there has been no indication of equipment problems. (For example, in the San Diego area all equipment following a diving fatality is analyzed for possible failure.) Rather, the inference is that human error—perhaps a result of exhaustion, fatigue, and panic—was the cause in the fatality.

An early sign common to most panic situations is rapid breathing, which is an indication of agitation.[35] Rapid, shallow breathing produces an inefficient exchange of oxygen and carbon dioxide leading to a sensation of air hunger that may further exacerbate the feeling of panic. It is frequently reported that a diver in a panic condition on the surface is seen to be struggling with his arms and legs to keep his head above water; the struggle results in the head being higher, but it also increases the work load on the body, as well as the heart and respiration rates. The struggling diver supporting the weight of his head (approximately 17 pounds) out of water can only support this work load for a matter of seconds; if he raises his shoulders out of the water he could well be supporting 30 to 35 pounds. The problem is compounded by exhaustion from his struggling. Divers have been reported to sink in a matter of seconds, or at the most, a minute or so. Implications for cardiac arrest have also been assumed as a consequence of some of these physiological events.

The first sign of panic is agitation.[41] A diver in control moves along smoothly with respiration and swimming movements controlled and regular. Also, a controlled diver is oriented toward the front or bottom in his diving environment, whereas an apprehensive diver, who may be approaching panic, is oriented toward the surface, frequently checking his orientation toward presumed safety. Another irregular type of movement in the panicking diver is that of bringing the knees forward and finning with short, jerky movements.[36] A diver in control will check his equipment to make certain that he has enough air, that his bottom time is carefully timed, and so on; but an agitated diver too frequently checks his equipment with almost a preoccupation with gauges.[35] Preventing panic is largely a function of good physical condition and adequate training, so that the diver develops competence and confidence in his skills. It is not uncommon to witness a diver venturing into an unfamiliar surf condition who fails not only to evoke appropriate behavior, but also fails to respond to pertinent directions given to him by his buddy. Often such behavior leads to failure to take such simple precautions as holding onto the face mask when the surf is about to break upon the diver. The subsequent loss of the face mask creates additional stress and results in the onset of panic in a minor emergency.

In the training of the diver, effective program sequences of diver training are crucial so that actual experience with the types of skills to be required are built into a diving program. In the prevention of panic, gaining positive buoyancy becomes a first priority for the anxious diver. The diver who still has a snorkel or regulator in his mouth should be made to float on his back with the mouthpiece removed to allow for greater air passage.[38] Floating on his back with his life vest inflated can provide a diver with rest and diminution of struggling, which thereby lessens the possibility of submergence through struggling.

A carefully trained, controlled diver in good physical condition with effective equipment adapted to exotic gases and pressure is a diver who can most optimally perform underwater.

REFERENCES

1. Bachrach AJ: Underwater performance, in Bennett PB, Elliott DH (eds): The Physiology and Medicine of Diving and Compressed Air Work. (ed 2) London, Bailliere Tindall, 1975, pp 264-284
2. Weltman G, Egstrom GH, Willis MA, et al: Underwater work measurement techniques: Final report. UCLA-ENG-7140 AD734014 1971
3. Zahuranec BJ (ed): Shark Research: Present Status and Future Directions. Washington, D.C., Office of Naval Research Report, April 1975
4. Bowen HM: Diver performance and the effects of cold. Hum Factors 10:445-464, 1968
5. Stang PR, Wiener EL: Diver performance in cold water. Hum Factors 12:391-399, 1970
6. Weltman G, Egstrom GH, Crooks TP, et al: Underwater work measurement techniques, 1969 studies. UCLA-ENG-7052 1970 (Biotechnol Lab Rep 48)
7. Vaughan WS Jr, Andersen BG: Effects of long-duration cold exposure on performance of tasks in Naval in-shore warfare operations. N0014-72-C-0309, Nr 197-019. Landover, Md, Oceanautics Inc, 1973, p 116

8. Egstrom GH, Weltman G, Baddeley AD, et al: Underwater work performance and work tolerance. UCLA-ENG-7243 pp 1-63, 1972 (Biotechnol Lab Rep 51)

9. Workman RD: Other medical problems associated with exposure to pressure, in Committee on Hyperbaric Oxygenation: Fundamentals of Hyperbaric Medicine, Washington DC, National Academy of Sciences; National Research Council, 1966, pp 110-114

10. Fenn WO: The physiological effects of hydrostatic pressure, in Bennett PB, Elliott DH (eds): The Physiology and Medicine of Diving and Compressed Air Work. Baltimore, Williams & Wilkins, 1969

11. Hunter WL Jr, Bennett PB: The causes, mechanisms, and prevention of the high pressure nervous syndrome. Undersea Biomed Res 1:1-28, 1974

12. Bachrach AJ, Bennett PB: Tremor in diving. Aerosp Med. 44:613-623, 1973, AD763994

13. Braithwaite WR, Berghage TE, Crothers JC: Postural equilibrium and vestibular response at 49.5 ATA. Undersea Biomed Res 1:309-324, 1974

14. Raymond LW, Spaur WH: (Abstrs) Biomedical Research and Underwater Breathing Apparatus Evaluation Dives 10 to 1600 feet. April 1-2, 1974 Conference. Bethesda, Md, Joint Technical Report, Naval Medical Research Institute, and Washington, D.C., Navy Experimental Diving Unit, 1974

15. Bennett PB: Neurophysiological, psychological, biochemical, and other studies, in: Experimental Observations on Men at Pressures between 4 Bars (100 ft) and 47 Bars (1500 ft). Report 1-71, Alverstoke, UK, Royal Naval Physiological Laboratory, 1971, pp 60-113

16. Biersner RJ: Human performance at great depths, in Lambertsen CJ (ed): Underwater Physiology, Proceeding of 4th Symposium of Underwater Physiology. New York, Academic Press, 1971, pp 479-485

17. Featherstone RM, Muehlbaecher C: The current role of inert gases in the search for anesthesia mechanics. Pharmacol Rev 15:97, 1963

18. Shilling CW, Willgrube WW: Quantitative study of mental and neuromuscular reactions as influenced by increased air pressure. Nav Med Bull 35:373-380, 1937

19. Miles S: Underwater Medicine. Philadelphia, Lippincott, 1969

20. Walsh JM: Amphetamine effects on timing behavior in rats and hyperbaric conditions. Aerosp Med 45:721-726, 1974, AD787006

21. Walsh JM, Bachrach AJ: Timing behavior in the assessment of adaptation of nitrogen narcosis. Bethesda, Md, Naval Medical Research Institute, 1971

22. Walsh JM, Bachrach AJ: Adaptation to nitrogen narcosis manifested by timing behavior in the rat. J Comp Physiol Psychol 86:883-889, 1974, A002411

23. Bennett PB, Blenkarn GD, Roby J, et al: Suppression of the high pressure nervous syndrome in human deep dives by He-N_2O_2. Undersea Biomed Res 1:221-237, 1974

24. Miller KW, Paton WDM, Smith RA, et al: The pressure reversal of general anesthesia and the critical volume hypothesis. Mol Pharmacol 9:131-143, 1973

25. Bennett PB: Elucidating anesthesia mechanisms: Current concepts and problems. Clin Trends Anesthesiol 5:1ff, 1975

26. Egstrom GH: Effect of equipment on diving performance, in Human Performance in Scuba Diving. Chicago, The Athletic Institute, 1970, pp 5-31

27. Bachrach AJ, Egstrom GH: Human engineering considerations in the evaluation of diving equipment, in: The Working Diver—1974. Washington, D.C., Marine Technology Society, 1974

28. Bachrach AJ, Egstrom GH, Blackmun SM: Biomechanical analysis of the U.S. Navy Mark V and Mark XII diving systems. Hum Factors 17:328-336, 1976

29. Kanwisher J, Lawson K, Strauss R: Acoustic telemetry from human divers. Undersea Biomed Res 1:99-109, 1974

30. Black SA, Quirk JT: Hydraulic tool systems for divers, in: Equipment for the Working Diver 1970 Symposium. Washington, D.C., Marine Technology Society, 1970

31. Bachrach AJ: Diving behavior, in: Human Performance in Scuba Diving. Chicago, The Athletic Institute, 1970, pp 117-138

32. Egstrom GH: UCLA-ENG Diving safety research project. NDAA-4-6-158-44021

33. Sand R: Diving fatalities in Puget Sound 1970-74, in: Man-in-the-Sea Symposium, Seattle, Washington, 22-23 March 1975. (Underwater Assoc Newsletter, May 1975)

34. Bachrach AJ: Panic, in: Oceans 2000. London, British SubAqua Club/World Underwater Federation, 1974

35. Bachrach AJ, Egstrom GH: Apprehension and panic, in British SubAqua Club Manual, London, British SubAqua Club (in press)

36. Bevan J: Diver panic—and how to beat it. Triton 18:311-312, 1973

37. Egstrom GH, Bachrach AJ: Diver panic. Skin Diver 20:36ff, 1971

38. Strauss MB: A program for panic prevention. Skin Diver 22:50-51, 1973

39. Egstrom GH, Weltman G: Underwater work performance and work tolerance: Final report. UCLA-ENG-7427, 1974

STUDY QUESTIONS

1. What conditions may predispose a diver to panic, and what may prevent panic?
2. Name two major factors in impaired diver performance.
3. Are dangerous marine animals, such as sharks, a significant hazard to divers?

J. Michael Walsh

14

Drugs and Diving

Drugs have become an integral part of modern day life, both as the miracle of medicine and as a source of social problems. Interest in drugs has generated volumes of research literature; however, knowledge of the effects of drugs under diving conditions remains extremely limited. Diver training programs uniformly reject the use of pharmacological agents in any form while diving; but, in spite of these warnings, many divers do take drugs routinely. Analgesics, antihistamines, alcohol, antimotion sickness preparations, and more recently, stimulant and euphoric-type drugs are being consumed by the diving population. At the same time, the number of scuba deaths is increasing at an alarming rate. How many of these accidental deaths are related to drug consumption is not known; however, it should be the concern of every physician who treats divers.

The purpose of this chapter is to discuss the drug-diving interaction, particularly with relevance to the "behavioral toxicology" of drugs in the underwater environment. The discussion will focus on providing background information, both physiological and psychological, to make the physician aware of the complexities involved in "hyperbaric pharmacology." The pharmaceutical toxicology of hyperbaric environments is beyond the scope of this chapter; those interested are referred to the review by Small and Friess.[1]

PHYSIOLOGICAL STATUS OF THE ORGANISM

To discuss the effects of drugs in a meaningful way, it is necessary to know something about the physiological state of the organism. Placing the organism in the underwater environment brings into effect a new complex of variables, each of which can be considered to exert a pharmacological effect itself. In the following paragraphs, I will attempt to outline some of the basic variables encountered by divers (e.g., pressure, breathing gases) that can result in substantial physiological changes in the organism.

Biological Effects of Pressure

High hydrostatic pressure, in and of itself, can produce considerable biological effects. According to Fenn,[2] enzymes, viruses, and toxins may become inactivated above 1000 atmospheres absolute pressure (ata). Pressure can affect the contractile mechanism of muscle,[3] and at very high pressures (300 ata), muscles become rigid and stiff. It has also been observed that pressure can be used to reverse the effects of anesthesia.[4] In a summary statement indicating the scope of the biological effects of pressure per se Fenn wrote:

> Gels are changed to sols, viscosity and the dissociation of electrolytes is increased, transference numbers are diminished, emulsions are inhibited, surface tension is decreased, pH is decreased, protein hydrolysis is favoured, and reaction rates may be increased or decreased depending on the volume changes. Most of these effects, however, are measurable only at pressures far higher than any likely to be encountered by divers. Nevertheless, the subjective sensations of a human diver and his performance measured by psychological tests are so exquisitely sensitive and involve such a tremendous series of complicated reactions that any slight abnormality might be readily detected. It would not be surprising, therefore, if pressure *per se* became the limiting factor in deep dives.[2]

Pressure—Gas Interaction

Although most of the effects of pressure per se are grossly exhibited only at very high pressures, it is likely that some changes do occur even at the relatively low pressures encountered in scuba diving. In addition, the effects of pressure become much more relevant for the diver's concern when they interact with the gases in the breathing mixture. As pressure increases, the partial pressures of the gases in the breathing mix (e.g., in air: N_2, O_2) also increase proportionately according to Dalton's law, which states, "The total pressure exerted by a mixture of gases is the sum of the pressures that would be exerted by each of the gases if it alone were present and occupied the total volume." The amount of each gas dissolved in the blood and tissues depends on the partial pressure. When the partial pressure increases, so does the amount of gas in solution. When the partial pressures of certain gases become sufficiently increased, serious disorders may occur, such as oxygen toxicity, nitrogen narcosis, and CO_2 poisoning.

There is great individual variation in the predisposition to disorders associated with gases at high partial pressures. Oxygen is generally thought to become toxic when the partial pressure exceeds 3 ata, although this varies with the individual and the work load. "Nitrogen narcosis" is the label applied to the behavioral changes that result from the respiration of air at elevated pressures (i.e., greater than 4 ata). These changes are characterized by a euphoric "intoxicated-like state" or "narcosis," a lack of neuromuscular coordination, amnesia, and a general slowing of cognitive functioning.[5-7] It is assumed that nitrogen narcosis results from the high tensions of N_2 in the tissues; but when air is breathed, the partial pressure of oxygen is also elevated, and this appears to interact synergistically with nitrogen.[8] The actual mechanisms for "oxygen toxicity" and "nitrogen narcosis" are presently unknown. Increased carbon dioxide retention due to the added work load of breathing under pressure, together with reduced gas exchange, may exacerbate both phenomena. The specifics of these hyperbaric anomalies are described in detail in other chapters (see Chapters 11, 12, and 13).

Other experiments with both humans and animals in the open sea and in hyperbaric chambers have indicated that metabolic, hormonal, neurological, and cardiovascular changes also occur while breathing air at depths as shallow as 90 feet (approximately 4 ata).[9-12] These changes are both immediate and delayed and, to a certain extent, attenuated in experienced divers. In general, the consensus has been that these clinical changes probably result as a generalized stress response to increased pressure and, in the case of humans, to anxiety over the diving situation.

In summary, the physiological status of the organism must be known to discuss intelligently the effects of drugs. The physiological status of the organism in diving conditions is very difficult to specify as there are a great number of variables operating and interacting. The basic assumption must be that the exposure of the organism to increased pressure and the concommitant changing partial pressures of breathing gases result in a modified organism. Therefore, the responses of that organism to both internal and external stimuli, either pharmacologically induced or encountered in the environment, may differ from those elicited under "normal" conditions.

EFFECTS OF DRUGS ON THE ORGANISM

The basic effect of a drug on the organism differs from pressure, in that with drugs no physical change occurs in the tissue. Drugs simply increase or decrease the sensitivity of cell function. Drugs come in many forms these days; they can be ingested, injected, inhaled, or applied topically.

Most drugs are distributed throughout the body in the water phase of the blood plasma. In order to act, therefore, unless it acts topically at the site of application, a drug must first enter the blood. It will then reach the tissues of each organ at a rate determined by the blood flow through the organ and by the rapidity of passage of the drug molecules across the capillary bed and into the cells of that particular organ.[13]*

This is a very complex, orchestrated series of processes, each one dependent on its precursor. The onset and time course of drug action are contingent on a myriad of factors. For example, the rate of absorption of the drug into the bloodstream is dependent upon the route of administration (i.e., intravenous, intramuscular, oral, etc.). Distribution of the drug molecules is dependent on blood flow and the permeability of capillary and cellular membranes for the specific drug molecules. Drug elimination is dependent on three processes: metabolism, storage, and excretion, which remove the drug from its sites of action and ultimately dispose of it.

A wide variety of variables can alter this orchestration and disturb normal drug action. Age, sex, weight, tolerance, hypersensitivity, and environmental factors are all common variables that cause a tremendous amount of biological variation in drug response—so much so that the effect of a drug is never identical in all individuals, or even in the same individual on different occasions. Some of these factors may qualitatively alter the effect of the drug so as to prohibit its use. "Others produce only quantitative changes in the usual effects of the drug and can be offset by appropriate adjustment of dosage. These variables must be taken into account before a drug is prescribed."[14] The purpose of this brief discussion is to review the essentials of drug mechanics and to stress the dependence of drug action on the physiological and environmental aspects surrounding the organism at the time of administration.

Pharmacological research in high pressure conditions has been concerned principally with the discovery of prophylactic agents for the prevention or reduction of high pressure disorders (e.g., decompression sickness, nitrogen narcosis, aseptic bone necrosis). Some investigators have used drugs as a tool in an attempt to define some of the basic mechanisms of these hyperbaric maladies. Relatively little has been done, however, to evaluate drugs per se for their efficacy or their relative safety for use with divers.

The pharmacological literature concerned with oxygen toxicity, decompression sickness, and nitrogen narcosis is too extensive to be dealt with here. The interested reader is directed to the recent review by Bennett.[15] The two kinds of evaluations (toxicological and behavioral) that are being done will be reviewed here to answer some of the questions about drugs that are relevant to the diving community.

---

*Reprinted by permission of John Wiley & Sons, Inc.

Toxicological Evaluations

Most of the toxicological work investigating drugs of a therapeutic nature has been conducted in the 19-20 ata (approximately 600 feet) range, substituting helium for nitrogen as the inert gas in the breathing mixture. Surprisingly, under these conditions, the acute toxicity for most drugs evaluated did not change. To cite a few examples: (a) Histopathic responses of tissue as well as serum haptoglobin levels indicated that the anti-inflamatory properties of cortisone were identical at 19 ata breathing helium-oxygen (He-O_2) as they were at sea level;[16] (b) pain thresholds indicated that morphine analgesia did not significantly differ at 19 ata from those animals tested at surface pressure;[17] (c) LD_{50}'s (i.e., the median lethal dose—where 50 percent of the subjects die following administration) for pentobarbitol, lidocaine, ethanol, and histamine in hyperbaric helium at 19 ata were no different from that at sea level pressures; however, the toxicity of tripelennamine was found to be significantly lower in guinea pigs, but not in rats.[18, 19] All of this work has presumably been focused toward the deep diving environment where the use of helium is a necessity. There appears to be a complete void in the literature regarding the acute toxicity of common therapeutic agents and other compounds interacting with compressed air, in the 2 to 7 ata range, which are the circumstances involved in most diving. It would appear that the research effort directed at deep diving is somewhat out of proportion with reality. During the 2-year period 1972-1973, 99 percent of all recorded dives made by the U.S. Navy (in excess of 125,000) were made to depths of 190 feet or less breathing air (See Fig. 14-1).[20] Less than one-tenth of 1 percent of these dives were made to 600 feet or greater. This lack of information about the toxicology of drugs at relatively shallow depths is unfortunate, but diving medicine is a burgeoning new field, and hopefully this information will be forthcoming soon.

Behavioral Evaluations

Probably the only systematic investigations of drugs primarily concerned with the environmental conditions encountered by the ordinary scuba diver have been the recent behavioral evaluations, which have focused on the behavioral toxicity of drugs. This work deals with the ability of a drug to interfere with the ongoing behavior of the organism; it provides the best answers presently available to the questions that form the crux of concern for the diver and his physician.

So far we have discussed the assumption that the physiology of the diver changes under pressure, that the altered physiology will modify drug action, and that there is somewhat conflicting evidence concerning the toxicology of drugs at increased pressure. Since nearly all drugs have multiple actions, the

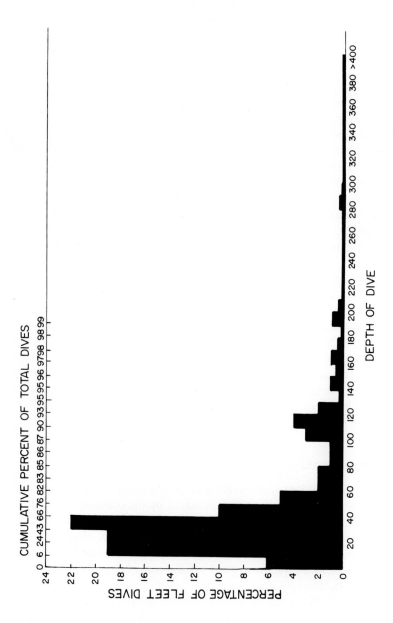

Fig. 14-1. Total percentage of recorded U.S. Navy dives plotted by the maximum depth of the dive for the years 1972-1973. (From Berghage et al., 1975)

ultimate effect is a composite of effects on different biological systems, which is perhaps best observed in the organism's behavior.

The broad concept of behavioral toxicology in man refers to objective changes in behavior and to subjective changes in attitudes and mood. Both kinds of behavioral toxicity pose potentially lethal situations for the diver. A diver who becomes drowsy or undergoes some loss of neuromuscular coordination due to the drug or drug-pressure interaction might have difficulty swimming to the surface. Another diver, without any symptom of physical defect, might experience a feeling of euphoria or well-being and may chance to enter dangerous areas that normally he would not attempt.

Experimental evidence of behavioral toxicology has been demonstrated using techniques of operant conditioning.[21] This technology of behavior has been used extensively by the pharmaceutical industry in the screening and assessment of the behavioral effects of drugs;[22] these same methods have been used effectively in the analysis of hyperbaric behavior.[23-25] In the hyperbaric experiments, complex patterns of behavior are developed in research animals. Once established, the behavioral baselines are used to assess the effects of both acute and chronic drug regimens under both normal and increased pressure conditions in a dry hyperbaric chamber. Dose-response curves are then generated at various depths using a variety of gas mixtures so that changes in behavior due to the interaction between drugs, gas, and pressure can be empirically determined (see example, Fig. 14-2).

The results of these studies indicate that the behavioral effects of drugs *do* change under pressure at depths as shallow as 50 feet. The effects of certain classes of drugs are potentiated, some are antagonized, and yet others yield entirely different effects than those observed under normal atmospheric conditions.[26, 27] It is difficult to make specific statements about general classes of drugs without going into detailed evaluation of each drug, at each dose level, and at each pressure level investigated. Suffice it to say that in all of the drugs evaluated in the author's laboratory (which includes amphetamines, barbiturates, autonomic blocking agents, major and minor tranquilizers, and MAO inhibitors), modulation of the dose-response curves has been consistently observed when the behavior was recorded under pressure. Depending on the drug, the dose-response curve may be displaced in either direction. That is, for one compound the behavioral effect of a 1-mg dose at depth may be equivalent to a 10-mg dose at surface; yet another drug may yield the opposite effect: a 1-mg dose at depth might be equal to a 0.1-mg dose under normal surface conditions.

The most persistent finding throughout these research efforts is that the behavioral effects of a drug under pressure are not predictable from its surface characteristics—a point clearly illustrated by the author's psychopharmacological evaluations of the amphetamines.[27] Dexedrine and methedrine were evaluated as potential prophylactic agents against the behavioral deficits

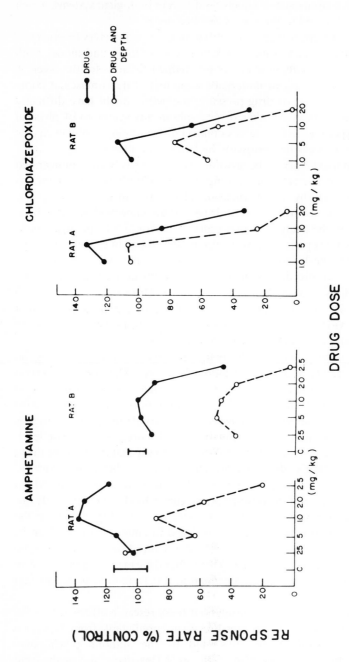

Fig. 14-2. Hungry rats were trained to press a lever to obtain food rewards. Changes in response rates for two animals (Rats A&B) are illustrated as a function of several doses of amphetamine (left portion of figure) and chlordiazepoxide (right portion of figure) at surface and at a depth of 250 feet on compressed air. Ranges of response rates during control sessions (c) are indicated as brackets. (Redrawn from JR Thomas, 1973.)

associated with nitrogen narcosis, since neurophysiological evidence indicated that nitrogen narcosis resulted from a generalized depression of central nervous system (CNS) activity. It was hypothesized that the introduction of a powerful CNS stimulant might antagonize some of the performance decrements. When the amphetamines were evaluated under the conditions of increased pressure, an increase rather than a decrease in behavioral dysfunction was observed. In fact, pressure interacted synergistically with amphetamine to produce behavior disruptions not evident with either drug or pressure alone. In terms of diver safety, this evidence suggests that a diver taking amphetamine could have serious behavioral problems at shallow depths, even when taking a dose that produces very little effect at surface.

The behavioral studies discussed have dealt with pressures in the 2- to 10-ata range with all of the drugs evaluated in subjects breathing compressed air. Further evaluations have been conducted[28] at 650 feet (approximately 20 ata) using a $He-O_2$ breathing mix. Changes in the dose-response curves were observed for amphetamine, chlordiazepoxide, and chlorpromazine, but to a lesser degree of magnitude than observed with the same doses at relatively shallow (250 feet) depths breathing air. The failure of toxicological investigators to show differences at these increased depths may simply reflect a lack of precision in their assessment techniques.

For those who are seeking pertinent information about drugs and diving, there are two obvious shortcomings in this basic research approach. First, although these studies were carried out under carefully controlled laboratory conditions, they were not done in the water, and the addition of that factor and its associated variables (e.g., cold, anxiety, fatigue) could certainly alter the effects of drugs. Second, animals, not humans, were used as subjects. It is most probable that differences between species do exist and that the interactions of drugs, pressure, and behavior would vary between humans and animals. However, for practical and ethical reasons this is the state of the art.

SUMMARY

So, where does all this leave the physician and his diver patient? The vital question still remains, "How will a drug, which under normal environmental conditions is safe for an individual, affect this individual's ability to function when he enters the water?" Unfortunately, for almost all drugs the answer is "we don't know." A start has been made, and some of the answers are emerging. It is known that when a diver enters the water a large number of variables come into play, each of which could alter the pharmacological action of a drug. It is also known that drugs under pressure are very unpredictable and can cause differential effects within an individual organism. Pressure, gas, age, sex, weight, cold, fatigue, anxiety, hypersensitivity—the question is enormously complex.

Physicians must be alerted to these possible drug interactions and those yet undescribed; they must exercise due caution in the prescription of drugs to divers. Diver self-medication may be responsible for many accidents. Misuse of prescription drugs is a major problem: drugs prescribed for a specific illness may be saved and used again by the same patient or by a friend. Nonprescription drugs purchased over the counter can contain powerful antihistamines, alcohol, codeine, and other compounds that may be especially dangerous for the diver. Many of these drugs carry warnings of behavioral toxicity (e.g., "may cause drowsiness," "do not operate machinery," "caution against engaging in operations requiring alertness"), which are generally unheeded in the everyday situation. Unfortunately, at 100 feet below the surface of the ocean, drowsiness or lack of alertness may cost a life. Physicians should make it a point to instruct their diving patients that drugs can cause decrements in their diving skills, subtle mood changes, and impaired judgment and that these events can result in mistakes which in the water may be fatal. Physicians and instructors must assume the responsibility for educating the diving community about drugs. A well-informed diver blended together with some good common sense may prevent diving accidents.

In summary, it is well known that divers do take drugs in various forms while diving in spite of the facts that warn against it. Ultimately, it is the responsibility of the diver's physician to condemn or condone these practices. For those who are looking for some general rules, the following guidelines may be useful: (a) It would be wise to avoid *all* drugs when diving; the condition that requires a diver to be on medication may well preclude diving for that period. (b) For those who must dive with medication, full warnings should be given that even the most benign compound may become behaviorally toxic under the increased pressures of nitrogen and oxygen and that any diving should be done with extreme caution. Physicians should consider restricting those on medication to shallow water diving only.

The revision of these "rules" together with the answers to numerous questions await further behavioral and toxicological research, as well as more extensive information about underwater physiology.

ACKNOWLEDGMENTS

From Bureau of Medicine and Surgery, Navy Department, Research Subtask MR041.01.01.0146. The opinions and statements contained herein are the private ones of the writer and are not to be construed as official or reflecting the views of the Navy Department or the naval service at large.

All animals used in experiments described from these laboratories were handled in accordance with the provisions of Public Law 89-44 as amended by Public Law 91-579, the "Animal Welfare Act of 1970" and the principles outlined in the "Guide for the Care and Use of Laboratory Animals," U.S. Department of Health, Education and Welfare Publication No. (NIH) 73-23.

REFERENCES

1. Small A, Friess SL: Toxicology of hypobaric and hyperbaric environments, in Hayes WJ (ed): Essays in Toxicology. New York, Academic Press, 1975
2. Fenn WO: The physiological effects of hydrostatic pressures, in Bennett PB, Elliott DH (eds): The Physiology and Medicine of Diving and Compressed Air Work. London, Bailliere Tindall, 1969, p 36
3. Goodall MC, Brown DES: Reversal of relaxing mechanisms in muscle fiber systems by hydrostatic pressure. Nature 178:1470-1471, 1956
4. Miller KW, Paton WDM, Smith RA, Smith EB: The pressure reversal of general anesthesia and the critical volume hypothesis. Mol Pharmacol 9:131-143, 1973
5. Behnke AR, Thomson RM, Motley EP: The psychological effects from breathing air at 4 atmospheres pressure. Am J Physiol 112:554-558, 1935
6. Miles S: Underwater Medicine. Philadelphia, Lippincott, 1969
7. Bennett PB: Inert gas narcosis, in Bennett PB, Elliott DH (eds): The Physiology and Medicine of Diving and Compressed Air Work. London, Bailliere Tindall, 1969, pp 155-182
8. Thomas JR: Combined effects of elevated pressures of nitrogen and oxygen on operant performance. Undersea Biomed Res 1:363-370, 1974
9. Schatte CL, Bennett PB: Acute metabolic and physiologic response of goats to narcosis. Aerosp Med 44:1101-1105, 1973
10. Davis FM, Charlier R, Saumarez R, Muller V: Some physiological responses to the stress of aqualung diving. Aerosp Med 43: 1083-1088, 1972
11. Martin KJ, Gray SP, Nichols G: Effect of a short simulated dive on selected blood constituents in man. Aerosp Med 44:516-522, 1973
12. Hardenbergh E, Buckles RG, Miles JA, et al: Cardiovascular changes in anesthetized dogs at 3 and 5 atmospheres absolute pressure. Aerosp Med 44:1231-1235, 1973
13. Goldstein A, Aronow L, Kalman SM: Principles of Drug Action: The Basis of Pharmacology (ed 3). New York, John Wiley & Sons, 1974, p. 129
14. Fingl E, Woodbury DM: General principles, in Goodman LS, Gilman A (eds): The Pharmacological Basis of Therapeutics (ed 4). New York, Macmillan Co, 1970
15. Bennett PB: Review of protective pharmacological agents in diving. Aerosp Med 43:184-192, 1972
16. Evans DE, Bailey GW, Dickson LG, et al: Anti-inflammatory properties of cortisone in rats exposed to helium-oxygen at 266 psig (600 feet sea water). Aerosp Med 41:1038-1041, 1970
17. Greenbaum LJ, Evans DE: Morphine analgesia in mice exposed to a helium-oxygen atmosphere at 266 psig. Aerosp Med 41:1006-1008, 1970

18. Small S: The effect of hyperbaric helium-oxygen on the acute toxicity of several drugs. J Toxicol Appl Pharmacol 17:250-261, 1970

19. Small A, McElroy HW, Ide RS: Acute toxicity of histamine and tripelennamine in animals exposed to hyperbaric helium. J Toxicol Appl Pharmacol 26:418-425, 1973

20. Berghage TE, Rohrbaugh PA, Bachrach AJ, Armstrong FW: Navy diving: Who is doing it, and under what conditions. Bethesda, Md, Naval Medical Research Institute, 1975

21. Ferster CB, Skinner BF: Schedules of Reinforcement. New York, Appleton-Century-Crofts, 1957

22. Thompson T, Schuster CR: Behavioral Pharmacology. Englewood Cliffs, NJ, Prentice-Hall, 1968

23. Walsh JM, Thomas JR, Thorne DR, Bachrach AJ: Differential performance changes under hyperbaric conditions. Aerosp Med 43:632-635, 1972

24. Walsh JM, Bachrach AJ: Adaptation to nitrogen narcosis manifested by timing behavior in the rat. J Comp Physiol Psychol 86: 883-889, 1974

25. Thomas JR, Walsh JM, Bachrach AJ, Thorne DR: Differential behavioral effects of nitrogen, helium, and neon at increased pressures, in Lambertson CJ (ed), Proceedings of the Fifth Symposium on Underwater Physiology (in press)

26. Thomas JR: Amphetamine and chlordiazepoxide effects on behavior under increased pressures of nitrogen. Physiol Biochem Behav 1:421-426, 1973

27. Walsh JM: Amphetamine effects on timing behavior in rats under hyperbaric conditions. Aerosp Med 45:721-726, 1974

28. Thomas JR: Personal communication

STUDY QUESTIONS

1. Changes in behavior resulting from drug-pressure interactions occur at depths as shallow as
   a. 10 feet
   b. 50 feet
   c. 100 feet
   d. 100 ata

2. As pressure increases with depth, the partial pressures of the individual gases in the breathing mixture
   a. Remain constant
   b. Increase
   c. Decrease
   d. Become additive
   e. None of the above

3. High partial pressure of gases can cause
   a. Nitrogen narcosis
   b. Oxygen toxicity
   c. Carbon monoxide poisoning

   d. a through c

   e. None of the above

4. Drug distribution is *most* dependent on?

   a. Metabolism

   b. Route of administration

   c. Blood flow

   d. Storage factors

   e. None of the above

5. The term behavioral toxicity refers to reduction in

   a. Motivation

   b. Motor coordination

   c. Judgment

   d. Purposive behavior

   e. All of the above

K.E. Cooper

15
Hypothermia*

To understand many of the problems facing underwater swimmers and divers, it is worth studying the effects of cold water immersion on unclad or lightly clad persons. From such study, further predictions can be made concerning the thermal problem of partially protected individuals in thermally hostile environments; this, in turn, can lead to more effective manipulation of the exposed individual's microclimate. In addition, they that habitually "go down to the sea in wet suits and occupy their business in cold waters" could contribute more to recreational water safety programs, given adequate knowledge of cold water immersion physiology.

HEAT LOSS

The first and most obvious problem to be faced in cold water immersion is heat loss. If the body is considered to be made up of a central core, maintained close to 37°C, and a peripheral shell made up of the limbs, the subcutaneous tissues, and the skin,[1] then it is obvious that body heat "content" can change a great deal before there is alteration in the "core" or "deep" body temperature. In other words, at any given deep body temperature, there can be widely varying states of body heat "storage." An implication of this is that a factor in survival during very cold water exposure will be the initial thermal state (or heat storage) of the body at the time of immersion.

Rates of body cooling also depend on subcutaneous fat thickness and

---

*A summary of practical points appears at the end of the chapter.

body shape.[2-4] Body cooling, at any one water temperature, is inversely related to mean subcutaneous fat thickness. Pugh and Edholm[4] noted, in many of those who swam the English Channel, that in addition to considerable fat thickness, they tended to have short limbs. However, a further factor that can accelerate cooling in water below 6°C is the occurrence of cold vasodilation in the extremities. The extent of this cold vasodilation is, in part, dependent on the core temperature and, thus, the better insulated the subject, the higher the core temperature, and the more likely he is eventually to experience severe cold vasodilation and peripheral heat loss from bare hands.

Studies by Hayward,[5] using infrared thermography, have shown that the chest wall, in the midaxillary line, and the groins are areas of very high heat loss; thus, in the design of protective clothing, these regions require special attention.

Any movement, which stirs the water in close vicinity of the skin, will increase heat loss by preventing the buildup of a warm boundary layer and creating turbulent eddies that will carry off heat. Keatinge[2] has demonstrated, with partially clothed subjects, that swimming very greatly increases the rate of fall of rectal temperature in water below 15°C. While the metabolic heat production may be increased by some four to six times by vigorous exercise, the stirring of the water during that exercise may increase heat loss far in excess of the increased metabolic rate; the result will be an effective loss of body heat and, eventually, a fall in core temperature. Similarly, shivering itself can, if sufficiently violent, increase heat loss to the point at which the heat gain it produces may be annulled. Some recent evidence[6] shows that, under some conditions, shivering can be inhibited by isometric muscle contractions of one forearm. Whether the reduction in heat loss due to inhibition of the shivering movements would balance the increased heat production occurring during vigorous shivering under the circumstances of their experiments has not yet been determined. It is also clear from the work of Keatinge[2] and the subsequent work of Hayward and co-workers[7] that even quite thin clothing will greatly prolong the survival time during immersion in very cold water.

Recent work of Hayward et al.[7] has shown that subjects wearing light clothing and kapok life jackets increase their metabolic heat production H_m (Kcal min^{-1}) while holding still, in a manner inversely related to water temperature (T_w°C). The best fit equation for their subjects is $H_m = 4.19 - 0.11$ T_w. They point out that this heat production increase is similar to that from exposure to air over the same temperature range when the velocity of air movement is increased above 5 mph. The rate of fall of rectal temperature in their subjects is given by the equation $C = 0.0785 - 0.0034\ T_w$, where C is the rectal temperature cooling rate in °C -min^{-1} and T_w is the water temperature in °C. In their experiments in water at 10.5°C, the cooling rate produced by swimming was 35 percent greater than holding still at a rate of swimming which would increase heat production to two and one-half times that of remaining still in the water. This group also predicted survival time of persons accidentally immersed in cold water, based on the assumption that incipient death would occur at a rectal temperature of 30°C, and developed the equation $T_s = 15 + 7.2/(0.0785 - 0.0034\ T_w)$, where T_s is the survival time in minutes and T_w is the water temperature. These measurements were made with the assumption that the subject was remaining still in the water and was lightly clad, wearing a standard kapok life jacket. The authors were careful to point out that there is considerable individual variation in this probable rate of cooling. As Haight and Keatinge[8] have pointed out, cooling can be much more rapid if there has been previous exhausting exercise combined with an intake of ethanol.

For the diver, the effects of body heat loss observed in the ordinary partially clothed swimming man are compounded. The sea temperature or water temperature at the surface would depend on the geographic location of the site of the dive, and in the Arctic, the surface sea temperature can be -1 to − 2°C. Further, in most climatic situations, the deeper the dive, the colder the water. A great deal of work has been done using direct and partitional calorimetry to determine further measures of heat loss. The diver, in water, will lose heat by convective heat transfer to the water, by conductive heat transfer, and in warming and saturating the inspired gas. For a detailed discussion of these studies, the reader is referred to a recent chapter by Webb[9] and papers by Beckman[10] and Craig.[11]

ADDITIONAL EFFECTS OF COLD WATER IMMERSION

During very sudden cold water immersion in unclothed or lightly clad subjects, there may be cardiac irregularities or even cardiac arrest.[2] An immediate effect of falling into really cold water is the gasping response in which, although the subject feels unable to breathe adequately, as much as 50 to 60 liters/minute of air may be moved in and out of the lungs. This gasp effect lasts 1 to 2 minutes and is followed by a sustained hyperventilation which may be between 15 and 48 liters/minute according to the subject, and the water temperature. The effect of these periods of hyperventilation is a very considerable reduction in arterial P_{CO_2}, and some subjects have experienced tetanic spasms during such periods of immersion. It is likely that under these conditions there would be a significant reduction in cerebral blood flow, which is linked closely to the arterial P_{CO_2} level, and this could result in a clouding of judgment or loss of consciousness.[12] In addition to this, the performance of sustained, but vigorous, isometric exercise in one limb can induce further hyperventilation which is superimposed upon the cold water hyperventilation.[13] Recent work has shown the interesting phenomenon that, in most subjects, preheating in a sauna greatly reduces both gasp and the early sustained hyperventilation responses.[6] It appears that the hyperventilation effect is determined by the skin temperature, and although it is not likely to be a problem in divers, there could be an added hyperventilation during a dive if the skin were to be cooled vigorously.

During cold water immersion, the limb muscle temperatures fall as do the temperatures of the nerves supplying them. The extent of this will depend on the water temperature, the degree of fat insulation over the muscles, and the amount of additional insulation supplied. Nevertheless, as a result of this cooling, muscle strength diminishes during a period of cold water immersion; in a series of nude subjects, it was found that after the first 5 minutes of immersion in water at 10°C the grip strength began to fall at a rate of approximately 1.8 percent/minute.[12] These effects are associated with considerable decrease in conduction velocity in the large fibers in the peripheral nerves, and also in an increase in the stimulus to twitch time from direct stimulation of the muscles. There may be a rise in blood pressure during the initial period of immersion corresponding with the cold pressor response. And, in addition, there is some evidence[14] that cold stimulation of the trigeminal area on the face, in addition to what is ordinarily thought of as the diving reflex, may produce relative bradycardia and also a potential fall in coronary artery blood flow.[15] An additional factor in reducing survival during acute cold water immersion may be the mentally disorganizing effect of many unpleasant peripheral stimuli at a high level, combined with fear, which may result in panic and deranged survival reactions.

PREVENTION OF HYPOTHERMIA

The main problem for the diver is prevention of hypothermia which, of course, becomes more difficult to treat as the dive depth increases. There should be the prevention of loss of muscle strength from limb cooling. Also, there is the problem, particularly in the Arctic, of providing adequate shelter to prevent precooling of the diver during transfer to the wet suit and to the diving hole, or during the transfer of the diver from the diving hole back into warming quarters. In addition, there is a further problem during prolonged dives to great depths of providing an adequate nutritional supply for the diver.

It is not a practical proposition to select for diving only those who have an ideal body build from the point of view of heat loss. Neither would such restriction obviate the problem in any general way. The only real solution is to provide the diver with external insulation appropriate to the thermal conditions of the water in which he will be exposed and to the degree of his own heat output and heat loss. As has been said before, the heat would be lost to the water by a conductive/convective means as well as from the respiratory tract. In addition, in cold water the urine volume voided increases quite con-

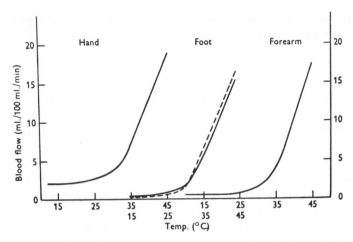

Fig. 15-1.   The effect of local temperature on blood flow in the hand, foot, and forearm. The ordinate indicates blood flow in ml blood per 100 ml tissue per minute. On the abscissa, there are three scales. The upper left-hand scale represents the local temperature of the forearm and the lower scale represents the temperature of the foot. The central solid line depicts the relationship between blood flow in the foot and local temperature as obtained from the average blood flow over the period 30-90 minutes after immersion of the foot at the water temperature indicated. The dotted line was obtained by using the maximum or minimum blood flow over a 15-minute period during the same time at the given temperature. (From Shepherd, 1963.[16])

siderably, and the total heat loss in urine voided during a long-term exposure at great depth could be a significant fraction of the body heat loss.

The conduction/convection transfer from the skin to the surrounding medium is proportional to the temperature grediant between them. In terms of heat loss from the body core, the rate at which heat is conducted through the skin from the core via the vascular system will be important. Once the heat has reached the skin, the thermal capacity and conductivity of the environment will become important as will be the rate of movement of the medium surrounding the skin. The relationship of skin blood flow to skin temperature is shown in Figure 15-1.[16] This shows that for different parts of the body the skin blood flow is related to skin temperature, and a sharp inflexion occurs at a critical temperature at which skin blood flow begins to rise rapidly. This onset of more rapid vasodilatation in the skin is different for different parts of the body, but it can be seen that at temperatures below about 29°C the peripheral blood vessels of the skin and superficial fat begin to constrict greatly. Thus, at these temperatures, there is less conduction of heat from the core to the periphery; but at the same time, discomfort may be induced since these temperatures are below the preferred distribution of skin temperature.[17] Again, it must be remembered that if skin temperature falls much below 10°C, there is the possibility of the induction of cold vasodilatation which can take place not only in the hands, but also in other skin areas.[18]

Wet Suits

The answer then lies principally in supplying additional insulation over the surface of the skin, and the accepted unit of clothing insulation is the CLO.[19] By definition, 1 CLO is that insulation which will transfer 5.56 KCal/m/hr/°C or in other words 0.18°C/KCal/m/hr. A nomogram relating water temperature, insulation of clothing, and rate of body heat loss during underwater swimming is given in Figure 15-2.[10] A quarter-inch foam neoprene wet suit for an underwater swimmer would have an insulation value in air of 1.48 CLO, in still water of 0.76 CLO, and in rapid disturbed water of 0.71 CLO. The efficacy of the insulation depends, in part, on the shape of the surface around which it is wrapped and also on compression of the material at any point.

The wet suit made of foam neoprene has many advantages, but at increasing depths the internal air cells of the foam become compressed, so that at great depths a considerable loss of insulation takes place. From another set of data on another type of quarter-inch foam neoprene wet suit, which at the surface had an insulation value of 0.59 CLO, had only an insulating value of 0.14 CLO at 165-foot depth. Furthermore, if the conditions of gas breathing used allow the gas to permeate the suit, then at great depths when helium is being used,[20] because of its very high thermal conductivity, there will be an additional heat loss through the suit. As Hayward[5] has recently pointed out, the distribution of insulation may have to be far more carefully regarded than previously, and particularly, added insulation must be provided over the chest wall in the axillary line and in the region of the groin.

A new development of the wet suit is the noncompressible variety made of hollow glass microspheres suspended in a mineral oil base and sandwiched between layers of foamed neoprene. This suit has very low compressibility, and it does retain its flexibility and thermal characteristics at considerable depths. In addition, another problem of compression suits, namely, change in buoyancy, is less likely to occur. Such a suit would be especially useful at very considerable depths. It does have some disadvantages which—in terms of expense, difficulty of tailoring, ease of tearing, high weight, and less flexibility than the ordinary neoprene suit—keep it still in the range of development.

The ordinary wet suit has limits on the depth for which it will be adequate; if the thickness is increased or the number of layers is increased to the point where adequate protection at very great depth would be provided in extremely cold water, it would be difficult for the wearer to move. In addition to this, it would have very high positive buoyancy at shallow depths which would make the dive more difficult. Furthermore, wet suits do allow chilling of the

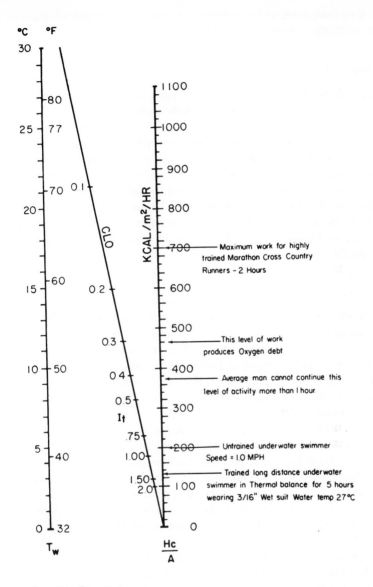

Fig. 15-2.   Nomogram relating water temperature, insulation of clothing, and rate of body heat loss during underwater swimming. (From Beckman, 1967.[10])

diver after leaving the water, and they can be uncomfortable when out of the water, particularly between repeat dives.

Dry Suit

An additional type of suit has been devised known as the dry suit, also made of neoprene. A valuable version is the variable volume type. It is a well-fitting neoprene suit that can be inflated by an inlet valve connected to the diver's air supply at the low pressure regulator fitting. An exhaust valve is also provided, and the diver can vary the buoyancy by varying the amount of air inside the suit. This suit allows more comfort when in the air between dives and, of course, provides a superior thermal insulation in the water as well. In addition, underwear can be worn beneath this suit, which will provide additional insulation. For details about the technical problems in the design of this, refer to *A Guide to Polar Diving*.[21] Such a suit may not be ideal at very great depths.

Heated Suits

Another approach to insulation is to provide what Kerslake (personal communication) has called dynamic insulation, by supplying heat continuously to the inner layer of the suit. The problems of this are the distribution of the heat within the suit and the source of power for the suit. While such a method can provide an additional degree of insulation in waters near 0°C, particularly during nonvigorous exercise or rest, the power requirement would be in the order of 0.7-1.0 kilowatts.

If the source of the electric power for such a suit were derived from batteries, considerable extra bulk would be involved in addition to the diving equipment. Other sources of power or heat involve the use of fuel cells, thermochemical reactions, and radioisotopes. These latter are in the development phase and still remain costly, for the most part. A simpler and more reliable approach has been to wear an undergarment with heating tubes distributed through it which are perfused with hot water supplied from the supply ship on the surface. Valves that control the rate and distribution of the flow of hot water through the suit can be placed on the outside of the dry suit. Problems include getting the right distribution of the heat supply over the body surface and avoiding burns, which[10] states can be produced at skin temperatures of 44°C, if maintained for 5 hours or longer. He recommends a maximal local skin temperature of 43°C and a thermal flux not in excess of 872 $W.m^{-2}$ during any continuous operation of this type of suit.

To maintain an adequate heat balance, the heat supply will have to exceed the conductive and convective heat loss from the skin by an amount equal to that lost to the gases being breathed. Attempts have been made to use a countercurrent flow system on the breathing equipment, so that the air entering the respiratory passages is preheated by the air leaving; but devices of this sort lead to complications in the breathing system and have not yet proved adequate in all respects.

Chambers and Habitats

Another major problem of deep diving is maintaining body temperature in a hyperbaric environment of the habitat and warming up divers in between trips out of their habitat. The first problem is to supply enough energy to keep the habitat warm. Assuming that can be done, the decision has to be made as to what the correct environmental temperature would be. In the hyperbaric gas mixture in the chamber, there is a low gas velocity and low diffusibility,[22] and this creates a sense of high humidity to the diver enclosed in the chamber. There is some preliminary biochemical evidence which suggests that the diver's metabolic rate, at rest, may be increased in a hyperbaric helium atmosphere. Despite this, there is evidence that an hyperbaric environment which is subjectively comfortable may be one in which there is a considerable heat drain from the diver. Webb invented a scale, which he entitled Convective Character, to express the temperature range of the comfort zone of different hyperbaric gas mixtures and fluids in a reasonable manner. The "convective character" of the gas mixture is derived from the density of the gas times the specific heat times the thermal conductivity divided by the viscosity, all in appropriate units; the numerical answer of this sum is related to the number derived for air at 1 atm. His scale of convective character extends from 1.0 for air to 167 for water. He points out that in a 1200-foot saturation dive, four subjects spent 6 days at this pressure and chose temperatures between 32.5 and 33.5°C as the comfort zone for their habitat. The convective character of that environment on the Webb scale was 144. He points out that the higher the pressure, the higher the convective character, and this correlates with the higher required comfort temperature and narrowing of the comfort temperature band. It is a useful empirical approach to the prediction of a good comfort zone.

There is evidence that in the hyperbaric environment weight loss occurs, and this appears to be related to the divers not wishing to eat enough calories to make up for the heat drain taking place.

In making excursions from a deep underwater habitat, the diver will become cold; it is extremely important to warn him completely between diving excursions from the habitat. It is best, if possible, not just to replenish the depleted heat stores but, if anything, to overload the heat stores slightly before the next dive. Heating in such an environment can be partly achieved by hot water showering.

TREATMENT OF HYPOTHERMIA

Usually, there is little evidence of problems of hypothermia until the body temperature has fallen below 35°C. Violent shivering may occur, particularly if the skin becomes cold; below 35°C, it is likely to become very severe. At lower temperatures, shivering may be replaced by muscle rigidity. An interesting recent study by Keatinge and associates[23] showed that some young people between the ages of 8 and 19 years, when in swimming pools with a water temperature of 20.3°C, came out of the water when their temperatures had fallen as low as 34.4°C after a swim. Below 34° to 35°C, some degree of mental impairment may occur, such as a slowing of mental processes, impairment of judgment, or inability to think rationally. At lower temperatures, consciousness may be lost. There seems to be a wide variation in the deep body temperature at which consciousness is lost, and there are reports in the literature of patients unconscious at temperatures of 32°C and wide awake at temperatures as low as 27°C.

The very low temperatures may occur as the result of dinghy accidents, and scuba divers in the vicinity should be aware of how to manage the situation. Even if the victim appears not to be breathing and appears not to have a heartbeat, it is worth attempting to rewarm him, for there have been a number of instances when apparently dead hypothermic subjects have recovered as a result of rewarming. The best accepted method of rewarming is the rapid process by immersion in hot water. The temperature of the water should be such that the operator can stand immersing his arm in it without being burned—this is usually about 43°C. It should be kept stirred and kept warm. It is best to immerse the subject for periods of half an hour at a time; be very careful to watch for a sudden collapse which might indicate faint since the subject is partially head up in the bath. Keeping the lower legs raised and covered may aid the venous return to the heart. Of course, other techniques could be devised in which a water perfused suit is used with additional external insulation; this might provide a carefully controlled device to induce a rise in temperature.

There has been some argument as to whether artificial ventilation is of value or is dangerous under these circumstances. Some think that intermittent positive pressure breathing may initiate reflex cardiac irregularities that would lead to ventricular fibrillation, and others maintain that ventilating the patient sufficiently to lower the arterial P_{CO_2} and raise the arterial P_{O_2} is an important aspect of the treatment. If they have been hypothermic for any period of time, there will be a metabolic acidosis superimposed on a respiratory acidosis; in such a situation, it may be advisable, if possible, to give intravenous sodium bicarbonate. In many situations, it is very difficult to perform this type of rewarming and, under those circumstances, the most rapid rewarming that can be achieved is the most valuable. The closed casualty evacuation bag can be used, as can immersion of one arm in water at

43°-44°C, while keeping the rest of the body well covered.

With the mild degrees of hypothermia which occur on excursion dives from a hyperbaric deep water habitat, Webb has suggested that a rough index of an adequate rewarming before attempting another dive would be to heat until the onset of sweating. Obvious peripheral vasodilatation and a marked rise in pulse rate may also denote a return of body temperature to near normal. It is, of course, extremely important not to get into a severe hypothermic condition in these exotic atmospheres, since the time for decompression is so long that access to sophisticated therapy at the surface would become impossible before the patient dies. It should be possible, though expensive, to have a pressurized capsule in which the hypothermic diver could be rapidly moved to a pressure chamber in a surface vessel for rewarming by skilled personnel.

If the cooling takes place close to a small hospital, then in-water rapid warming is the best way to treat the victim; this should be undertaken with careful monitoring of blood pressure, blood gases, and electrocardiogram. If the hospital is sufficiently far from the site of the accident, which would involve too prolonged a transport to expert supervision, it is probably safer to attempt rapid rewarming if a hot bath can be found close to the disaster site. Once again, in the diving situation, if there is a "mother" ship, the hot tub properly instrumented and stirred should be on board, so that these emergencies can be dealt with immediately.

ADAPTATION TO COLD

There is a considerable amount of unmeasured, hearsay evidence to suggest that a process of habituation to cold takes place. The experience of many, at the beginning of the summer, in swimming in the sea is that of unpleasantness and the short duration of the swim. Later in the season, after repeated swimming, the immersion becomes a pleasant experience without there having been any significant change in the water temperature. Within some communities, there is evidence that those who spend a considerable time in the water are able to do so more readily, with less ill effect, than those who are not habitually exposed to cold water immersion. For example, Korean Ama diving women as compared with the rest of the Korean population.[24] Again in studies on the Ainu people in one of the Japanese islands, Itoh[25] has shown evidence for a degree of adaptation to cold. Within any one population, there are considerable variations in the responses to immersion in cold water. In the author's experience, some subjects will shiver violently within a few minutes of immersion in water at 16°C and continue to shiver even before there is a significant drop in rectal temperature. Other subjects can sit in the water below 10°C without any shivering. It is also interesting that subjects shivering in cold water may have their shivering inhibited by performing an isometric forearm muscle contraction at 30 percent of maximum voluntary contraction. The onset of shivering also can be delayed considerably by preheating in a sauna.

The adaptations that may take place to modify the effects of cold water on the body may be local or generalized. There have been reports [14, 25-29] of modifications to the cold vasodilator response in groups of people whose work habitually brings their hands in contact with cold water. In addition, the cold pressor responses have also been shown to be modified in people who habitually expose their limbs to cold; this may be an habituation effect. In addition, the actual level of cold vasodilation is dependent upon the thermal condition of the rest of the body; thus, interpreting some of the results in this field becomes difficult without further knowledge of the state of the thermal equilibrium of the rest of the body. There has been evidence that there are sensory changes during exposure to cold, such as defects in the two-point discrimination test,[30] which are less marked in cold acclimated man than in the warm acclimated person. In addition, the process of habituation in animals has been shown to involve changes in some of the low frequency components of the electroencephalogram related to the hippocampal and the amygdalar regions.

In studies of whole body adaptation, another important aspect has been raised by Hong[24]. These workers demonstrated that in Korean women divers, who habitually expose themselves to cold, there were modifications of the peripheral blood flow, possibly in the behavior of countercurrent heat exchange systems, which could alter the effect of thermal insulation from the body core to the surface in an advantageous way. In addition to this, there is evidence from the work of Itoh[25] that the basal metabolic rate of cold-adapted Japanese differs from that of the noncold-adapted Japanese, in being negatively correlated to the level of plasma free fatty acid. They suggested that the turnover rate of plasma free fatty acid is increased markedly in the cold-adapted people under study. They produced evidence that in this particular ethnic group who are exposed habitually to cold free fatty acid is rapidly converted to ketone bodies in the liver; in this way, they differ very much from the Eskimo who has high plasma free fatty acid levels, but low ketone body levels. The Ainu people in Japan appear to respond with great sensitivity to endogenous noradrenaline, such that a small dose of noradrenaline produces a marked elevation in oxygen consumption. Plasma free fatty acid and ketone bodies and oxygen consumption were virtually unaffected in the non-Ainu Japanese controls. Much remains to be done on the subject of habituation and adaptation to cold before these studies can be applied directly to divers in pretraining them for periods of cold exposure in deep dives. Nevertheless, a very fruitful study would be to investigate the possibility that some training program could be instituted which would give them an advantage in heat conservation and heat production over the untrained individual.

SUMMARY OF PRACTICAL POINTS

It would be fitting to end this chapter with practical advice to those who are at risk of exposure to cold water. First of all, for those other than scuba divers or deep divers, no one should go into cold water in situations where there is danger of a capsize, or sudden immersion, without wearing a life jacket that will

1. Support an unconscious person with the head out of water.
2. Provide additional thermal protection, particularly in the regions of the sides of the chest and the groin. Clothing worn in addition will provide added thermal insulation.

In the capsize situation, unless wearing a life jacket and within a fairly reasonable distance of shore, no one should attempt to swim to shore in water below 8°C. In water at 10°C or above, providing an adequate life jacket is worn, it is probable that most people could swim 3/4 mile before succumbing to hypothermia. Without a life jacket, the victim should stay with the capsized craft and, under no circumstances, attempt to swim to the shore. During immersion, treading water will increase the cooling rate by an average of some 34 percent above that which would occur if the subject was able to keep still. The drown-proofing maneuver in which the victim floats with lungs full of air and the head face down in the water and raises the head out of the water four or five times a minute to breathe has frequently been recommended. Since the face is an area from which a tremendous amount of heat may be lost, the drown-proofing maneuver is probably dangerous in very cold water. In addition, if any sudden stimulus to hyper-ventilation occurs, having the face in the water would lead to inhalation of water. It is recommended that in very cold water, the drown-proofing maneuver not be used. In any situation where prolonged immersion in cold water is likely, the subject should never swim since this increases the cooling rate dramatically. The best maneuver for one person is to keep the arms close to the side of the chest to prevent heat loss from this area, to keep the knees up, and to float within the life jacket with the head out of the water in a fetal position. If more than one person is in the water, huddling together while floating in life jackets decreases the cooling rate.

Alcohol should not be taken under conditions where the subject is likely to fall into very cold water, or, where exposure is likely to occur following prolonged severe exercise, since this will accelerate the cooling rate. There is some evidence that taking glucose may provide a substrate that will help to maintain the metabolic rate and keep the body temperature up. The reader is referred to a pamphlet published by Hayward[31] for very valuable advice to those at risk of cold water immersion

With regard to the resuscitation of subjects who have been rendered hypothermic, the best method of rewarming is rapidly, in a tub of water at about 44°C (or as hot as the first aid personnel can stand on the forearm). It may help to keep the feet elevated above heart level and carefully wrapped up during this immersion; a reasonable monitoring of body temperature should be done once consciousness is reached to prevent severe overheating. If rewarming proceeds to the point where forehead sweating is generated, it is probable that the rewarming is adequate and should stop at that point. Under conditions where it is not possible to immerse the subject in a hot bath, it is probably best to wrap the subject in as much insulative covering as feasible and, if they are available, add warm water bottles separated from the skin by several layers of cloth to prevent local burns. In addition, sometimes it is possible to immerse a hand, or hand and forearm, in a well-stirred heated water bath at 42°-44°C, while keeping the rest of the body covered, to get heat absorbed using the hand and forearm as a heat exhanger. In any instance, if a hot bath is available close to the scene of the accident and the ambulance drive to a hospital is an hour or more, it is probably better to start the rewarming by short term immersion locally before going on to the hospital. In hospital, correction of blood gas tensions and blood electrolyte imbalances during the period of rewarming are important and the correction of the severe combined metabolic and respiratory acidosis can safely take place with intravenous bicarbonate.

In the case of divers, the best way of tackling the problem of hypothermia is that of preventing it. This involves adequate insulation, the timing of dives and rewarming following excursion dives during prolonged sojourns in deep-diving chambers. The general principle of rewarming, should hypothermia occur, is the same as when it occurs on the surface. However, the problem may be complicated by the difficulties of decompression. In all instances where hypothermia has occurred, even though it appears that breathing has stopped and there is no cardiac action, it is worth attempting rewarming and resuscitation: for, as mentioned before, there are a number of instances in which patients have recovered when they have appearantly been dead in the hypothermic state. The nursing rules that apply to unconscious patients, e.g., prevention of inhaled vomitus, must be applied in cases of hypothermic coma, as they would in any other form of unconsciousness.

REFERENCES

1. Aschoff J, Wever R: Naturwissenschaften 45: 477, 1958
2. Keatinge WR: Survival in Cold Water. Oxford, Edinburgh, Blackwell Scientific Publ, 1969
3. Pugh LGCE: in Rahn H (ed): Physiology of Breath-Hold Diving and the AMA of Japan, p. 25, Publ No 1341. Washington, D.C., National Academy of Sciences, National Research Council, 1965

4. Pugh LGC, Edholm OG: Lancet 2:761, 1955
5. Hayward JS, Collis M, Eckerson JD: (1973). Aerosp Med 44(7) 708, 1973
6. Cooper KE, Martin S: 1975, Unpublished observations
7. Hayward JS, Eckerson JD, Collis ML: Can J Physiol Pharmacol 53:21, 1975
8. Haight JSJ, Keatinge WR: J Physiol (Lond) 229:87, 1973
9. Webb P: Cold exposure. In Bennett, Elliot (ed). Physiology and Medicine of Diving and Compressed Air Work. Bennett and Elliot 1970 (in press)
10. Beckman EL: Milit Med 132:195, 1967
11. Craig AB Jr: (1971): Heat exchange between man and the watered environment in Lambertson CJ (ed): Underwater Physiology. New York, London, Academic Press, 1971, p. 425
12. Cooper KE, Martin, Sheilagh, Riben P: J Appl Physiol (in press)
13. Cooper KE, Petrofsky J, Lind AR: 1975, Unpublished observations
14. Leblanc J, Hildes JA, Heroux O: J Appl Physiol 15:654, 1960
15. Gooden BA, Stone HL, Young S: J Physiol (Lond) 242:405, 1974
16. Shepherd JT: Physiology of the Circulation in Human Limbs in Health and Disease. Philadelphia and London, Saunders Co, 1963
17. Kerslake D McK: RAF Instit Aviat Med FPRC/Memo 213, 1964
18. Clarke RSJ, Hellon, RF, Lind AR: J Physiol (Lond) 137:1-85, 1957
19. Burton AC, Edholm OG (eds): Man in a Cold Environment. London, Edward Arnold Ltd, 1955
20. Raymond LW, Bell WH, Bowdi KR, Lindberg CR: J Appl Physiol 24:678, 1968
21. Jenkins WT: A Guide to Polar Diying. Arlington, United States Office of Naval Research, 1974
22. Webb P: Aerosp Med 44(10) 1152, 1973
23. Keatinge WR, Sloan REG: J Physiol (Lond) 226:1-55, 1972
24. Hong SK: Heat exchange and basal metabolism of Ama. In Physiology of Breath-Hold Diving and the Ama of Japan (H. Rahn. ed.) pp 303-314 Publ. 1341. Nat. Acad. Sci—Nat. Res. Council, Washington, D.C.
25. Itoh S: Physiology of Cold-Adapted Man, Vol. 7. Sapporo, Japan, Hokkaido University Medical Library Series, 1974
26. Paik KS, Kang BS, Han DS, et al: J Appl Physiol 32(4) 446, 1972
27. Glaser EM, Hall MS, Whitton GL: J Physiol (Lond) 146:152, 1959
28. Belding HS: in Burton AC, Edholm (eds): Man in a Cold Environment. London, Edward Arnold Ltd, 1955, p 190
29. Krog J, Aluik M, Lund-Larsen K: Fed Proc 28:1135, 1969
30. Mackworth, J. Appl. Physiol., 5. 533, 1953
31. Hayward, 1975. Pamphlet. University of Victoria, B.C. Canada.

STUDY QUESTIONS

1. What main factors influence the rate of cooling of a person immersed in cold water?
2. When rewarming a severely hypothermic patient in the hospital, what measurements should be made and what physical and biochemical disor-

ders may need correcting?

3. What is the best method of rewarming a hypothermic patient?
4. Apart from hypothermia, what may cause death during sudden immersion in cold water?
5. Does the heat production during very vigorous swimming in extremely cold water adequately replace the heat loss into the cold water from the body?

Bruce W. Halstead

16

Hazardous Marine Life

With the rapid expansion of mankind's recreational, economic, and military activities in the marine world, there is presented an ever increasing opportunity for encounters with hazardous marine organisms. Although a great deal of folklore, myth, and misinformation has prevailed over the centuries concerning dangerous marine animals, it has only been within the last few years that serious scientific research has been devoted to the subject. The purpose of this chapter is to present a brief summary of factual data on hazardous marine organisms and some practical medical measures that physicians can employ to deal with problems relating to contact with these organisms.

Although dangerous marine organisms are essentially cosmopolitan in their distribution in the oceanic world, they are more concentrated in warm temperate and tropical seas. The area with the greatest variety and numbers of noxious creatures is unquestionably the vast Indo-Pacific region, which extends from Polynesia westward to the Indian Ocean, and roughly between latitudes 35° north by 35° south. However, a number of dangerous European species are found as far north as latitude 50°.

Hazardous marine life can be conveniently grouped as (1) traumagenic, (2) stinging, (3) poisonous to eat, and (4) shocking. Although most noxious organisms are animal in nature, a few of them are plants. The primary objectives in dealing with hazardous marine life are to be intelligently aware of their existence, to respect their territorial rights, and to avoid needless unpleasant contact with them.

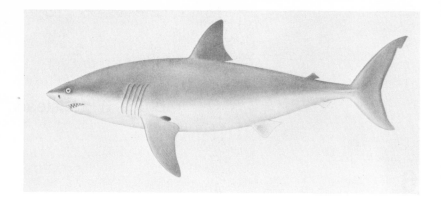

Fig. 16-1.   Great white shark (*Carcharodon carcharias*). Oceanic, widespread in all tropical and temperate oceans. Attains a length up to 36 feet. Most dangerous of all sharks, savage, aggressive, fast-swimming (M. Shirao).

TRAUMAGENIC MARINE ORGANISMS

Sharks

Sharks are among the most feared of the dangerous marine organisms known to man (see Fig. 16-1). Unfortunately, there is an amazing lack of reliable scientific data on the biology of sharks potentially dangerous to man. The following resume is based largely on data compiled and analyzed by Gilbert and Baldridge and their associates, working with the worldwide Shark Attack File, housed at the Mote Marine Laboratory, Sarasota, Florida.[1, 2] Although numerous data deficiencies exist within this file, it continues to be the most authoritative source of data presently available on the subject of shark attacks on human beings. The Shark Attack File is based on a series of 1165 case histories compiled during the years 1941 through 1968.

General. There are about 250 species of sharks known to ichthyologists, but only 27 species have definitely been implicated in attacks on man. Sharks range in size from about 18 inches, in some of the smaller species, to the giant whale shark which attains a length of greater than 50 feet. Fortunately, the whale shark feeds on minute marine organisms. All sharks are carnivorous, but their danger to man depends largely upon their dentition and size, combined with their aggressiveness. Even a small shark can inflict significant injuries.

The means employed by sharks in detecting food entails the use of a number of sensory systems, some of which are highly developed. The intelligence of a shark is generally considered to be of a comparatively low order. Although the visual acuity of sharks is poorly adapted for distinguishing details and color, they are well equipped for differentiating an object, especially one that is moving, from its background. The musculature of the eye permits the shark to maintain a constant visual field even when the shark is twisting, turning, or moving ahead. In brief, the eyes of sharks are an effective device for directing their predatory activities. Sharks have a remarkably acute sense of smell. Olfaction enables a shark to detect blood and food in the water. Sharks also have gustatory chemoreceptors that provide them with a sense of taste, which permits them to discriminate between food and other objects. The gustatory receptors undoubtedly play a part in shark feeding. Sharks also have another set of chemoreceptors in the skin, which are sometimes referred to as the "common chemical sense." These epidermal chemoreceptors provide the shark with the ability to perceive substances of an irritating nature. Although all of these teleceptors are important factors in the detection of food, probably the most important organ utilized by sharks in detecting moving prey is their hearing apparatus. Fish struggling, or a swimmer or diver moving in the water, produce low-frequency sound waves or vibrations which quickly attracts sharks. Sharks perceive sound by means of the labyrinth, the lateral line, and a group of specialized sensory receptors known as the ampullae of Lorenzini. With the use of these highly sensitive teleceptors, sharks have a phenomenal ability to detect low frequency vibrations in the waters. Moreover, they are able to home in on their prey with almost unerring accuracy.

The feeding habits of sharks generally follow one of two patterns: (1) *normal feeding pattern,* which occurs when a single or several sharks are in a relatively subdued state in quest of food. During this behavior period, they are relatively slow and purposeful in their movements. (2) The *frenzied or mob feeding pattern* most commonly occurs as a result of a catastrophic event, such as after an explosion, dumping of garbage, sinking of a ship, plane crash, in which large quantitites of food and blood suddenly appear in the water. During this frenzied activity, sharks become extremely erratic, snapping savagely at anything in sight, with rapid darting swimming movements. At this time, sharks are completely fearless and most repellent measures become ineffective. Even cannibalism has been observed during these frenzied states. Sharks tend to select a single individual out of a collection of people and then direct their attention to that person. If the attacking shark is not in a frenzied state, the shark usually confines his attention to the victim and does not molest the rescuer.

On the basis of the data presently available, it is difficult to provide reliable generalizations concerning shark behavior as it relates to attacks on man. The following observations are presented with reservation, but do provide some insight as to the nature of the beast. It must be kept in mind that shark attacks are dependent upon a combination of conditions which bring humans in contact with sharks. Consequently, most shark attacks are usually related in some way with the aquatic recreational pursuits of people.

Environmental factors. Most shark attacks have occurred between latitudes 47° south and 46° north. The most northerly unprovoked shark attacks occurred in the upper Adriatic Sea, and the most southerly attack took place off South Island, New Zealand. About 54 percent of the attacks have taken place in the Southern Hemisphere.

The extent to which people make recreational use of the sea depends upon weather conditions and time of day. Therefore, it is not surprising that most attacks have occurred during the daylight hours in warm weather, where the water temperature is above 68° F (20°C). Studies show that there is greater danger during late afternoon and at night, when large sharks are most actively feeding.

Murky water is considered to be hazardous because it fails to provide adequate visibility. Attacks can sometimes be avoided if the person can see the shark in time to take preventive measures. Areas considered to be especially dangerous include deep water channels and drop-offs which expose the diver to deep water where one is more likely to encounter large sharks. The documented accounts reveal that most attacks occurred within 100 feet of the shore, where the greatest density of bathers is usually found. The water depth in which these attacks took place was 5 feet or less. However, it is generally agreed that the further out one goes from shore, the greater the chance for an attack.

Sharks have a prediliction for attacking bright, contrasting, or reflective objects. Any movement upon the part of a swimmer or diver which results in low frequency vibrations in the water also serves as an attractant to sharks.

Medical aspects: Most attacks are made by solitary sharks. The majority of the victims are attacked suddenly, violently, and without warning. Since most victims suffer only one or two discrete bites, it is doubtful that most of these attacks are motivated by hunger. The bite of a shark frequently leaves a parabolic-shaped wound. Bites from sharks are severe and death most frequently results from massive tissue loss, hemorrhage, and severe primary shock. Bites are most commonly inflicted on the arms and legs. The biting force of some sharks is estimated to be more than 7 tons/square inch. With a biting force of this magnitude, one can appreciate the amount of damage that may result from a single bite. The case fatality rate in a series of 1150 shark attacks was about 35 percent. Severe skin abrasions may be received by brushing up against the skin of sharks.

Treatment: Because of massive hemorrhage and the danger of shock, immediate rescue and first aid are imperative. In some instances it may be desirable to attempt to control bleeding while the victim is still in the water, by manually constricting a severed artery or by packing the wound with a piece of cloth. As soon as the victim is removed from the water, bleeding must be controlled. The possibility of contaminating the wound is of minor interest at this point. Use whatever material is readily available for a pressure bandage: gauze, cotton, shirt, pants, sweater, bathing suit, gunnysack, etc. If a large vessel is the main source of the bleeding, tie it off by using a piece of string, suture, thread, shoelace, or whatever is available. Time is of the essence, and all efforts must be made to count. If it is not possible to tie off the bleeder, force gauze or improvised bandage material into the open wound and apply pressure. Tourniquets can be dangerous under emergency conditions, and must be used with caution. Pressure bandages are safer, and usually more effective.

It is frequently advisable to administer advance first aid to the patient while on the beach or boat, prior to transferring to the hospital. This has the advantage of permitting the patient's condition to stabilize and increases the chance of survival. With the bleeding temporarily controlled, the patient should be placed with the head lowered, kept warm, and a unit of plasma administered intravenously before further movement. When working in shark-infested waters, a Feinberg Shark Pack should be kept readily available at all times. This pack consists of the following:

Normal saline—1 liter
Human plasma—500 ml
Plasma diluent
Intravenous sets (2)
Morphine, coramine, epinephrine ampules
Syringe
Swabs, bandages
Alcohol
Tourniquets

Initial surgical procedures should be as conservative as possible. Remove dressings after anesthesia has been induced and swab all lesions with sterile throat swabs which should be inserted deeply into any lesions. The swabs should be plated out immediately for the organisms' antibiotic sensitivity. Some species of marine bacteria have been found to be extremely virulent and resistent. Check bone defects by x-ray. Debride only obvious necrotic tissue, and, at this time, do not attempt to remove all of the tissue involved. If the blood supply is intact, even the most infected and lacerated limb may be saved and returned to function. Do not attempt tendon repair unless the wound is clean. If the bowel is involved, resect widely and exteriorize. It is recommended that early skin grafting be done whenever possible in order to preserve nerves, tendons, vessels, joints, and even muscles. Intravenous therapy should not be prolonged, and intensive physiotherapy should be instituted as soon as possible.

Prevention: Although there are no surefire methods of preventing a shark attack, there are some procedures that can be used to minimize the possibility. Unless a person is thoroughly familiar with sharks in a specific locality, the behavior of sharks will be found to be unpredictable. Every precaution must be taken to avoid an attack.

A person should always swim with a companion or remain with a coherent group of bathers or divers. If you isolate yourself, you become a prime target for an attack. A buddy gives you a better chance of becoming aware of a shark in sufficient time to take defensive measures.

Try to avoid waters known to be frequented by dangerous sharks. If a large shark is sighted, it is best to get out of the water, but make your exit with slow purposeful movements. Erratic, irregular movements tend to excite a shark. Face the shark at all times and do not turn your back on the brute. Some sharks seem to have an aversion toward facing people.

Do not provoke a shark by spearing, holding on to the tail, riding, etc. Even a small shark can inflict serious injury.

Blood is an attractant to sharks. Keep out of the water if you have an open sore or wound. Women should avoid swimming in shark waters during their menstrual periods.

Try to avoid murky or turbid water because of limited visibility. Refrain from swimming far from shore in deep water, in deep water channels, or at drop-offs which are areas frequented by large sharks.

Check the water carefully before jumping or diving off a boat. Avoid swimming at dusk and at night when sharks are searching for food.

Do not tether captured fish, dead or alive, about your person. Throw the fish into a boat or anchor them at some distance from where you are operating.

In selecting diving and swimming gear, it is wise to avoid bright colors and shiny objects.

If you are scuba diving and a shark approaches, it is advisable to remain submerged if possible. It is helpful if one can move to a defensive terrain with a coral reef or some other immovable object at one's back. You then have the opportunity to fend off a frontal attack with the use of a camera, spear, pole, or shark billy. This technique has proved to be effective on a number of occasions. When diving, it pays to be continually vigilant. Whatever you do, do not place the shark in a trapped position between yourself and any obstacle such as the beach, reef, or a boat. Try to remain calm and take full advantage of weapons available to you. Use any object at hand to ward off a shark, but

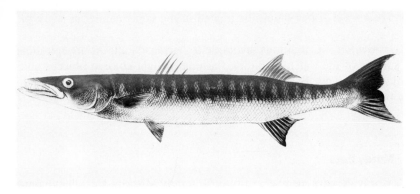

Fig. 16-2.   The great barracuda (*Sphyraena barracuda*) attains a length of 8 feet. It can inflict serious wounds (from Kumada).

try not to wound or aggravate the animal. Sharks often seem to react with increased vigor to efforts at sticking it with pointed objects. Once actual contact has been made, fight the shark as best you can. The skin of sharks is rough and can produce severe lacerations. Avoid hitting the shark with your bare hands. If possible, hit the shark with an object on the snout, eyes, or gills. There are pros and cons about using a powerhead as a defensive weapon. At the right time and place in the hands of the right person the powerhead is an effective instrument, but under the wrong circumstances—for example, a frenzied attack in a school of sharks—the powerhead may not only be useless but may greatly aggravate the situation.

Barracuda

The great barracuda (*Sphyraena barracuda*) (Fig. 16-2) has been known to attack man. There are about 20 species of barracudas, but only one of them has been incriminated in human attacks. *S. barracuda* is found throughout all tropical seas. This fish is said to attain a length of 8 feet or more, but it is rare to encounter a specimen much over 5 feet. The mouth of the barracuda is large and filled with enormous knifelike teeth. Barracuda are swift, solitary swimmers, striking rapidly and fiercely. Although barracuda are frequently encountered by divers, they seldom attack. However, when barracuda do attack, they usually make only a single strike.

Medical aspects: The wound produced by a barracuda appears as a straight or V-shaped laceration, since their jaws consist of two nearly parallel rows of teeth. This is in contradistinction to the crescent-shaped bite of a shark. Aside from this one difference, the medical problems remain about the same as that of a shark attack, namely, blood loss and primary shock.

Treatment: Bites should be treated in the same manner as shark bites.

Prevention: Conditions favorable to barracuda attacks are splashing at the surface of the water, turbidity, flashing or light-colored objects, and irregular movements. Barracuda will also strike at any speared fish that a diver may be carrying.

Moray Eels

Moray eels are members of the fish family Muraenidae, which contains about 20 species. They are found in all tropical and subtropical seas, and a few species are found in warm temperate waters. Some of the larger species attain a length of 10 feet. Their powerful muscular bodies are covered by a tough leathery skin that cannot be readily penetrated by a knife. Morays are bottom dwellers, commonly found lurking in holes and writhing snakelike through crevices, or under rocks or corals in quest of food. Moray eels are notoriously powerful and vicious biters, but seldom attack unless provoked. Most accidents occur as a result of a diver poking his hand into a hole in the coral containing the gaping mouth of a moray eel.

Medical aspects: Morays can inflict severe lacerations with their narrow vicelike muscular jaws which are armed with strong, fanglike teeth. Unlike sharks and barracuda, a moray will tenaciously hold on, tearing the flesh in an almost bulldoglike fashion.

Treatment: Bites should be handled in a manner similar to shark bites. Usually the damage is not as severe.

Prevention: Don't stick your hand into an unexplored hole in the rocks or coral until you have made certain that a moray eel is not present.

Giant Grouper

Giant grouper or seabass are members of the fish family Serranidae. Some of the larger species may attain a length of 12 feet and a weight of more than 500 pounds. They are found in tropical and temperate seas. These fish tend to be curious, bold, and voracious feeders. Although usually not aggressive in the sense of a shark, they may be dangerous because of their large size, cavernous jaws, and fearless attitudes. Grouper are frequently found lurking around rocks, in caverns, or in old wrecks.

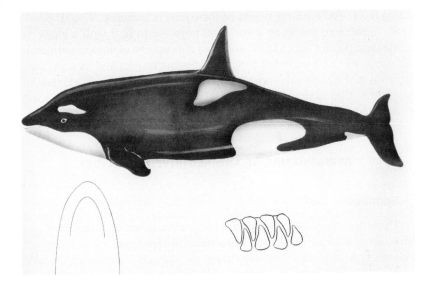

Fig. 16-3. The killer whale (*Orcinus orca*) attains a length of about 20 feet. Although no longer considered as a "ferocious killer," it must be treated with respect (Hon).

Sea Lions

Sea lions are usually rather docile, but during the mating season the males may become quite aggressive. Several accidents have occurred in which divers have been seriously bitten. Sea lions have large conical teeth and are quite capable of inflicting nasty wounds.

Killer Whales

Although the killer whale (*Orcinus orca*) (Fig. 16-3) has long been designated as a "ruthless and ferocious killer," more recent studies fail to justify this reputation. Part of the reason for this sudden shift in people's attitude toward the killer whale is their contact with these magnificent animals living in oceanariums. The killer whale is the largest of the living dolphins. They are found in all oceans ranging from tropical to polar latitudes. They usually travel in pods of up to 40 individuals. They are predators, fast swimmers, and feed on an incredible range of creatures, including large invertebrates such as squid, fish, birds, seals, walrus, and even some of the larger whales. They have a powerful set of jaws equipped with a formidable array of cone-shaped teeth that are directed toward the throat and are thus adapted for grasping and holding food. The crushing power of these jaws is immense. The killer whale is quite capable of snapping a seal or a porpoise in half with a single bite. Despite their playful antics in the secluded atmosphere of an oceanarium, they must continue to be regarded with considerable respect and as a potentially dangerous marine animal, even though most experts are convinced that killer whales do not go in search of humans. However, a case of mistaken identity by the killer whale could be tragic.

STINGING MARINE ANIMALS (INVERTEBRATES)

Sponges

There are many different species of sponges, some of which are capable of producing a severe dermatitis when handled. Sponges should therefore be handled with caution. The treatment of sponge dermatoses is largely symptomatic. There are no specific antidotes and the nature of the dermatopathic agents is unknown.

Coelenterates (Hydroids, Corals, Jellyfish, etc)

The coelenterates include the hydroids, jellyfish, and corals. Since there are several thousand species of coelenterates, most of whom are equipped with a stinging apparatus, it is not possible to deal with the subject in any degree of depth. Consequently, only a few of the more common stingers have been selected as representative of the group as a whole.

Hydroids. Members of this group vary in morphology from a feathery plume-like organism, *(Pennaria lytocarpus)* to the colonial siphonophore Portuguese man-of-war *(Physalia)* (Fig. 16-4), or the stony coral-like Fire Coral *(Millepora).*

Scyphozoa. This group includes the larger medusae or jellyfish, such as the deadly sea wasps and other larger species (*Chironex, Cyanea, Chiropsalmus*).

Anthozoa. Included within this group are the sea anemones, stony corals, and alcyonarians or soft corals. Probably the most important anthozoans, as far as venomologists are concerned, are members of the genera *Sagartia, Actinia, Anemonia, Actinodendron,* and *Triactis.*

The venom apparatus of coelenterates consists of the nematocysts or stinging cells which are largely located on their tentacles. Contained within the fluid-filled capsular nematocyst is the hollow, coiled, thread tube. The

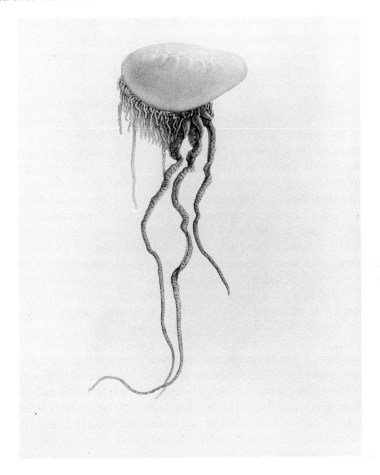

Fig. 16-4. Portuguese man-of-war (*Physalia utriculus*). Float size is up to about 5 inches in length. Can inflict an extremely painful wound, but rarely fatal (M. Shirao).

fluid within the capsule is the venom. Discharge of the nematocyst may be stimulated by either physical contact or by a chemoreceptor mechanism which causes the operculum to spring open like a trapdoor and the thread tube conveying the venom to be everted. The sharp tip of the thread tube penetrates the skin of the victim and the venom is thereby ejected. When a person comes in contact with the tentacles of a coelenterate, he brushes up against thousands of these stinging nematocysts and is thereby envenomated.

Medical Aspects. The symptoms produced by coelenterate stings vary according to the species, the site of the sting, and the person. In general, those stings caused by hydroids (*Pennaria,* and *Lytocarpus*) and hydroidcorals

(*Millepora*) are primarily local skin irritations. *Physalia* stings may be very painful. Symptoms resulting from scyphozoans vary greatly. The sting of most jellyfish is too mild to be of any medical significance, whereas *Cyanea, Chiropsalmus,* and *Chironex* are capable of inflicting very painful local and generalized symptoms. The sea wasp *Chironex fleckeri* is the most venomous marine organism known and may produce death within 30 seconds in humans. Sea anemones (*Sagartia, Actinia, Anemonia, Actinodendron,* and *Triactis*) are capable of producing severe skin ulcerations.

Symptoms most commonly encountered from coelenterates vary from an immediate, mild, prickly or stinging sensation like that of a nettle sting, to a burning, throbbing, or shooting pain which may render the victim unconscious. In some cases, the pain is restricted to an area within the immediate vicinity of the contact, or it may radiate to the groin, abdomen, or armpit. The area coming in contact with the tentacles usually becomes reddened followed by a severe inflammatory rash, blistering, swelling, and minute skin hemorrhages. In severe cases, in addition to shock there may be muscular cramps, abdominal rigidity, diminished touch and temperature sensation, nausea, vomiting, severe backache, loss of speech, frothing at the mouth, the sensation of constriction of the throat, respiratory difficulty, paralysis, delirium, loss of consciousness, convulsions, and death.

Treatment. Treatment should be directed toward accomplishing three objectives: relieving pain, alleviating effects of the poison, and controlling primary shock. Morphine is effective in relieving pain. Intravenous injections of calcium gluconate have been recommended for the control of muscular spasms. Oral antihistaminics and topical creams are useful in treating the rash. Dilute ammonium hydroxide, sodium bicarbonate, olive oil, papain, boric acid solution, alcohol, and a variety of soothing lotions have been used with varying degrees of success. Artificial respiration, cardiac and respiratory stimulants, and other forms of supportive measures may be required. Generally speaking, there are no known specific antidotes. However, the Commonwealth Serum Laboratories, Melbourne, Australia, have recently developed an antivenin for use against sea wasp stings.

Sea wasp antivenin is prepared by hyperimmunizing sheep with the venom of the jellyfish. The preparation contains concentrated immunoglobulins which have the power of specifically neutralizing this venom. The administration of the antivenin is supplementary to first aid measures which are of the utmost importance if a patient has been severely stung. First Aid measures consist of the following: (1) Apply a tourniquet immediately to the thigh or upper arm if stinging has occurred on the limbs. (2) Apply alcohol in any form to any piece of tentacle adhering to the skin. Do not attempt to remove tentacle by rubbing with sand, towel, or other means until the alcohol has been applied to render the nematocysts inactive. (3) If breathing is impaired, apply artificial respiration—mouth-to-mouth, if necessary. Antivenin should be administered to any victim of suspected sea wasp envenomation who, following the application of the above first aid measures, continues to have difficulty in breathing, swallowing, or speaking, or is in severe pain. The antivenin should not be used for minor stingings. The object of treatment with antivenin is to neutralized the venom as soon as possible. The preferred route of administration is intravenous—administer the antivenin slowly. The intramuscular route can be used if the intravenous route is not possible. *Sea wasp* antivenin is supplied in ampules of 20,000 units. The contents of one ampule of antivenin is the usual initial dose by the intravenous route (three ampules if the intramuscular route is used). There is a risk of serum reaction and the usual precautions in injecting an antivenin should be employed.

Prevention. The tentacles of some jellyfish may trail a great distance from the body of the animal. Consequently, jellyfish should be given a wide berth. Tight-fitting woolen or nylon underwear or a diver's wet suit are useful in affording protection from jellyfish stings. Jellyfish washed up on the beach, even though appearing dead, may be quite capable of inflicting a serious sting. The tentacles of a jellyfish may cling to the skin. Care should be exercised in the removal of the tentacles, or additional stings will be received. Whenever possible, alcohol or dilute ammonia should be applied to the tentacles and the lesions immediately upon envenomation. Nematocysts may adhere to the skin and, as long as they do, stingings will continue. Care should be exercised in removing the tentacles or additional stings will be received. Use a towel, rag, seaweed, stick, or handful of sand, but not your bare hands. Swimming soon after a storm may result in multiple severe stings from remnants of damaged tentacles floating in the water. Upon being stung, the victim should make every effort to get out of the water as soon as possible, because of the possible danger of drowning.

Coral Cuts

Stony coral have calcareous outer skeletons with razor-sharp edges that are capable of inflicting nasty wounds. These injuries are generally superficial, but they are notoriously slow in healing and often cause prolonged disability. The primary reaction to a coral cut, sometimes referred to as "coral poisoning," is the appearance of red welts and itching around the wound. This soon develops into a cellulitis, which may be followed by an ulcer with a septic sloughing base surrounded by a painful reddened area.

Treatment. This consists of prompt cleansing of the wound, removal of foreign particles, removal of dead tissue, and the application of antiseptic agents. In severe cases, it may be necessary to give the patient bed rest with elevation of the limb, kaolin poultices, magnesium sulfate in glycerin solution dressing, and antibiotics. Antihistaminic drugs given orally, or applied locally to the wound, may be helpful.

Prevention. When working around coral reefs, one should take every precaution to avoid contact with coral. Do not handle coral with bare hands. Wear heavy leather, plastic covered, or cotton gloves, rubber-soled canvas shoes, heavy booties, or a completely soled flipper. Divers should wear wet suits or a heavy nylon suit over the entire body in order to prevent scratches which can develop into festering sores. Lacerations and abrasions should be immediately treated with a suitable antiseptic or antibiotic agent.

Mollusks

Venomous mollusks consist primarily of two groups of organisms, cone shells and octopuses.

Cone shells. There are about 400 species of univalve mollusks which are members of the genus *Conus*. They derive their name from their cone-like shape. Most of them, but not all, possess a highly developed venom apparatus. There are about 18 species that have been incriminated in human envenomations, and some of these have produced fatalities. Only three representative species are presented herein, viz, *Conus marmoreus, C. textile,* and *C. striatus* (Fig. 16-5). The venom apparatus consists of a set of radular teeth associated with a venom bulb, duct, and a radular sheath. The radular teeth which are housed in the radular sheath are released into the pharynx and then to the proboscis, where they are grasped for thrusting into the flesh of the victim. The teeth are impregnated with venom just prior to discharge.

Medical aspects. Stings produced by cone shells are of the puncture wound variety. Localized ischemia, cyanosis, numbness in the area about the wound, or a sharp stinging or burning sensation are usually the initial symptoms. Numbness and tingling begin at the wound site and may spread rapidly involving the entire body and especially about the lips and mouth. In severe cases, paralysis may be present. Respiratory distress is usually absent. Coma may ensue, and death is believed to be the result of cardiac failure.

Treatment. Symptomatic. There are no specific antidotes. Artificial respiration may be required.

Prevention. Live cone shells should be handled with care, and an effort should be made to avoid coming in contact with the soft parts of the animal.

Octopuses. Octopus bites in human beings are relatively rare, but

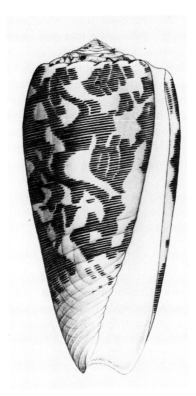

Fig. 16-5.   Striated Cone (*Conus striatus*). Attains a length of about 4 inches. Stings from cone shells can be fatal (K. Tomita).

several fatalities have been reported involving the Australian blue-ringed or spotted octopus, *Octopus (Hapalochlaena) maculosus* and *O. (H.) lunulatus*. The venom apparatus of the octopus is comprised of the so-called anterior and posterior salivary glands, salivary ducts, buccal mass, and the mandibles or beak. The mouth of the octopus is situated in the center of the oral surface of the arms or tentacles, surrounded by a circular lip, fringed with fingerlike papillae. The mouth leads into a pharyngeal cavity having a thick muscular wall. This entire muscular complex is known as the buccal mass, which is surrounded and concealed by the muscular bases of the arms. The buccal mass is furnished with two powerful chitinous jaws, whose shape resembles that of a parrot's beak. These jaws are able to bite vertically with great force, tearing the captured food held by the suckers before it is passed onto the rasping action of the radula. The secretions from the salivary glands are toxic and are discharged from the ducts into the pharynx.

   Medical aspects.   Octopus bites usually consist of two small puncture wounds produced by the chitinous jaws. Most octopus bites result in a localized burning or tingling sensation that may spread to involve the entire appendage. Bleeding is frequently profuse for the size of the bite. Swelling, redness, and heat commonly develop in the area about the wound. Recovery is usually uneventful without treatment. However, bites from *Octopus maculosus* and *O. lunulatus* may be of a more serious nature, and may cause generalized symptoms such as dryness of the mouth, dysphagia, ataxia, vomiting, respiratory distress, aphonia, loss of consciousness, and death.

Treatment. Symptomatic. Artificial respiration may be required.

Prevention. Octopuses should be handled with gloves. Most octopus bites, including the fatalities, have resulted from handling small specimens, usually less than 6 inches in span.

Annelid Worms

Some of the marine segmented worms are equipped with sharp parapodial bristlelike setae capable of inflicting stings. Some marine worms possess strong chitinous jaws and are able to produce painful bites. Wounds from annelid worms may result in a cellulitis. Treatment is symptomatic.

Echinoderms

Contact with the venomous spines of the crown-of-thorns starfish (*Acanthaster planci*) may result in painful wounds accompanied by redness, swelling, numbness and paralysis. *Acanthaster* is an inhabitant of the Indo-Pacific region. Sea urchins may inflict painful wounds by means of their spines or globiferous pedicellariae. Sea urchins of the genus *Diadema* (Fig. 16-6) have long slender, hollow, sharp spines that are dangerous to handle. The acute tips permit ready entrance of the spines deep into the flesh but, because of their extreme brittleness, they break off readily in the wound and are difficult to remove. The aboral spines of *Asthenosoma* are developed into special venom organs enveloped by a single large gland. The point is sharp and serves as a means of introducing the venom. In the sea urchin *Toxopneustes* and related species, the test or shell of the animal is covered by short spines interspersed with small, delicate, seizing organs known as globiferous pedicellariae. They are comprised of two parts: a terminal, swollen, conical head, armed with a set of three calcareous pincerlike valves or jaws; and a supporting stalk. The outer surface of each jaw is covered by a large venom gland. When a foreign body comes in contact with the pedicellariae, it is immediately seized. The pedicellariae do not release their hold as long as the object moves. If the moving object is too strong to be held, the pedicellariae may

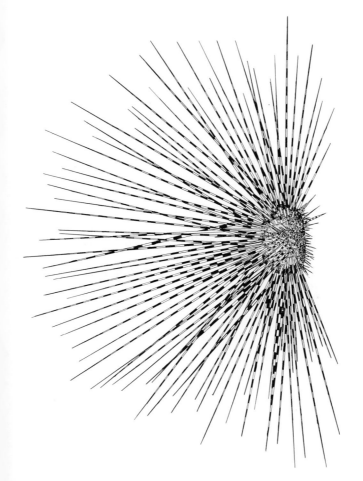

Fig. 16-6.　Long-spined sea urchin (*Diadema setosum*). Spines attain a length of over 12 inches. The spines are needle sharp and can penetrate gloves or flippers, and usually break off in the wound. Because of their friable nature, they are difficult to remove. The spines are thought to be poisonous (R. Kreuzinger).

be torn from the shell, but they will continue to bite and to envenomate the victim.

Medical aspects.   Penetration of the needle-sharp sea urchin spines may produce an immediate and intense burning sensation. The pain is soon followed by redness, swelling, and an aching sensation. Numbness and muscular paralysis have been reported. Secondary infections are not uncommon. The sting from sea urchin pedicellariae may produce an immediate, intense, radiating pain, faintness, numbness, generalized muscular paralysis, loss of speech, respiratory distress, and in severe cases, death.

Treatment.   Symptomatic. Detached pedicellariae clinging to the skin must be immediately removed or they will continue to envenomate the victim. Sea urchin spines are extremely difficult to remove from the flesh because of their brittleness. The spines of some species will be readily absorbed within 24 to 48 hours, whereas others must be surgically removed. There may be some discoloration of the area about the wound due to the purple dye that is leeched out of the spine, but this is of no consequence.

Prevention.   Do not attempt to handle sea urchins having long needlelike spines. Sea urchin spines can readily penetrate most gloves, shoes, and flippers. Care should be taken in handling any tropical species of short-spined sea urchin without gloves, because of the pedicellariae. A diver working at night in coral areas must exercise extreme care because of the danger of coming in contact with sea urchins.

VENOMOUS FISH

Stingrays

The stingrays (Fig. 16-7) comprise one of the largest and most important groups of venomous marine animals. Stingrays are common inhabitants of tropical, subtropical, and warm temperate seas. A few species are found in brackish and freshwaters. Rays are swimmers of moderate depths and are most common in shallow water areas, such as sheltered bays, shoal lagoons, river mouths, and sandy areas between patch reefs. They may be observed lying on top of the sand or partially submerged in it, with only a portion of the body protruding. The venom apparatus, or sting, of stingrays is an integral part of the caudal appendage. There are four different anatomical types of stingray venom organs that are recognized, but space does not permit a detailed discussion of them. In general, the venom apparatus consists of the serrate spine and the enveloping sheath of skin, and the caudal appendage to

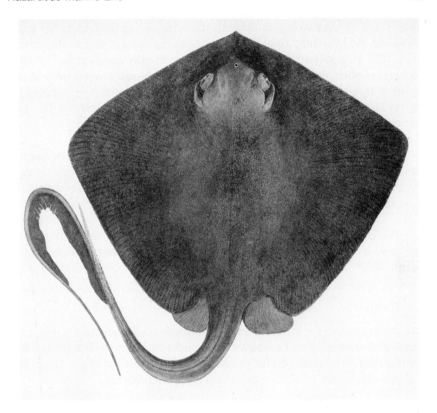

Fig. 16-7.   Stingray (*Dasyatis sephen*). Width of disk about 20 inches. Note large sting projecting from tail (G. Coates).

which the spine is attached. The vasodentinal spine is edged on either side by a series of sharp retrorse teeth. Along either edge, on the underside of the spine, there is a deep groove. These are known as the ventrolateral-glandular grooves. Lying within these grooves are the venom glands which are covered in the intact sting by the integumentary sheath. Thus, the grooves tend to protect the soft glandular material that lies within them, and even if all of the integumentary sheath is worn away, the venom producing tissue continues to remain within these grooves.

Medical aspects.   Stingray wounds are extremely painful. The pain may be sharp, shooting, spasmodic, or throbbing in character. Generalized symptoms of fall in blood pressure, vomiting, diarrhea, sweating, tachycardia, muscular paralysis, and death have been reported. Bacterial contamination of the wound is frequent. Stingray wounds are either of the laceration or puncture type. Penetration of the skin and underlying tissue is usually accomplished without serious damage to the surrounding structures, but withdrawal of the sting may result in extensive tissue damage due to the serrate spine. The area about the wound initially has an ashy appearance, but later becomes swollen, cyanotic, and then reddened. Although stingray injuries occur most frequently about the ankle joint and foot, as a result of stepping on the ray, instances have been reported in which the wounds were in the chest and elsewhere on the body.

Treatment. There is no known specific antidote. It should be kept in mind that stingray venom contains a cardiotoxin and may seriously damage the cardiovascular system of the victim. See below the "Treatment of Venomous Fish Stings."

Prevention. Stingrays are commonly found buried in the sand or mud, and there is always the danger of stepping on one. This danger can be largely eliminated by shuffling one's feet along the bottom.

Catfish

Although most species of catfish are freshwater inhabitants, there are a number of marine forms capable of inflicting serious stings. One of the most painful stings is produced by the oriental catfish (*Plotosus lineatus*). The dorsal and pectoral spines of many catfish species are venomous.

Medical aspects. Catfish stings are generally described as an instantaneous stinging, throbbing, or scalding sensation which may remain localized or radiate up the affected limb. The area about the wound becomes pale immediately after being stung. The pallor is followed by a cyanotic appearance, redness, and swelling. In severe cases the swelling may be very severe, accompanied by numbness and later gangrene of the area about the wound. Improperly treated cases frequently result in secondary bacterial infections of the wound. Deaths have rarely been reported.

Treatment. See the section on the treatment of fish stings.

Weeverfish

Weevers are small marine fish, members of the family Trachinidae, and are among the most venomous fish of the temperate zone. They are capable of inflicting extremely painful wounds. Weevers are inhabitants of flat, sandy, or muddy bays. They usually bury themselves in the soft sand or mud with only the head partially exposed. They may dart out rapidly, striking an object with unerring accuracy with either their venomous opercular or dorsal spines.

Weevers are found in the Mediterranean Sea and European coastal areas. The venom apparatus of the weeverfish consists of the dorsal and opercular spines and their associated glands.

Medical aspects. Weever envenomations result in instant pain, described as an intense burning or crushing sensation, initially confined to the immediate area of the wound, then gradually spreading throughout the affected limb. The pain gets progressively worse until it reaches an excruciating level, generally within 30 minutes. The severity is such that the victim may scream, thrash wildly about, and lose consciousness. In most instances, morphine fails to give relief. Untreated, the pain usually subsides within 24 hours. Tingling, followed by numbness, finally develops about the wound. Other symptoms consist of headaches, fever, chills, delirium, nausea, vomiting, dizziness, sweating, cyanosis, joint aches, loss of speech, slow heart beat, palpitation, mental depression, convulsions, respiratory distress, and death. The skin about the wound, at first, is blanched, but soon becomes reddened, hot, and swollen. The swelling may become quite extensive with severe ecchymoses. Secondary infections are common. Gangrene may be a complication. Recovery varies from days to months, depending upon the degree of involvement.

Treatment.   Symptomatic. See the section on the treatment of fish stings.

Prevention.   Weeverfish stings are most commonly encountered while wading or swimming along sandy coastal areas. Since they are frequently buried in the sand, one should be careful when swimming close to the bottom because of the danger of encountering these fish. Persons wading in waters inhabited by weevers should wear adequate footwear. Skin divers should avoid coming close to these fish because they can easily be provoked into stinging. Never under any circumstances attempt to hold a live weever. Even when dead, weever spines may inflict a painful wound.

Scorpionfish.

The scorpionfish are exceeded only by the stingrays as an important group of piscine stingers. They are all members of the family Scorpaenidae. Scorpionfish are widely distributed throughout tropical and temperate oceans. Venomous scorpionfish have been divided into three groups on the basis of the structure of their venom organs: (1) Zebrafish (*Pterois*); (2) Scorpionfish proper (*Scorpaena*); and (3) Stonefish (*Synanceja*). There are a number of different genera and species in each of these basic groups. Zebrafish are among the most beautiful and ornate of coral reef fish. They are generally found in shallow water hovering about in a crevice or at times swimming un-

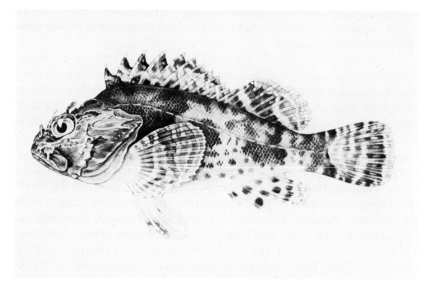

Fig. 16-8.   California scorpionfish (*Scorpanea guttata*). Attains a length of about 18 inches. This is representative of a large number of other species of scorpionfish, all of which possess venomous dorsal and anal spines (M. Shirao).

concernedly in the open. The scorpionfish proper (Fig. 16-8) are largely shallow water, bottom dwellers, found in bays, along sandy beaches, rocky coastlines, or coral reefs, from the intertidal zone to depths of 50 fathoms or more. Because of their morphology and coloration, they are well camouflaged and difficult to detect and their background. They conceal themselves in crevices, among debris, under rocks, in seaweed, etc. Stonefish are largely shallow-water dwellers, commonly found in tidepools and shallow reef areas. They have the habit of lying motionless in coral crevices, under rocks, in holes, or buried in sand and mud. They appear to be almost fearless of any intruder. Anatomically, the venom organs of scorpionfish differ from one group to the next. Generally, the venom organs consist of their dorsal, pelvic, and anal spines, and their associated venom glands. The zebra fish type have long slender delicate spines. The scorpionfish type have moderately stout spines. The stonefish type have heavy robust spines covered by a thick warty integumentary sheath.

Medical aspects. The pain from scorpionfish stings is usually described as immediate, intense, sharp, shooting, or throbbing, and radiates from the affected part. However, the character of the pain varies greatly with the amount of venom delivered and the species of scorpionfish. Probably the most severe pain is produced by *Synanceja,* the stonefish, and may persist for several days. Pain caused by the stonefish is sometimes so severe as to cause the victim to thrash about, to scream, and to lose consciousness. The area about the wound becomes ischemic, and then cyanotic, surrounded by a zone of redness, swelling, and heat. Sloughing of the tissues about the wound may occur. The area about the wound may become numb and the skin some distance from the wound painful to touch. Complete paralysis of the limb may ensue. Other symptoms that may be present include delirium, convulsions, various nervous disturbances, nausea, vomiting, lymphangitis, joint aches, fever, respiratory distress, cardiac failure, and death. Complete recovery from stonefish stings may require months and may have an adverse effect on the general health of the victim.

Treatment. There is stonefish antivenin that has been developed by the Commonwealth Serum Laboratories, Melbourne, Australia. This antivenin can be used in the treatment of other scorpionfish stings. The initial dose of the antivenin is 2 ml intramuscularly and in severe cases it can be administered intravenously. If the symptoms persist, a second dose of 2 ml can be given. Also see section on the treatment of fish stings.

Prevention. Most scorpionfish stings result from the person removing them from the hook or nets and being jabbed by their venomous spines. Stonefish are especially dangerous because of the difficulty of detecting them amid their surroundings. Placing one's hands in crevices or in holes likely to be inhabited by scorpionfish should be done with caution.

Miscellaneous Venomous Fish

There are numerous other kinds of venomous fish such as ratfish, sharks, toadfish, surgeonfish, rabbitfish, stargazers, carangids, scats, but space does not permit a review of these various groups. However, stings from this miscellaneous group are less frequent and generally less severe in their consequences.

Treatment of Venomous Fish Stings

In treating fish stings, care should be directed toward alleviating pain, combating the effects of the venom, and preventing secondary infections. The pain from fish stings is produced by a combination of factors, namely, trauma from the offending spine, venom, and the introduction of slime and other irritating foreign substances into the wound. Stingray and catfish spines have retrorse barbs along the margins of the spines that may produce severe lacerations. Wounds of this type should be promptly irrigated with cold saltwater or sterile saline if such is available. Fish stings of the puncture-wound type are usually small in size, and removal of the venom is more difficult. Suction, if instituted promptly, may be of limited value. It may be necessary to make a small incision across the wound in order to irrigate it satisfactorily. Keep in mind that the venom tissue is part of the integumentary sheath of the spine and that a portion of the sheath may become lodged in the wound and may continue to envenomate the victim even though the spine has been removed. The use of a ligature in most fish envenomations is of questionable value.

The injured limb should be soaked in hot water for about 30 minutes. The water should be maintained at as high a temperature as the victim can tolerate without injuring the tissues. If the wound is on the face or body, use hot moist compresses. The heat will have an attenuating effect on the venom, and it contributes greatly to the relief of pain. Infiltration of the wound area with 2 percent Xylocaine may be useful. Morphine or demerol may be required. Following the soaking procedure, debridement and further cleansing of the wound may be desirable. Lacerated wounds should be closed with dermal sutures. If the wound is large, a small drain should be left in it for a day or two. Antibiotic and tetanus antitoxin may be required. The primary shock that follows immediately after the stinging generally responds to simple supportive measures. However, secondary shock resulting from the action of stingray venom on the cardiovascular system requires immediate and vigorous therapy. Treatment should be directed toward maintaining cardiovascular tone and the prevention of any further complications. Respiratory stimulants may be required.

SEA SNAKES

Sea snakes (Fig. 16-9) are true snakes and have their bodies covered by scales. They have no limbs or ear openings and breathe with lungs. Sea snakes are further characterized by having a body more or less compressed posteriorly with a flat, paddle-shaped tail. There are about 50 species of sea snakes which inhabit the tropical and warm temperate Pacific and Indian Oceans. Sea snakes are usually found in sheltered coastal waters and around river mouths, but, at times, may be found migrating in great numbers far out at sea. With their compressed, oarlike tails, sea snakes are well adapted for locomotion in their marine environment. Swimming is accomplished by lateral undulatory movements of the body. They have a remarkable ability to move backward or forward in the water with equal rapidity, but are awkward on land. Sea snakes are able to remain submerged in the water for hours at a time. They capture their food underwater, which consists mainly of fish swallowed whole. A considerable portion of time is spent feeding on, or around, rocks or corals on the bottom.

Sea snakes are generally docile. However, aggressiveness varies some-

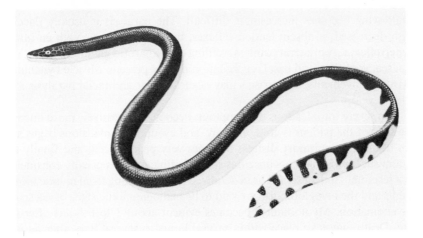

Fig. 16-9.   Yellow-bellied sea snake (*Pelamis platurus*). Attains a length of about 36 inches. This is the most widely distributed of all the sea snakes, ranging from the eastern Pacific to the Persian Gulf. It is capable of inflicting a fatal bite (M. Shirao).

what from one species to the next and with the season of the year. During the reproductive season, the males of some species become aggressive and dangerous to handle. Most sea snake bites occur while handling nets, sorting fish, wading, washing, or accidentally stepping on the snake. Fortunately, sea snakes have a rather weak, but well-developed venom apparatus consisting of two to four maxillary fangs and a pair of associated venom glands. The fangs of most sea snakes are short and easily torn from their sockets, so envenomation may not take place even though the person has been bitten. Nevertheless, it should be kept in mind that sea snake venom is extremely potent and, thus, should be handled with great care.

Medical aspects.   Symptoms resulting from envenomation by sea snakes characteristically evolve rather slowly, taking up to several hours before definite symptoms develop. It is believed that the length of the latent period varies with the amount of venom injected and the sensitivity of the victim. Aside from the initial prick, there is no pain or reaction at the site of the bite. The victim may even fail to connect the bite with his illness. The initial symptom may be merely a feeling of a mild euphoria, malaise and nervousness. A sensation of thickness of the tongue and a generalized feeling of stiffness of the muscles gradually develops. The usual complaint during the initial phase is "aching, stiffness, or pain" upon movement. There may be little indication of actual weakness at this time. The paralysis that soon follows is usually generalized, but of the ascending type, beginning with the legs and shortly thereafter involving the trunk, arm, and neck muscles. Speaking and swallowing becomes increasingly difficult. The paralysis is usually flaccid, with decreased or absent tendon reflexes, but may be spastic with an initial hyperreflexia. A bilateral painless swelling of the parotid glands may develop. Nausea, vomiting, and nasal regurgitation may be present. Muscle twitchings, twisting movements, and spasms may occur. Ocular and facial paralysis may later develop.

In severe intoxications the symptoms become progressively more intense: the skin of the patient is cold, clammy, and cyanotic; convulsions begin and are frequent; respiratory distress becomes very pronounced; and finally the victim succumbs in an unconscious state. Failing vision is usually considered as a terminal clinical sign. The generalized pains resulting from muscle movements and the myoglobinuria are said to be pathognomonic signs of sea snake envenomation. Myolobinuria becomes evident about 3 to 6 hours after the bite. Death may take place within several hours to several days after an untreated envenomation. The overall case fatality rate is estimated to be about 3 percent.

Treatment.   In the first aid treatment of sea snake bites, it should be kept in mind that the venom is absorbed rapidly. Hence, suction is of value only if it can be applied within the first few minutes following the bite. It is generally advisable to leave the bite alone. The affected limb should be immediately immobilized and *all exertion must be avoided.* The patient should lie down and keep the immobilized part below the level of the heart. A tourniquet should be applied tightly enough to occlude the superficial venous and lymphatic return. Apply the tourniquet to the thigh in leg bites or above the elbow in upper limb bites. It should be released for 90 seconds every 10 minutes. A tourniquet is of little value if applied later than 30 minutes following the bite, and it should not be used for more than 4 hours. The tourniquet should be eliminated as soon as antivenin therapy has been started.

If sea snake or polyvalent antivenin containing a krait (Elapidae) fraction is available, it should be administered intramuscularly, either in the buttocks or at some other site distant from the bite. The antivenin should be given only after the appropriate skin or conjunctival test has been made. However, there are many physicians who believe that the antivenin should be administered intravenously without concern for the side effects. They feel that any hypersensitivity can be controlled with the use of adrenalin and cortisone. Usually one unit (vial or ampule) is sufficient until the patient can be transported to the hospital.

Keep the patient warm. He should not be given alcoholic beverages, but may be given water, coffee, or tea. Keep calm and reassure the patient. Do not make the patient walk or exert himself. Attempt to get the offending snake for identification, since this may have an important bearing on the need for further treatment. A delay in instituting proper medical treatment can lead to serious consequences.

The first step in treatment is to determine if envenomation has actually occurred. In most instances, by the time the patient reaches the physician, the 1-hour test period has elasped, so there should be some clinical evidence of poisoning if any is to develop. If there is no evidence of intoxication, the patient should be carefully observed for another hour or two and then released.

If there is evidence of intoxication, antivenin must be administered without further delay. Follow the instructions enclosed with the antivenin container. The Commonwealth Serum Laboratories produce sea snake antivenin. The intramuscular route is considered to be safer, but is less effective. A portion of the first ampule should be injected subcutaneously, proximal to the bite, surrounding the wound, or in advance of the swelling. Antivenin should never be injected into a finger or toe. Avoid injecting large amounts of antivenin into the injured part. A second portion of the antivenin should be injected into a large muscle mass at some distance from the bite. The last portion should be given intravenously. When used intravenously, the antivenin should be administered by the drip method over a period of 1 hour. Intravenous antivenin is indicated if the patient is in shock. The antivenin can be added to physiological saline solution and given in a continuous drip. Subsequent doses can be added to the saline solution. The incidence of sensitivity reactions is said to be lessened when the antivenin is combined with hyaluronidase (10 ml of antivenin with 1000 units of hyaluronidase) and given intramuscularly. If hypersensitivity reactions occur, they can usually be controlled with adrenalin subcutaneously, with or without antihistaminic drugs.

In severe cases of intoxication, 3 to 4 or more ampules of antivenin may be required. If envenomation has taken place, antivenin therapy should be instituted as soon as possible, but may be given up to 8 hours after the bite. Supportive measures such as blood transfusions, plasma, vasopressor drugs, antibiotics, antitetanus agents, and oxygen, may be required. Corticosteroids are the drugs of choice in combating delayed allergic reactions provoked by the antivenin.

Prevention.   In most instances, sea snake attacks have resulted because of provocation of the snake. Individuals wading and divers working around rocky crevices, piers, and old tree roots inhabited by sea snakes should be aware of the potential danger. Most attacks have occurred among fishermen working with their nets in the vicinity of river mouths. Despite the reputed docility of sea snakes, an attempt should be made to avoid handling or coming in contact with them.

MARINE ANIMALS POISONOUS TO EAT

There is a vast array of marine animals which are known to be poisonous to eat. The animals involved include dinoflagellates, coelenterates, mollusks, echinoderms, crustaceans, fishes, turtles, and a variety of marine mammals. Although these organisms are poisonous to eat they can be readily avoided and do not constitute quite the underwater hazard that most of the organisms do that are discussed in this chapter. Nevertheless, there is one form of oral intoxication that should be brought to the attention of anyone working in tropical waters, and that is *Ciquatera fish poisoning.* More than 300 different species of tropical reef fishes and a variety of invertebrates are capable of causing ciquatera. This biotoxication is treacherous because most of the organisms involved are usually edible under ordinary circumstances. It is believed that these organisms become poisonous as a result of their food habits, the toxicity cycle beginning probably with poisonous marine algae upon which they have been feeding. Ciquatera is characterized by a sensation of tingling about the lips, tongue and throat, followed by numbness, usually within a period of 30 hours after ingestion of the food. Gastrointestinal disturbances may be present. Extreme exhaustion and muscular weakness are common. A pathognomonic symptom of ciquatera poisoning is the paradoxical sensory disturbance in which there is a reversal of temperature sensation— a hot object feels cold and a cold object feels hot. A variety of other neurological disturbances may also be present. The overall case fatality rate is believed to be about 12 percent. Treatment is symptomatic. There are no known specific antidotes.

There are a number of other types of marine oral intoxicants, but since this subject goes beyond the intent of the present work the reader is referred to the monograph on *Poisonous and Venomous Marine Animals of the World,* 3 volumes, (Halstead, 1965, 1967, 1970) U.S. Government Printing Office, Washington, D.C., or the forth-coming abriged edition, soon to be published by Darwin Press, Princeton, N.J., under the same title.

MARINE ANIMALS THAT SHOCK

Electric fish constitute a relatively minor health hazard, but the medically oriented diver should be aware of their existence. There are a number of different types of electric fish, but only two groups are marine. The others inhabit freshwaters. The marine electric fish include the stargazers (*Astroscopus*) and the electric rays (*Torpedo* and its relatives). The electric rays are the ones most likely to be encountered. Electric rays are found in all temperate and tropical oceans. They are sluggish, feeble swimmers, spending most of their time lying on the bottom partially buried in mud or sand. The

electric organs are situated on each side of the anterior part of the disk between the anterior extension of the pectoral fin and the head, extending from
about the level of the eye backward past the gill region. Usually, outlines of
the electric organs are externally visible on both the ventral and dorsal sides.
The organs are comprised of columnar prismlike structures separated by
loose connective tissue, forming a network similar to the cells of a
honeycomb. The ventral side of the ray is electrically negative, whereas the
dorsal side is positive. The production of an electrical discharge is believed to
be a simple reflex action, the result of tactile stimulation. A ray can deliver a
series of discharges, but he becomes progressively weaker, until finally exhausted. After a period of time, the ray recuperates and is again able to produce a discharge. Rays can deliver a voltage up to 220 volts. Contact with a
large ray may result in a shock sufficient to knock over and temporarily disa-
ble a man, which may resulting in his drowning. Recovery from the shock is
usually uneventful.

REFERENCES

1. Gilbert PW: Sharks and Survival. Boston, D.C. Heath and Co., 1963
2. Baldridge HD: Shark Attack Against Man. Mote Marine Laboratory, Sarasota,
   Florida. Technical Report, Office of Naval Research, U.S. Navy, 1973

FURTHER READING

Halstead BW: Dangerous Marine Animals. Cambridge, Md, Maritime Press, 1959
Halstead BW: Poisonous and Venomous Marine Animals of the World. Washington,
   D.C., U.S. Government Printing Office. Vol. I, Invertebrates, 1965; vol. II, Ver-
   tebrates, 1967; vol. III, Vertebrates—continued, 1970
Halstead BW: Poisonous and Venomous Marine Animals of the World. Abridged
   edition (updated).Princeton, N.J., Darwin Press, 1976 (in press)

STUDY QUESTIONS

1. What is the most important sense used by sharks to detect prey?
2. What should initial aid for shark bite include?
3. Barracuda are attracted by silver or light-colored objects.
   a. True
   b. False
4. What is the most frequent cause of moray eel bite?
5. The sting of the sea wasp is similar to that of the insect wasp.
   a. True
   b. False

6. What is the treatment for coral cuts?
7. The embedded spines of some sea urchins are resorbed within a few days and do not require surgical excision.
   a. True
   b. False
8. Treatment for the sting of a stingray includes soaking the limb in cold water for 30 minutes.
   a. True
   b. False
9. The bite of a sea snake causes severe pain and local reaction.
   a. True
   b. False

Robert Elsner

17

Diving Adaptations in Marine Mammals

While man faces the prospect of deep and prolonged dives with some trepidation, it is instructive to note that many species of marine mammals perform such dives frequently, repetitively, and apparently without concern. The performances of some species result in dives of great length and depth. It is well established that some species of marine mammals are capable of routine dives to depths which result in compressions in excess of 50 atm. Free dives of antarctic Weddell seals *Leptonychotes weddelli,* verified by a retrieved depth recorder, have been measured to a depth of 600 meters. Six sperm whales *Physeter catodon* have been found entangled in deep sea cables at 900 to 1000 meters. The depth records of several species of diving mammals have been reviewed by Kooyman and Andersen.[1]

Our knowledge of the natural history of diving has been much expanded through the investigations by Kooyman and his colleagues on Weddell seals in the antarctic. The animals were captured on sea ice near shore and were then transported several miles distance to a site known to be located far from any breathing holes. At that place, an instrument for recording depth was attached to the seal and it was released through a prepared hole cut in the ice. The instrument package could then be retrieved when the seal returned to breathe. By using this technique, several hundred free dives have been observed involving many seals.

The general pattern of dive profiles (Fig. 17-1) suggests two distinct kinds of behavior, in addition to very brief and shallow dives which appear to be a matter of exploring the immediate neighborhood of the hole. The maximum depth record of 600 meters coincides with the bottom at that site. Deep

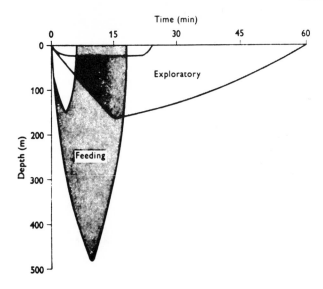

Fig. 17-1. Diving profiles of Weddell seals showing a comparison of feeding and exploratory dives.[2]

dives of 200 to 400 meters appeared to be associated with feeding. They were usually of short duration, about 8 to 15 minutes, and the dive rate averaged 55 meters/minute.[2] Longer dives were exploratory in nature, did not exceed 200 meters in depth, and often involved swimming considerable distances from the site. Such dives occasionally resulted in escape to a distant breathing hole.

Various species of marine mammals are differently adapted for maneuver within the submarine world. All, however, possess in some degree streamlined body contours and specialized appendages for efficient underwater propulsion. Some species, such as the sea lions, fur seals, and some of the smaller cetaceans, are well adapted for tracking down their prey by virtue of acrobatic and fast swimming in relatively short diving times. Some dolphins, for example, can sustain speeds of 20 knots for long periods. Certain other species, such as seals of the family Phocidae (the true or earless seals represented by harbor, Weddell, and elephant seals) and some of the large whales, perform the same feats by diving for very long periods and swimming at relatively slow speed.

Certain physical characteristics of the marine environment and of the diving situation impose conditions upon the submerged marine mannal to which it is fitted by virtue of specific physiological and morphological adaptations. These include sufficient breath-holding time to permit underwater propulsion to great depth. The environmental factors of temperature, light, and pressure determine the features of other adaptations. Most examples here will be drawn from the well-studied phocid seals.

DIVING DURATION

The adaptations that lead to a capability for long, apneic dives have been investigated for more than a century and have received considerable attention in recent years. Success depends largely upon circulatory mechanisms for conservation of oxygen reserves by selective vasoconstriction leading to preferential perfusion of heart and brain.

The resting, nondiving, oxygen consumption of seals and porpoises is generally higher than that of terrestrial animals of comparable size. Therefore they might not be expected to have an advantage in oxygen economy during dives. Some seal species, however, begin a dive with considerably larger oxygen stores than land mammals, mostly in the form of circulating hemoglobin. Greater red cell mass and blood volume combine to increase relative blood oxygen stores by two to three times compared with man. The maximum diving time of a well-trained man is perhaps 2 to 3 minutes, and the comparable time on a single breath for a harbor seal is about 20 minutes and for the Weddell seal, 60 minutes. However, differences in diving time between men and seals do not correspond with the differences in oxygen storage, and it is this inconsistency that requires an explanation.

Cardiovascular Adaptations

It has been known for some time that the cardiovascular system plays a major role in adaptation to diving in marine mammals. Irving and Scholander, some 35 years ago, found that this cardiovascular adaptation amounts to the conservation of stored oxygen by selective vasoconstriction. Over the long period of the dive, oxygen is spared by this mechanism for use mainly by those vital tissues which lack extended anaerobic capability: brain and heart. Simultaneously, there occurs an abrupt and marked slowing of the heart rate, the well-known diving bradycardia. More recently this concept has been verified by direct measurements of blood flow in some major arteries during diving.

Fig. 17-2 shows the results of an experiment on a diving seal. It is clear that the blood flow in major circuits, such as the renal artery and abdominal aorta, falls nearly to zero and remains much reduced throughout the dive. The drastically slowed heart rate is also evident.[3] These changes are among the more profound seen in any physiological state. At the same time, the central arterial blood pressure is maintained remarkably constant.

A probable contributor to the maintenance of arterial blood pressure is a structural adaptation seen in most marine mammals. It consists of an enlargement of the root of the aorta, thick-walled and highly elastic in nature. It can contain approximately the entire stroke volume of the heart, and its stretching in systole presumably stores the kinetic energy of cardiac contraction for the

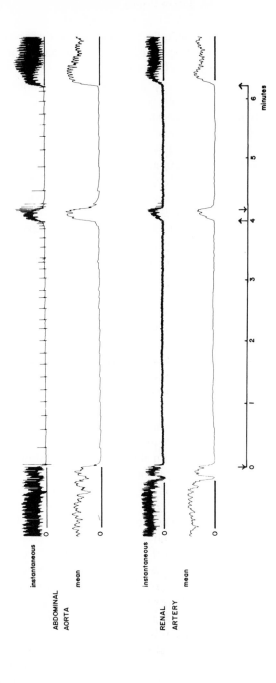

Fig. 17-2. Blood flow in the abdominal aorta and renal artery of a harbor seal in an experimental dive. The animal was surfaced for 10 seconds at 4 minutes and then redived.[3]

later slow expulsion of blood into the constricted arterial tree, which thus maintains pressure during the long diastolic phase. It is now clear that these cardiovascular adaptations are extensions of similar responses demonstrable in a wide variety of other animals, including man, and that they are characteristic of responses to asphyxia.[3]

Venous System

The venous system of phocid seals is remarkable in its special adaptations. The venous drainage from the brain depends only in part upon the jugular veins and passes mainly through a complex venous route lying mostly within the spinal canal. The *extradural intravertebral* vein extends throughout the length of the spinal canal giving off branches via the azygous system to the superior vena cava and having connections also to the inferior vena cava. This latter structure is often bifurcated and considerably enlarged compared to its counterpart in terrestrial species. A large hepatic sinus exists in the inferior vena cava just below the diaphragm. At the diaphragm, it passes through a muscular sphincter.

Several lines of evidence suggest that the venous blood flow returning to the heart is restricted during diving by action of the muscular sphincter. In some recent work, x-ray contrast medium was injected into the inferior vena cava of a seal and its disappearance was watched in subsequent radiographs with and without experimental diving. During the dive, the sphincter constricted, and the rate of disappearance of contrast medium from the inferior vena cava was slowed.[4]

Some Acid-Base Consequences

About 35 years ago, Scholander discovered that during a dive lactic acid accumulated in the ischemic muscle tissues as they converted to anaerobic metabolism but this increased lactate production failed to appear in the circulating blood in any great quantity until after the dive.[5] This finding was one of the first pieces of evidence upon which the concept of selective vasoconstriction was based. While oxygen in circulating arterial blood was depleted by the brain and heart, and to some limited extent by other tissues, carbon dioxide steadily accumulated. The increased circulating hemoglobin characteristic of the seal provides an advantage in buffering the accumulation of hydrogen ions; nonetheless, a steady fall in pH occurs. There is often a further fall in pH immediately after the dive when lactic acid is flushed from the tissues.

Cerebral Tolerance to Hypoxemia

The question arose of what might happen to a seal that was forced to dive for an extremely long period and required to tolerate the accompanying low level of arterial oxygen, increased carbon dioxide, and low blood pH. What little information was available for terrestrial animals suggested that when the arterial partial pressure of oxygen falls to about 20 mm Hg, consciousness can no longer be maintained. The onset of this disturbance of brain function is heralded by characteristic "slow wave" activity in the electroencephalographic pattern.

The electroencephalogram of harbor and Weddell seals during long periods of experimental asphyxia has been recorded. Samples of carotid artery blood were drawn and were analyzed for partial pressures of oxygen and carbon dioxide and for pH. The characteristic EEG changes were seen in these animals only when arterial oxygen pressure was reduced below 10 mm Hg. Changes in CO_2 and pH values had little influence on the end point.[6,7] It was therefore clear that these seals have greater cerebral tolerance for hypoxia than do terrestrial mannals. This evidence also suggested that in some seal divers there may be another explanation for their long diving times in addition to the mechanisms of enhanced oxygen storage and circulatory redistribution.

Anaerobic metabolic processes in the brain of the harbor seal were examined with particular regard to the late stages of a maximum dive. Blood samples were drawn from the arterial circulation and also from the intravertebral vein at the point where it exists from the skull. Blood flow was also measured at that latter site. In the last few minutes of these dives an increased cerebral production of lactic acid was observed. These results indicated that during advanced asphyxial hypoxia the seal brain tolerates a decrease in oxygen consumption, and part of its energy is obtained by anaerobic mechanisms resulting in the production of lactic acid.[7] Although similar events may occur in the brain of terrestrial mammals, it would be difficult to observe them because of the very brief tolerance to asphyxia in those species.

DEEP DIVING

The adverse effects of increased pressure associated with deep diving would be likely to become apparent in the air cavities of the animal. These include the lungs, trachea, middle ear, and other sinuses. If the contents of these gas cavities could not become equilibrated with ambient pressure, the soft tissue structures within and lining them would be subjected to pressure differentials sufficient to produce edema, blood vessel rupture, and other discomfort—a condition familiarly known to human divers as "squeeze."

Marine mammals known to be deep divers have been found to have structural adaptations which afford protection against this condition. Sinus cavities are reduced in size or totally absent in some species. The thorax of many diving mammals is unusually flexible because of the looseness or lack of connection between the ribs and sternum. The extremely oblique location of the diaphragm also contributes to the facility with which equilibration is achieved between ambient hydrostatic pressure and the pressures within the thorax. Tracheal rings of cartilage are incomplete in some diving mammals, and the trachea is flattened and flexible. Most seals dive with a relatively small lung volume, and the residual air during the dive can be contained within the dead space of the major airways. The lungs become almost completely collapsed in deep dives and frequent compression atelectasis and reexpansion appear to be well tolerated.[8] Tissues lining the sinuses of the middle ear contain venous channels which can become filled with blood and thus reduce the volume of the air space.

Bends in Marine Mammals

The diving marine mammal is much less likely to be troubled by decompression sickness than is the human diver with his continuous source of breathing air at ambient, elevated, hydrostatic pressure. However, the rapid changes of pressure that occur during repetitive deep diving could induce the gradual accumulation of nitrogen within tissues with the consequences of bends. Since the blood flow distribution of the apneic diving mammal is restricted mainly to the brain and heart, nitrogen diffusing from the lungs to the blood will be constrained within those parts of the body. Under these circumstances, if all lung nitrogen were absorbed, its resulting tension within the heart and brain could lead to bubble formation.[2]

Attempts have been made to discover special tissue modifications in marine mammals which might limit the absorption of nitrogen or mitigate the effects of its absorption. However, the solubility of nitrogen in seal blood does not differ significantly from that of human blood.[2] Distribution of nitrogen throughout tissues in which it might be preferentially absorbed, as the blubber, can be ruled out because of the widespread peripheral vasoconstriction that takes place during dives. The susceptibility of marine mammals to decompression sickness is not yet entirely clear, although some animals have been accidentally killed in compression experiments in which blood bubble formation has been observed. There remains the possibility that nitrogen may be excluded from the circulation by reducing its absorption from the lungs.

Pulmonary adaptations. Scholander[5] suggested that diving mammals may be protected against bends by displacement of lung air from the easily compressible alveoli into less compressible nonabsorptive airway structures.

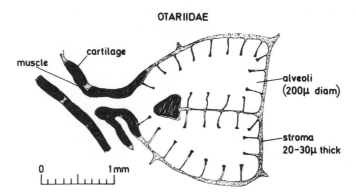

Fig. 17-3.   Diagram of terminal airways and alveoli of sea lion and fur seal lungs.[16]

This concept is favored by the unusual ability of marine mammals to empty their lungs[9] and by the low resistence to flow within their airways.[10] Figure 17-3 shows a diagrammatic sketch of the terminal airways and alveolar structure representative of sea lions and fur seals (family Otariidae). The stiffening of terminal airways suggested by their armored construction, besides aiding lung collapse during dives, is probably helpful in shortening expiration time during brief breathing intervals at the surface. The ratio of dead space to lung volume is large, and the small airways of many marine mammals are reinforced by unusual amounts of cartilage and smooth muscle which extend to the alveoli.[11]

Recent experiments of Kooyman and his co-workers[12] reveal the effectiveness with which nitrogen absorption in blood is prevented in some marine mammals. Harbor seals and elephant seals were compressed in a hydraulic chamber to pressures of up to 28 atm. Nitrogen tensions in arterial and central venous blood remained low, especially in the early stages of compression.

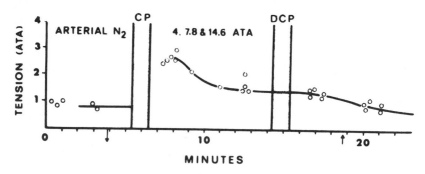

Fig. 17-4.   Nitrogen pressure in arterial blood during deep dives in elephant seals. Compression of two animals to 4, 7.8, and 14.6 ata. Beginning and end of dives indicated by arrows. CP, compression; DCP, decompression.[16]

Figure 17-4 shows the results of experiments in which elephant seals were dived in a pressure chamber. During compressions up to 14.6 ata, arterial blood nitrogen pressure did not exceed 3 ata, which was apparently insufficient to produce bends symptoms under these conditions.

COLD EXPOSURE

A combination of factors determines the need for deep-diving marine mammals to have protective adaptations against cold exposure. The deep body temperature of these species differs little from that of terrestrial mammals. Most marine mammals inhabit cold polar seas for at least a part of their lives, but even tropical oceans, which have relatively warm surface water, are much cooler at depths encountered during dives. In addition, the heat transfer characteristics of water are such as to induce about 25 times greater heat loss than in air of similar temperature.

While man is at a distinct disadvantage thermally, and in other respects, during water immersion, many species of marine mammals live throughout the world's oceans—in especially great concentrations in polar regions—and manage to survive and to thrive throughout lifetimes in cold water. We would do well to examine some of the simple physiological and morphological adaptations which permit such accommodation in a hostile environment for mammalism temperature regulation. All but a very few of the marine mammal species of the world depend upon a thick layer of relatively fixed fat subcutaneous insulation to protect their deep body cores from heat loss to cool water. These species vary enormously in body size, from a few pounds of certain newborn seals to the biggest living creature, the blue whale of 60 or more tons. The polar bear and sea otter do not possess well-developed blubber layers and must depend upon air trapped in their thick fur. Since air is readily compressible, the hydrostatic pressure of moderately deep dives profoundly reduces this layer of insulation and drastically interferes with both diving depth and duration. Some newborn seal species must similarly depend upon their fur for protection until rapid accumulation of subcutaneous fat permits full development of their aquatic behavior. The situation of scuba diving man is very similar to that of the fur-protected mammal. The typical wet suit, while providing suitable protection at the surface, contains air cells that are readily compressed and thereby suffer considerable reduction in insulating quality.

While marine mammals of the world appear generally to need to conserve heat while in water, they may encounter situations when heat dissipation is required. Such might be the case in seals hauled out on sunny beaches. In these conditions, their flippers become warmed by the transfer of heat from deeper structures through the mechanism of increased circulation. Dolphins and whales, as well as seals, have circulatory structures well suited to the ready transfer of blood to their appendages.[13] Those species are also equipped with what appear to be well-engineered countercurrent blood flow structures permitting limited circulation in the appendages while conserving heat. The features of thermal adaptation in marine mammals have been reviewed recently by Irving.[14]

VISION AND NAVIGATION

Deep diving mammals are faced with problems of decreased visibility associated with depth and turbidity, both of which might effect their success in orientation, navigation, and food seeking. There is anatomical evidence for both specialized sensory apparatus for echo location, as well as for adaptations in structure and function of visual components to compensate for conditions of reduced light.[1,15]

Consider the navigational problems to be solved by a Weddell seal finding its way back in dim light or darkness to a breathing hole a few inches in diameter, under sea ice several feet thick, after an exploratory excursion of 30 minutes, from a distance of perhaps 2 miles (swimming speed about 5 knots). Consider further that the seal at some point had to make the decision to turn back toward the breathing hole in order not to exceed the half-time of its diving time! Clearly, it possesses specialized sensing and navigating equipment which we might well envy.

REFERENCES

1. Kooyman GL, Andersen HT: Deep diving, in Andersen HT (ed): The Biology of Marine Mammals. New York and London, Academic Press, 1969, p 65-92
2. Kooyman GL: Deep diving behavior and effects of pressure in reptiles, birds and mammals. Symp Soc Exp Biol 26:295-311, 1972
3. Elsner R, Franklin DL, Van Citters RL, Kenney DW: Cardiovascular defense against asphyxia. Science 153:941-949, 1966
4. Elsner R, Hanafee WN, Hammond DD: Angiography of the inferior vena cava of the harbor seal during simulated diving. Am J Physiol 220:1155-1157, 1971
5. Scholander PF: Experimental investigations on the respiratory function in diving mammals and birds. Hvalrad Skr 22:1-131, 1940
6. Elsner R, Shurley JT, Hammond DD, Brooks RE: Cerebral tolerance to hypoxemia in asphyxiated Weddell seals. Respir Physiol 9:287-297, 1970
7. Kerem D, Elsner R: Cerebral tolerance to asphyxial hypoxia in the harbor seal. Respir Physiol 19:188-200, 1973
8. Kooyman GL, Hammond DD, Schroeder JP: Bronchograms and tracheograms of seals under pressure. Science 169:82-84, 1970
9. Irving L, Scholander PF, Grinnell SW: The respiration of the porpoise, *Tursiops truncatus.* J Cell Comp Physiol 17:145-168, 1941

0. Olsen CR, Hale FC, Elsner R: Mechanics of ventilation in the pilot whale. Respir Physiol 7:137-149, 1969
1. Denison DM, Kooyman GL: The structure and function of the small airways in pinniped and sea otter lungs. Respir Physiol 17:1-10, 1973
2. Kooyman GL, Schroeder JP, Denison DM, et al: Blood nitrogen tensions of seals during simulated deep dives. Am J Physiol 223: 1016-1020, 1972
3. Elsner R, Pirie J, Kenney DW, Schemmer S: Functional circulatory anatomy of cetacean appendages, in Harrison RJ (ed): Functional Anatomy of Marine Mammals, vol 2. New York and London, Academic Press, 1974, p 143-159
4. Irving L: Aquatic mammals, in Whittow C (ed): Comparative Physiology of Thermoregulation, vol 3. New York and London, Academic Press, 1973, p 47-95
5. Norris KS: The echolocation of marine mammals, in Andersen HT (ed): The Biology of Marine Mammals. New York and London, Academic Press, 1969, p 391-421
6. Kooyman GL: Respiratory adaptations in marine mammals. Am Zool 13:457-468, 1973

STUDY QUESTIONS

1. Among seals, dive duration is extended, to some degree, by
   a. Greater red cell mass
   b. Greater blood volume
   c. Greater tolerance to tissue hypoxia
   d. Selective vasoconstriction
   e. All of the above
2. During a dive, which of the following organs remain(s) well perfused?
   a. Brain
   b. Kidney
   c. Heart
   d. a and c above
   e. All of the above
3. During a dive, lactic acid rises considerably in the circulating blood.
   a. True
   b. False
4. Diving mammals do not get "lung squeeze" because
   a. They inspire deeply before a dive
   b. The thorax collapses readily
   c. All airways collapse readily
   d. All of the above
5. Diving mammals do not get the bends because
   a. Alveoli collapse and air is pushed into airways where it is not absorbed by blood

  b. Nitrogen from the lungs is preferentially absorbed by subcutaneous fat

  c. The solubility of nitrogen in their blood is less than that of terrestrial mammals.

6. The core temperature of diving mammals remains high because

  a. They are insulated either by subcutaneous fat or air trapped within fur

  b. They swim only in warm water

  c. Countercurrent blood flow to appendages helps to decrease heat loss

  d. The skin is highly perfused during swimming

  e. a and c above

  f. All of the above

Suk Ki Hong

18
The Physiology of Breath-Hold Diving

There are perhaps millions of people in this world who are engaged in amateur breath-hold dives for recreation. They are usually equipped with a face mask (or goggles) and a snorkel and dive to a shallow depth for a short period of time. On the other hand, there are many thousands of professional divers who dive to deeper depths for a longer period for certain underwater activities. The latter group includes Navy divers, women divers of Korea (Hae-Nyo) and Japan (Ama), sponge divers in Greece, and pearl divers in the Tuamotu Archipelago. These divers learned the art of diving through many years of hard training, in order to increase both the depth of diving and the bottom time with minimal risks. In fact, they attracted considerable interest from many physiologists during the last 20 years and contributed extensively to the understanding of the physiology of breath-hold diving.

Unlike in the case of a scuba (self-contained underwater breathing apparatus) diver, a breath-hold diver can afford to stay under water usually for less than 2 minutes. During such a short period of diving time, however, profound changes in certain physiological functions take place. This chapter will mainly deal with the changes in cardio-respiratory functions and the potential hazards associated with breath-hold diving. Because of the high thermal conductivity of water, the body heat balance is also disturbed if the water temperature is below thermoneutral level (about 35°C or 95°F). However, various physiological problems directly associated with the regulation of body temperature in water will not be dealt with in this chapter, but are referred to in Chapter 15.

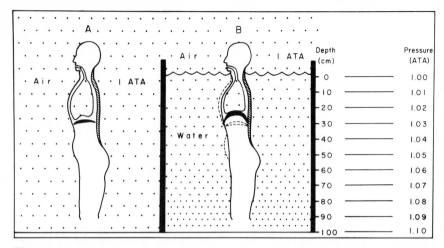

Fig. 18-1.   Distribution of pressure surrounding a man (A) standing in air and (B) immersed in water to the neck. The density of dots reflects the magnitude of pressure. The broken curves over the chest and below the diaphragm in (B) indicate the positions of the chest wall and the diaphragm standing in air.

EFFECTS OF IMMERSION IN WATER TO THE NECK

A breath-hold dive is usually preceded by immersion of the body in water to the neck (head-out immersion). In fact, average breath-hold divers are likely to spend more time floating on the water surface (i.e., immersed to the neck) than totally submerged underwater. It is, therefore, important to recognize some of the important physiological changes attendant to immersion to the neck.

When a person is in air, the pressure surrounding the body is no different from one region to another, and is equal to the pressure within the lungs (see Fig. 18-1A). This is no longer true in the case of immersion up to the neck. As illustrated in Figure 18-1B, the body below the neck is now under the influence of the atmospheric pressure (1 ata), plus the hydrostatic pressure which is directly proportional to the vertical distance from the water surface. Thus, the pressure distribution over the body is no longer uniform. Since the subject still keeps his head above the water and breathes the outside air, the intrapulmonary pressure must be equal to 1 ata. Consequently, the subject is forced to engage in "negative pressure breathing." Since the hydrostatic pressure level over the chest is not uniform, it is not easy to calculate exactly the degree of this negative pressure breathing. By studying the magnitude of the shift in the relaxation pressure (or the total respiratory pressure) observed during head-out immersion, the degree of negative pressure breathing was estimated to be approximately 20 cm H_2O[1].

Primarily due to this intrapulmonary negative pressure, coupled with a greater compression of the abdomen by the hydrostatic pressure, the expiratory reserve volume decreases by about 70 percent during head-out immersion as compared to standing in air.[1-3] In contrast, the vital capacity decreases relatively less during immersion,[3, 4] which indicates an increase in the inspiratory capacity. Several investigators also found a slight, but significant, reduction in residual volume,[2, 4] which they attribute to an increase in the intrathoracic blood volume (see following discussion). More importantly, Hong et al.[1] observed a 60 percent increase in the work (both elastic and dynamic) of breathing during immersion, which is partly due to an increase in the nonelastic airway resistance reported by Agostoni et al.[2]

The end-expiratory intrathoracic pressure, estimated by measurement of the intraesophageal pressure, increases slightly from approximately $- 5$ cm H_2O while standing in air to $- 2$ cm H_2O during immersion.[2, 5] On the other hand, the abdominal pressure below the diaphragm, estimated by the intragastric pressure minus 11 cm H_2O, increases greatly from $- 6$ cm H_2O in air to $+ 12$ cm H_2O during immersion.[2, 5] These findings indicate an increase in the transdiaphragmatic pressure from nearly zero in air to 14 cm H_2O during immersion. Since venous return is determined by this pressure gradient between the extra- and intrathoracic regions, such an increase in the transdiaphragmatic pressure during immersion is likely to increase venous return. This facilitation of venous return during immersion is further aided by the high density of water which eliminates the usual blood pooling in the peripheral veins in air. (In this respect, a state of immersion in water is analogous to a gravity-free state.) Moreover, the temperature of water in which divers are immersed is usually much lower than thermoneutral (35°C or 95°F), e.g., 26°C or 80°F even in subtropical Hawaii; hence, one would expect a strong peripheral vasoconstriction in water. This would also bring about a further increase in the central blood volume at the expense of the peripheral volume.

The magnitude of the increase in the intrathoracic blood volume during head-out immersion has been indirectly estimated to be in the order of 500 ml.[1, 6] Recently, Arborelius et al.,[6] using a dye-dilution technique, reported a 30 percent increase in the cardiac output and stroke volume during immersion in 34°C water. The same authors also reported an increase in the right atrial pressure from $- 2$ mm Hg in air to $+ 16$ mm Hg during immersion, which reflects an increase in venous return. The latter observation suggests that the heart (and the intrathoracic blood vessels) is distended as a result of the pronounced blood shift, and may be under considerable strain. Fortunately, however, an excessive congestion of the heart during immersion is prevented because of the collapse of the large veins as they enter the chest.[7]

The increase in the intrathoracic blood volume appears to be responsible for so-called immersion diuresis. In a hydropenic subject, the urine flow increases by four-to fivefold during immersion; however, the osmolal clearance increases only slightly, if at all. These results are consistent with a hypothesis that inhibition of antidiuretic hormone (ADH) due to stimulation of volume receptors in the wall of the left atrium is responsible for this diuresis.[8] Recent studies by Epstein et al.[9] and Kurata et al. (unpublished) in the author's laboratory indeed proved this hypothesis to be correct. Interestingly enough the immersion diuresis also appears to be partly due to inhibition of the renin-aldosterone system.[10] At any rate, one would expect a varying degree of dehydration depending upon the duration of immersion. Another important consequence of this increase in intrathoracic circulation during immersion has been reported recently by Balldin and Lundgren.[11] They found that immersion (especially in warm water) enhances the rate of nitrogen elimination during oxygen breathing, which may have some bearing on the risk of decompression sickness.

As mentioned earlier, the abdomen is compressed to a greater degree as compared to the chest during head-out immersion. According to Johnson et al.[5] in the author's laboratory, the intragastric pressure at the end of normal expiration increases from + 5 mm Hg in air to + 20 mm Hg during immersion, while the intraesophageal pressure at the superior limit of the distal esophageal sphincter increases from − 1 to only + 4 mm Hg. Hence, the gastroesophageal pressure gradient increases from 6 mm Hg in air to 16 mm Hg during immersion, thus predisposing the subject to gastric reflux. In fact pyrosis and regurgitation of gastric contents have been reported by some swimmers. However, in normal subjects who have a competent distal esophageal sphincter, the sphincter pressure also increases by 13 mm Hg during immersion, so that there is no danger of reflux. Drugs that diminish distal esophageal sphincter pressure, and thus its competency, should be avoided during immersion. Individuals with severe gastroesophageal reflux may be at risk from aspiration of gastric contents with occupation or recreation involving water immersion.

In summary, a person immersed in water to the neck is subjected to a reduction in the functional residual capacity, an increased work of breathing, an increase in the intrathoracic (including the heart) blood volume, and dehydration, and, in addition, is predisposed to gastric reflux.

ALVEOLAR GAS EXCHANGES DURING BREATH-HOLD DIVING

The basic pattern of alveolar gas exchange during a breath-hold dive is quite different from that during simple breath-holding in air. This is due to the fact that the diver undergoes compression during descent, followed by decompression during ascent. Well-trained professional divers hyperventilate

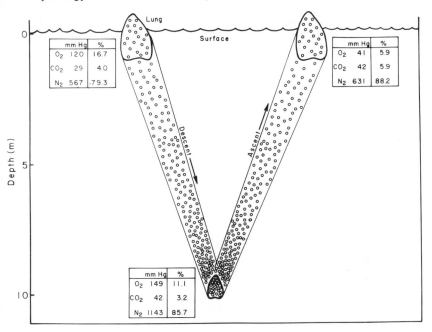

Fig. 18-2. Alveolar gas composition (%) and pressures immediately before descent (upper left), on the bottom, and immediately after returning to the water surface (upper right). Note a progressive reduction in the lung volume coupled with an increase in the gas density (or pressure) during descent, which are reversed during ascent. (Data on the alveolar gas are from Hong et al.[12])

mildly, take a deep breath (a lung volume equivalent to about 80 percent of the vital capacity), close the glottis, and then start a descent. The composition of alveolar gas at this point is given in Figure 18-2, along with that at depth (10 m or 30 feet) and upon return to the surface. These values are taken from studies on Ama during actual diving in the ocean.[12]

Typically, the alveolar gas at the very beginning of dive is composed of 4 percent CO_2 (P_{CO_2} = 29 mm Hg), 17 percent O_2 (P_{O_2} = 120 mm Hg), and 79 percent N_2 (P_{N_2} = 567 mm Hg), which is only slightly different from the normal composition. During descent, the lung volume decreases due to compression of the chest, which results in increases of partial pressures of O_2, CO_2, and N_2. Since the gas pressures of the mixed venous blood should not change during the first 20 seconds (circulation time) of compression, one would expect diffusion of all three gases from the alveolus to the blood. As shown in Figure 18-2, the concentrations of both O_2 and CO_2 of the alveolar gas obtained when the diver reached the bottom are considerably lower than the corresponding values at the beginning of dive, which reflects a net transfer of these gases from the alveolus to the blood. The alveolar concentration of

N_2 on the bottom is slightly higher than that before descent, despite the fact that N_2 must also be removed from the alveolus to the blood during descent. This is attributed to a much faster rate of diffusion of CO_2 and O_2 as compared to N_2, which has a very low solubility in blood plasma. As a result of rapid removal of O_2 and CO_2 during compression, the alveolar concentration of N_2 progressively increases during descent.

It is important to note that the P_{O_2} of alveolar gas on the bottom is as high as 150 mm Hg, which assures an adequate delivery of O_2 to the blood. In other words, as long as the diver is on the bottom, there is a sufficient P_{O_2} gradient between the alveolus and blood to maintain a continuous diffusion of O_2 into the blood.

Normally, CO_2 is transferred from the blood to the lungs. As just stated, this direction of CO_2 transfer is reversed during descent because the alveolar P_{CO_2} becomes greater than the mixed venous blood P_{CO_2} due to compression of the chest. Therefore, large amounts of CO_2 are retained in the blood with a resultant increase in P_{CO_2}. It is interesting to note that the P_{CO_2} of the arterial blood is now greater than that of mixed venous blood, as long as CO_2 is diffusing into the blood. It is this retention of CO_2, with attendant increase in P_{CO_2} of the blood, that gives the signal to the diver to return to the surface.

Once the diver leaves the bottom for the surface, the lungs will expand rapidly due to decompression. Consequently, the alveolar P_{O_2} decreases progressively, thus continuously decreasing the diffusion gradient for O_2. As shown in Figure 18-2, the alveolar concentration of O_2 at the time of return to the surface is only 6 percent, with P_{O_2} of 42 mm Hg. The latter value is equal to the P_{O_2} of the mixed venous blood, which indicates that there is no diffusion gradient for O_2 between the alveolus and the blood at this point, and thus the diver is in a critical state of hypoxia. In fact, the normal direction of O_2 transfer could be completely reversed during ascent if the diver stayed on the bottom longer. Such a reversal of O_2 transfer has indeed been demonstrated.[13] CO_2 retained in the blood during descent (and on the bottom) now leaves the blood for the lungs as alveolar P_{CO_2} decreases continuously during ascent and a favorable diffusion gradient between the blood and the alveolus is re-established. However, not all CO_2 retained in the blood during descent (and on the bottom) is eliminated into the lungs during ascent, and the process of excess CO_2 elimination continues even after the return to the surface. A small amount of N_2 that entered the circulation and tissue during descent and on the bottom will also leave slowly, according to the reversed diffusion gradient.

The pattern of alveolar gas exchange during a breath-hold dive as described thus far is distinctly different from that during simple breath-holding in air. In the latter case, the alveolar P_{O_2} decreases continuously during breath-holding,[14] but is higher than that at the end of a breath-hold dive of comparable duration.[12] This is due to the faster removal of alveolar O_2 during

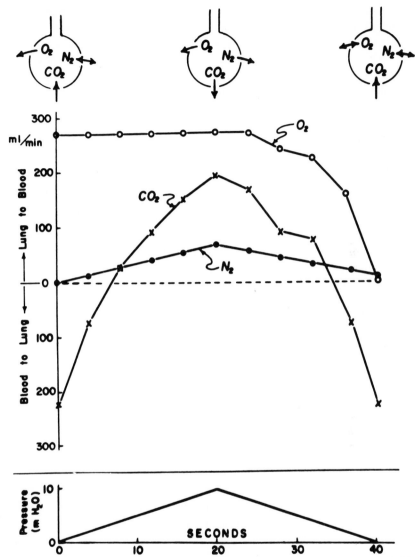

Fig. 18-3.   The rate of alveolar O_2, CO_2, and N_2 exchange during a breath-hold dive to 10 meters (Graph from Hong et al.[12])

descent and on the bottom. Even during simple breath-holding in air, there is a theoretical possibility that the direction of CO_2 transfer could be reversed, but the amount of CO_2 transferred in the reverse direction is much less than that during a breath-hold dive.

Since the amount of N_2 transferred from the alveolus to the circulation during a breath-hold dive is very small, there is no real danger for developing decompression sickness. However, it is theoretically possible to accumulate enough N_2 if the diver repetitively dives to considerable depths with very short surface intervals. In fact, Paulev, by making about 60 breath-hold dives to 20 meters in 5 hours, developed what appeared to be decompression sickness. Each dive lasted about 2.5 minutes with surface intervals of less than 2 minutes. He reports: "During the last two hours I had progressive symptoms of nausea, dizziness . . . . Within one-half an hour after the end of the diving, I got pains in the left hip joint . . . . Two hours after the end of the diving, severe chest pains began. The paresthesia developed in the right hand together with blurring of vision. Three hours after the diving, a colleague found me markedly pale and exhausted as in impending shock . . . . As the symptoms were in progress, I was placed in the recompression chamber. At 6 ATA I felt an immediate relief with regard to the dizziness and nausea. In a few minutes the bends and the partial paresis had disappeared . . . ."[15] The pearl divers of the Tuamotu Archipelago make repetitive dives to a depth of 30-40 meters (each dive lasting about 1.5-2.5 minutes) for about 6 hours a day during the diving season, and 10-30 percent of divers are known to develop what they call "Taravana" (*tara*, to fall; *vana*, crazily) by the end of the day. "Taravana" symptoms include vertigo, nausea, partial or complete paralysis, temporary unconsciousness, and in extreme cases, death.[16] Although the etiology of "Taravana" is not fully understood, many diving scientists suspect that it may be related to the retention of N_2.

A seemingly complicated pattern of alveolar gas exchange during a breath-hold dive may be summarized as follows: The transfer of O_2 from the lungs to the blood is not disturbed until ascent starts. It is during this ascending phase that the diver could run into a critical state of hypoxia. The normal direction of CO_2 transfer from the lungs to the blood is reversed during descent and on the bottom which results in a significant retention of CO_2 in the blood (hypercapnia). During ascent, the retained CO_2 is transferred to the lungs. A small amount of N_2 also enters the circulation during the descent, which is reversed during ascent. Based on certain assumptions, the rate of alveolar exchange of O_2, CO_2, and N_2 during a breath-hold dive to 10 meters has been calculated[12] and is shown in Figure 18-3.

DANGER OF EXCESSIVE HYPERVENTILATION BEFORE DIVING

Approximately 7000 deaths by drowning occur yearly in the United States. If we knew the events leading to drowning, lives could be saved. By interviewing swimmers who lost consciousness underwater, but somehow survived, Craig was able to reconstruct events possibly contributing to drowning.[17, 18] He noted that all of the survivors hyperventilated before going underwater and also that the swimmers usually noted the urge to breathe, but had little or no warning that he was going to "pass out." Most of these survivors also stated that they had some goal in mind, or were in competition with others. Based on this and other information, Craig concluded that a combination of hyperventilation, breath-holding, and exercise could lead to loss of consciousness.

Most underwater (breath-hold) swimmers have learned that hyperventilation will increase their breath-holding time. The rate of elimination of CO_2 from the body increases as a function of ventilation and, in fact, the alveolar P_{CO_2} (and hence arterial blood P_{CO_2}) is inversely proportional to the alveolar ventilation. Therefore, it will take a longer time for blood P_{CO_2} to reach a breaking point when breath-holding is preceded by excessive hyperventilation, which thereby extends the breath-holding time. However, one has to remember that any extension of breath-holding time is associated with a further reduction in blood P_{O_2}. It is true that hyperventilation slightly increases the level of alveolar and arterial P_{O_2}. However, this does not appreciably increase the blood O_2 content because the oxyhemoglobin saturation in the arterial blood is almost 100 percent during normal ventilation, with the arterial P_{O_2} being 100 mm Hg. Therefore, the rate of fall in blood P_{O_2} during breath-holding is about the same with or without preparatory hyperventilation. This is why the alveolar (or arterial blood) P_{O_2} at the breath-hold breaking point is lower with preliminary hyperventilation than without (Table 18-1).

In the case of breath-holding with air at 1 ata, the subject terminates breath-holding as a result of increased P_{CO_2} coupled with reduced P_{O_2}. In general, the respiratory center (or chemoreceptors) is far more sensitive to a rise in P_{CO_2} than to a fall in P_{O_2}. However, when the level of P_{O_2} in the blood decreases to about 50 mm Hg, the ventilation begins to increase rapidly, indicating that the respiratory center is stimulated. On the other hand, in case of breath-holding with O_2 at 1 ata, the breath-holding is terminated by the high P_{CO_2} alone because P_{O_2} of the blood does not decrease to 50 mm Hg. Therefore, one can hold a breath longer, with a greater accumulation of CO_2, following O_2 breathing than air breathing.

A situation similar to breath-holding with O_2 exists during breath-hold diving. While the diver stays on the bottom with a breath held, the urge to breathe (or the signal to return to the surface) will come almost solely from the high P_{CO_2} of blood, since the blood P_{O_2} level is maintained high due to compression. Until the P_{CO_2} reaches a critical level, the diver will stay on the bottom and continuously consume O_2. By then, the diver has barely enough O_2 in the body to return to the surface, as indicated by a very low alveolar P_{O_2} at the end of the dive (see Fig. 18-2). When a dive preceded by vigorous hyperventilation, the initial level of blood P_{CO_2} is lowered; hence, the diver can certainly stay longer on the bottom before the P_{CO_2} level increases to a critical

Table 18-1

Effects of Hyperventilation on the Breath-Holding (BH) Time and Alveolar Gas Pressure at the Breaking Point in Resting and Exercising Man.[18]

Measurements	Resting		Exercising	
	Without hyperventilation	With hyperventilation	Without hyperventilation	With hyperventilation
BH time (sec)	87	146	62	85
End-tidal P_{CO_2} (mm Hg)				
Before BH	40	21	38	22
Breaking point	51	46	54	49
End-tidal P_{O_2} (mm Hg)				
Before BH	103	131	102	130
Breaking point	73	58	54	43

level. However, remember that the diver's O_2 store in the body is essentially the same with or without vigorous hyperventilation. Therefore, while the diver succeeds in extending the bottom time, the valuable O_2 store is further depleted, thus endangering the safe return to the surface!

The situation just described is further aggravated if the diver is engaged in strenuous activity. It has been shown by many investigators that the level of P_{CO_2} at the breath-hold breaking point is higher during exercise than at rest (Table 18-1). This means that the exercising diver could further extend the bottom time. Since the rate of O_2 consumption increases with exercise, the diver would further deplete the valuable O_2 store more rapidly during this period of extended bottom time. One can, therefore, visualize the occurrence of critical hypoxia leading to loss of consciousness or even to death, when a breath-hold dive is combined with vigorous preparatory hyperventilation and a high rate of O_2 consumption.

CARDIOVASCULAR CHANGES DURING BREATH-HOLD DIVING

More than a century ago, Paul Bert of France observed pronounced bradycardia during diving in the duck. Since then, the same phenomenon has been observed in all diving animals. According to Irving and Scholander, this bradycardia is a reflex phenomenon which is accompanied by an intense peripheral vasoconstriction, a drastic reduction in the cardiac output, and a significant reduction in O_2 consumption. In other words, this reflex serves to extend the duration of a breath-hold dive.[19, 20]

Human breath-hold divers also show a distinct bradycardia during dives.[21, 22] As shown in Figure 18-4, the heart rate begins to decrease with the onset of the dive, and finally reaches a minimal level in 20-30 seconds. Usually, the lowest heart rate during a breath-hold dive is equivalent to 60-70 percent of the predive level. Figure 18-4 also indicates that the same heart rate response is observed even during a breath-hold surface swim or a simple breath-hold whole-body immersion at the water surface. Evidently, the response is independent of pressure or physical exercise. In fact, it has been shown subsequently that a breath-hold immersion of the face alone gives rise to the same bradycardial response observed during an actual breath-hold dive,[20] and hence most of the current knowledge on diving bradycardia in man is derived from such face immersion studies.

As in the case of diving mammals, the diving bradycardia in man is also associated with intensive peripheral vasoconstriction.[23, 24] It is, however, generally agreed that the observed bradycardia is not directly coupled to vasoconstriction.[23, 25] The most interesting aspect of diving bradycardia in man is its dependence on the water temperature. Regardless of whether one is

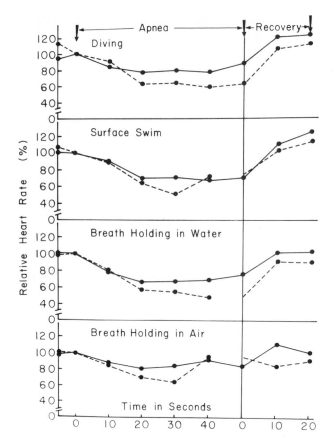

Fig. 18-4.   Relative changes in the heart rate during various breath-hold maneuvers in summer (solid lines; water temperature, 27°C) and winter (broken lines; water temperature, 10°C). (From Hong et al.[21])

engaged in actual breath-hold diving or breath-hold face immersion, the degree of bradycardia increases with the decrease in water temperature.[23, 26] However, the relationship between the two variables is not linear, and it is only when the water temperature is below 15°C (59°F) that the degree of bradycardia increases linearly with the reduction in temperature. Moreover, the degree of bradycardia observed during breath-hold face immersion is the same as that during breath-hold whole-body immersion in water of comparable temperature.[27] These findings indicate that the cutaneous cold receptors on the face play a very important role in the development of diving bradycardia. Although some investigators claim that the nasal region is involved in this mechanism, others failed to confirm such findings. The lung volume at the onset of breath-hold face immersion is also known to alter the degree of bra-

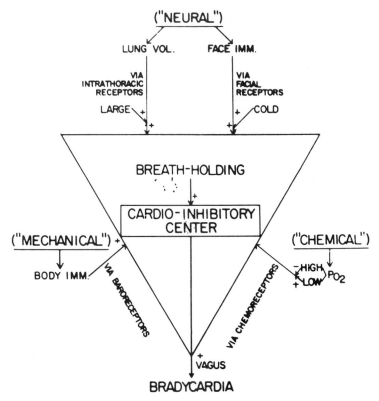

Fig. 18-5.   Schematic model of factors modifying apneic bradycardia: + indicates potentiation; − indicates attenuation of bradycardial responses. Triangle symbolizes the different types of stimuli modifying the basic bradycardia accompanying apnea, per se. (From Moore et al.[30])

dycardia.[23] However, its mechanism is entirely unknown.

A mechanical theory has been proposed by Craig[28, 29] as the alternative to the neural theory just described. This theory is based on the observation that the degree of bradycardia during breath-hold face immersion increases with a decrease in the intrathoracic pressure, and vice versa. This finding has been interpreted to mean that the venous return increases with a decrease in the intrathoracic pressure, which, in turn, decreases the heart rate through a baroreflex mechanism. Undoubtedly, this mechanism is involved in determining the degree of bradycardia, but cannot be considered the sole mechanism for diving bradycardia because the degree of bradycardia can be still manipulated by changing the face immersion water temperature without changing the intrathoracic pressure.[23]

Recently, a chemical factor has been added to the mechanism. Moore *et al.*[29] in the author's laboratory observed that the degree of bradycardia is significantly attenuated when a breath-hold face immersion is preceded by a single breath of pure O_2. Other studies[27] carried out in this laboratory also support the same conclusion. Curiously, however, these investigations failed to show any effect of high P_{CO_2}.

The current state of the art concerning the mechanism of diving bradycardia is schematically illustrated in Figure 18-5. The bradycardia is triggered by the act of breath-holding which, through unknown mechanisms, activates the cardioinhibitory center in the central nervous system and then the vagus nerve. This basic response to breath-holding is subject to either potentiation or attenuation by neural, mechanical, and chemical factors.

Unlike in the diving animals, arterial blood pressure seems to increase while cardiac output decreases only slightly during breath-hold face immersion in man.[26, 31] Moreover, there is no convincing evidence to indicate that there is an O_2 conserving mechanism operating in man during breath-hold diving.

One of the most intriguing findings with regard to diving medicine is the occurrence of cardiac arrhythmias during breath-hold diving. This is also in contrast to diving animals who display a marked bradycardia, but never show any cardiac arrhythmias during diving. In man, it is common to find various types of arrhythmias even during simple breath-holding. Interestingly enough, the incidence of cardiac arrhythmias during diving also increases significantly when the water temperature is low. In a study conducted on Korean women divers,[21] the incidence of cardiac arrhythmias (e.g., abnormal P waves and nodal rhythms, idioventricular rhythms, premature atrial beats, and premature ventricular beats) is 43 percent in the summer (water temperature of 27°C or 81°F), as compared to 72 percent in the winter (water temperature of 10°C or 50°F). It thus appears that diving in cold water is associated with a greater bradycardia and a higher incidence of cardiac arrhythmias. To what extent these changes contribute to fatal diving accidents is yet to be determined.

MAXIMAL DEPTH OF BREATH-HOLD DIVING

Until recently, it was thought that lung volume decreases continuously during descent until it is reduced to residual volume. It was felt that further reduction would cause lung squeeze, and the theoretical maximal depth of a breath-hold dive was the depth at which the lung volume is reduced to the residual volume. For instance, if a diver has a residual volume of 1.5 liters and his total lung capacity is 6.0 liters, Boyle's law tells us that the lung volume will be reduced to the residual volume at a depth of 30 meters (100 feet or 4 ata).

Recently, however, several divers far exceeded the limit calculated on the basis of the total lung capacity (TLC)/residual volume (RV) ratio. For instance, Jacques Mayol whose TLC and RV are, respectively, 7.22 and 1.88 liters, dived to a depth of 231 feet. If one assumes that he started the dive with TLC, then the theoretical maximal depth of dive was 27 meters or 90 feet (TLC/RV = 7.22/1.88 = 3.7 ata or 27 meters). Another example may be found in Robert Croft, a U.S. Navy diver, who dived 240 feet despite his TLC/RV ratio of 7.0 (= 9.1/1.3). These records raise questions about the validity of the generally held notion that the maximal depth of a breath-hold dive is determined by TLC/RV ratio. There must be additional factors to be considered.

As discussed earlier in this chapter, the intrathoracic blood volume increases during immersion in water to the neck. Although the issue is not completely settled, several investigators[2, 4] reported a significant reduction in the residual volume during immersion. If indeed the residual volume decreases during either head-out immersion or breath-hold diving, one would expect a substantial increase in the TLC/RV ratio. For instance, in the case of Jacques Mayol, if the intrathoracic blood volume increased by 1.0 liter during diving, his residual volume would be reduced from 1.88 to 0.88 liters, thereby increasing the TLC/RV ratio to 8.2 (= 7.22/0.88) and the maximal depth to 72 meters (or 230 feet). In other words, his record depth of 231 feet can be accounted for by an 1.0 liter increase in the intrathoracic blood volume. The most crucial question is, therefore, "Does the intrathoracic blood volume increase by 1.0 liter during diving?"

There is at least one report related to this question. Schaeffer et al.[32] estimated the thoracic blood volume during the open-sea dives to 130 feet, by using the impedance plethysmograph, and found that about 1 liter of blood was forced into the thorax. Other evidence for this shift of blood into the thorax during breath-hold diving has been published by Craig.[33] He asked the subject (RV = 2.0 liters) to fully expire and to dive. Surprisingly, the subject dived to a depth of 4.75 meters without developing a significant difference between the ambient pressure at depth and the intrathoracic pressure. These results indicated to him that the subject's RV must have been compressed from 2.0 liters at the surface to 1.4 liters at depth; also, this change of 0.6 liters could be due to a shift of blood from the peripheral to the central circulation.

These findings indicate that the TLC/RV ratio increases during the dive due to a reduction of RV associated with an increase in the intrathoracic blood volume; hence, the diver can reach a depth considerably deeper than that predicted by the TLC/RV ratio determined at the surface.

REFERENCES

1. Hong SK, Cerretelli P, Cruz JC, et al: Mechanics of respiration during submersion in water. J Appl Physiol 27:537-538, 1969
2. Agostoni E, Gurtner G, Torri G, et al: Respiratory mechanics during submersion and negative pressure breathing. J Appl Physiol 21:251-248, 1966
3. Hong SK, Ting EY, Rahn H: Lung volumes at different depths of submersion. J Appl Physiol 15:550-553, 1960
4. Craig AB Jr, Ware DE: Effect of immersion in water on vital capacity and residual volume of the lungs. J Appl Physiol 23:423-425, 1967
5. Johnson LF, Lin YC, Hong SK: Gastroesophageal dynamics during immersion in water to the neck. J Appl Physiol 38:449-454, 1975
6. Arborelius M, Balldin UI, Lilja B, et al: Hemodynamic changes in man during immersion with the head above water. Aerosp Med 43:592-598, 1972
7. Rahn H: The physiological stresses of the Ama, in Rahn H (ed): Physiology of Breath-Hold Diving and the Ama of Japan. National Association of Science, National Research Council Publ 1341, 1965, pp 113-138
8. Gauer OH, Henry JP, Sieker HO, et al: The effect of negative pressure breathing on urine flow. J Clin Invest 33:287-296, 1954
9. Epstein M, Pins D, Miller M: Suppression of ADH by water immersion in normal man. Physiologist 17:218, 1974
10. Epstein M, Saruta T: Effect of water immersion on renin-aldosterone and renal sodium handling in normal man. J Appl Physiol 31:368-374, 1971
11. Balldin UI, Lundgren CEG: Effects of immersion with the head above the water on tissue nitrogen elimination in man. Aerosp Med 43:1101-1108, 1972
12. Hong SK, Rahn H, Kang DH, et al: Diving pattern, lung volumes, and alveolar gas of the Korean diving women (Ama). J Appl Physiol 18:457-465, 1963
13. Lanphier EH, Rahn H: Alveolar gas exchange during breath holding with air. J Appl Physiol 18:478-482, 1963
14. Hong SK, Lin YC, Lally DA, et al: Alveolar gas exchanges and cardiovascular functions during breath holding with air. J Appl Physiol 30:540-547, 1971
15. Paulev P: Decompression sickness following repeated breath-hold dives, in Rahn H (ed): Physiology of Breath-Hold Diving and The Ama of Japan. National Association of Science, National Research Council, Publ 1341, 1965 pp 221-226
16. Cross ER: Taravana-Diving syndrome in the Tuamotu diver, in Rahn H (ed): Physiology of Breath-Hold Diving and the Ama of Japan. National Association Science, National Research Council, Publ 1341, 1965, pp 207-219
17. Craig AB Jr: Underwater swimming and loss of consciousness. JAMA 176:255-258, 1961
18. Craig AB Jr: Causes of loss of consciousness during underwater swimming. J Appl Physiol 16:583-586, 1961
19. Irving L, Scholander PF, Grinnel SW: The regulation of arterial blood pressure in the seal during diving. Am J Physiol 135:557-566, 1942
20. Scholander PF: Physiological adaptation to diving in animals and man. Harvey Lect 57:93-110, 1961-62
21. Hong SK, Song SH, Kim PK, et al: Seasonal observations on the cardiac rhythm

during diving in the Korean Ama. J Appl Physiol 23:18-22, 1967

22. Scholander PF, Hammel HT, LeMessurier H, et al: Circulatory adjustment in pearl divers. J Appl Physiol 17:184-190, 1962
23. Song SH, Lee WK, Chung YA, et al: Mechanism of apneic bradycardia in man. J Appl Physiol 27:323-327, 1969
24. Brick I: Circulatory responses to immersing the face in water. J Appl Physiol 21:33-36, 1966
25. Murdaugh HV Jr, Cross CE, Millen JE, et al: Dissociation of bradycardia and arterial constriction during diving in the seal *Phoca vitulina.* Science 162:364-365, 1968
26. Kawakami Y, Natelson BH, DuBois AB: Cardiovascular effects of face immersion and factors affecting diving reflex in man. J Appl Physiol 23:964-970, 1967
27. Moore TO, Lin YC, Lally DA, et al: Effects of temperature, immersion, and ambient pressure on human apneic bradycardia. J Appl Physiol 33:36-41, 1972
28. Craig AB Jr: Heart rate responses to apneic underwater diving and to breath holding in man. J Appl Physiol 18:854-862, 1963
29. Craig AB Jr: Effects of submersion and pulmonary mechanics on cardiovascular function in man, in Rahn H (ed): Physiology of Breath-Hold Diving and the Ama of Japan. Washington, D.C., National Association of Science, National Research Council, Publ 1341, 1965 pp 295-302
30. Moore TO, Elsner R, Lin YC, et al: Effects of alveolar P_{O_2} and P_{CO_2} on apneic bradycardia in man. J Appl Physiol 34:795-798, 1973
31. Hong SK, Moore TO, Seto G, et al: Lung volumes and apneic bradycardia in divers. J Appl Physiol 29:172-176, 1970
32. Schaefer KE, Allison RD, Dougherty JH, et al: Pulmonary and circulatory adjustments determining the limits of depths in breath-hold diving. Science 162:1020-1023, 1968
33. Craig AB Jr: Depth limits of breath-hold diving. (an example of Fennology). Respir Physiol 5:14-22, 1968

STUDY QUESTIONS

Select one *most* likely answer.
1. During immersion to the neck in thermoneutral water
   a. The venous return decreases
   b. The pulmonary arterial pressure does not change
   c. The right arterial pressure increases
   d. The stroke volume decreases
   e. The cardiac output does not change
2. Which of the following attenuates the apneic bradycardia in man?
   a. Immersion in cold water
   b. Increase in intrathoracic pressure
   c. Peripheral vasoconstriction
   d. Decrease in arterial P_{O_2}

3. During breath-hold diving, the following changes in cardiovascular functions are often observed in man, *except*
   a. Bradycardia
   b. Cardiac arrhythmias
   c. Decrease in arterial blood pressure
   d. Decrease in cardiac output
4. During breath-hold diving, the diver is most likely to suffer from hypoxia
   a. During descent
   b. Upon reaching the bottom
   c. While staying on the bottom
   d. During ascent

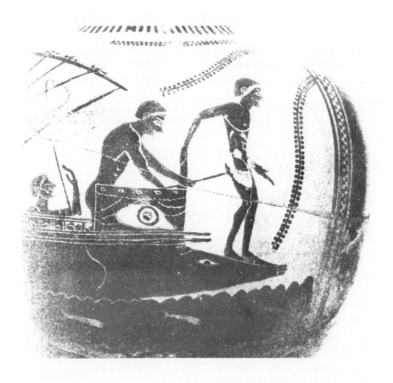

This sixth-century B.C. vase shows a Greek diver about to descend, probably in search of sponges. From *History of Diving,* U.S. Navy Diving Manual, 1973.

James Vorosmarti, Jr.

19
SATURATION DIVING

Saturation diving refers to that type of diving in which the time of exposure at a depth is sufficiently long for the inert gas tension in body tissues to equilibrate with the inert gas tension of the ambient atmosphere; in other words, the tissues are "saturated" with inert gas. Theoretically, this means that, no matter how long a diver remains at one depth, the subsequent decompression to reach one atmosphere safely will require the same amount of time. Although the practical application of this theory is recent, the concept dates back to the work of J. S. Haldane early in this century. Of no practical interest at that time, the concept never came to fruition. The need for reaching deeper depths for military and commercial reasons provided the impetus in the 1950s for reexamining and investigating this concept. The first experiments in saturation diving were undertaken in 1957 at the U.S. Naval Submarine Research Laboratory to prove, using animals, the safety of long exposures to normoxic mixtures of helium-oxygen at depth. Shortly after this series, successful human dives followed in the same laboratory. The first at-sea saturation dives were conducted almost simultaneously in September 1962. Conshelf I exposed 2 men for 7 days at a pressure of 6.06 ata. From that time, more and more saturation dives have been done for experimental and operational reasons. At the present time, this technique has become a fairly routine procedure to depths of 250 meters in shore-based chambers and, in the near future, will be a common procedure at sea, particularly in support of offshore oil development. By 1975, the deepest exposure has been to 600 meters in a shore-based chamber complex at the Comex facility in Marseilles, France.

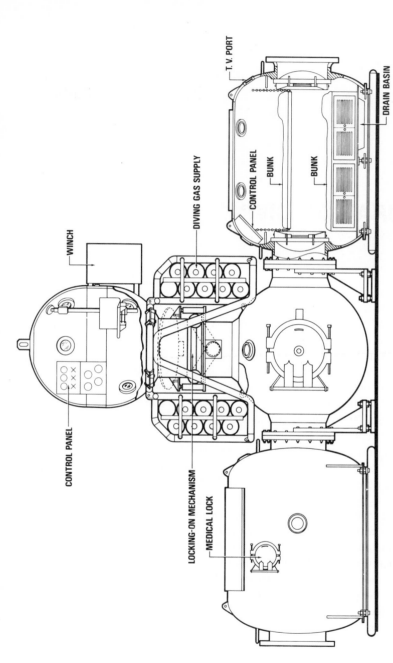

WINCH

CONTROL PANEL

LOCKING-ON MECHANISM

MEDICAL LOCK

DIVING GAS SUPPLY

T. V. PORT

CONTROL PANEL

BUNK

BUNK

DRAIN BASIN

Fig. 19-1. Line drawing of a typical operational saturation diving complex with diving bell attached. It is small because it is designed to be moved easily from one job to another. The overall length is approximately 27 feet and the diameter of the two larger chambers about 6 feet. The cylinders shown end-on around the trunk of the bell are for breathing gas for the divers when in the water. (Courtesy of U.S. Navy.)

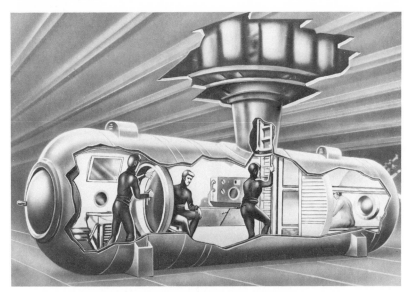

Fig. 19-2. An artist's conception of the U.S. Navy Mark II deep-diving system which is a much larger system permanently installed aboard a diving and salvage ship. The picture shows a diver about to climb the ladder through the trunk to the diving bell which is above on the main deck of the ship. (Courtesy U.S. Navy.)

The primary reason for the interest in the saturation technique is the extremely long decompression needed after even a fairly short bottom time dive to deep depths. It is obviously impossible to subject a diver to more than a few hours decompression in the water. A common method of doing this sort of diving involves the use of a bell and chamber complex. The divers enter the bell which is lowered to the work area and then pressurized to the ambient pressure. The divers leave the bell to do the job and, when finished, reenter the bell and are hoisted aboard the ship to finish their decompression in the chamber. This is satisfactory for doing a quick inspection or a job that requires only a short amount of time, but this technique is economically unviable for longer jobs, or for jobs requiring intermittent work over a period of several days. In these cases, saturation diving is the method used because the divers can stay at pressure and work in the water as many times as required without having to undergo lengthy and commercially unproductive decompressions. The technique is similar to that just described for bell diving with some minor changes. The divers are compressed in the chamber to which the bell is locked so that they are at pressure before entering the bell and being lowered to the work site. Since they must live in the chamber for much longer than required for single dives, the chamber design must be more sophisticated and the support for the system more complex. Fig. 19-1 is a schematic representation of a typical small operational saturation diving chamber-bell com-

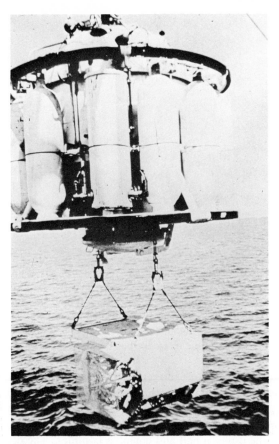

Fig. 19-3.   The diving bell of the U.S. Navy Mark II deep-diving system being lowered into the sea. The cylinders around the
bell contain breathing gas for the divers. The cylinder with the
flat ends contains batteries for electrical power. The large
square mechanism hanging from the bottom is a combination
anchor clump and winch. Once this is placed on the bottom, it
is possible for the bell to winch itself up or down so that the
bell does not have to be repositioned each time it returns to the
bottom.

plex. One should not be misled by the simplicity of this figure. It shows none
of the gas storage cylinders for chamber support, life support system, nor control systems needed to ensure successful operations and the safety of the personnel in the chamber. (See also Figs. 19-2 and 19-3.)

ATMOSPHERE CONTROL

The necessity of a closed artificial atmosphere in saturation diving makes strict atmosphere control a basic consideration. The standards in general use for the atmospheric components are as follows: O_2, 0.25 to 0.5 bar; CO_2, less than 0.005 bar, with the balance made up of helium with a small amount of nitrogen from the residual air in the chamber. This small amount of nitrogen is permissible and, in the practical sense, impossible to get rid of unless the air can be evacuated prior to the introduction of the helium-oxygen mixture. The oxygen level in the chambers can be easily raised to the correct level either by pressurizing the chamber with air or alternatively with pure oxygen until this level is reached.

Needless to say, the oxygen and carbon dioxide levels must be constantly monitored. There are instruments of adequate accuracy and reliability available commercially for these analyses. Their accuracy must be frequently checked by calibration. Accuracy is doubly important in instruments that measure the volume percentage of the gas at the surface, rather than the actual partial pressure, since the result must be multiplied by a factor of the depth to determine the partial pressure. For example, the correct oxygen percentage to provide 0.4 bar partial pressure at 250 meters is 1.54. An erroneous reading of only 0.24 percent below this would indicate that partial pressure is 0.338 bar and that additional oxygen should be added, when it is not needed.

To make up for the oxygen used metabolically, the pure gas is injected either into the chamber or into a moving stream of gas in the life-support system, if this is external. In any case, the oxygen must be thoroughly mixed with the chamber gas as it is added or it, being heavier than helium, will pool in lower regions of the chamber. Carbon dioxide is removed by passing the chamber atmosphere over standard absorbent material, once again in the chamber or in an external system. Since carbon dioxide will also pool in low areas, the flow of gas through the chamber must be adequate to prevent this. In the case of oxygen pooling, the author can recall one instance when a chamber was being pressurized with helium after the correct oxygen partial pressure had been established. The automatic oxygen addition system began adding oxygen with no apparent increase in the chamber oxygen level. It was found after sampling various areas of the chamber that the added oxygen had pooled in the lowest part of the chamber where it had reached a level of 10 percent. Depending on the final depth of the chamber, of course, this oxygen level could cause acute oxygen toxicity very shortly. During the U.S. Navy Sealab II experiment, it was found that carbon dioxide levels in the bunks were reaching very high levels. This was caused by the curtains around each bunk preventing the adequate circulation of gas necessary to remove the carbon dioxide produced by the occupant.

This closed environment also forces the consideration of atmospheric contaminants for several reasons. The first of these is a practical problem in that the only way to rid the chamber of them is to flush it with a fresh gas supply—a very expensive proposition, at least, and perhaps impossible because of an inadequate gas supply, particularly if aboard a ship. The second reason is that it is unknown whether the toxic effects of even common contaminants change due to pressure. It must be assumed that since the physiological effects of oxygen, carbon dioxide, and carbon monoxide are based on partial pressure and not volume percentage, toxic elements will behave in the same manner. Third, the threshold limit values for constant exposure in the majority of cases are not known even at atmospheric pressure.

One potential problem in long deep dives could be carbon monoxide. This is produced by the divers themselves in the amount of 8 to 10 cc/day/man through the normal metabolism of hemoglobin. Depending upon the volume of the chamber, it is conceivable that this substance could reach dangerous levels on dives of several weeks duration.[1] Although, in most chambers, human waste is locked out almost immediately, some units may have sanitary holding tanks. These tanks must not be vented to the chamber atmosphere since degradation products include ammonia, carbon dioxide, chlorine, sulfur dioxide, hydrogen sulfide, indole, and skatole. Since mercury is very toxic and vaporizes readily in the higher than normal temperatures required in saturation systems, mercury thermometers and electrical switches utilizing mercury are strictly forbidden in case they may be broken. Freon of several types has been found as a contaminant in saturation systems. It has been introduced during cleaning procedures of piping systems or from leaks in the refrigeration units of the life support system.

It is stressed that the only effective way of handling trace contaminants in a closed diving system is to prevent their entrance into it.

TEMPERATURE AND HUMIDITY CONTROL

The thermal conductance of helium is about six times that of air, and the thermal capacity about five times that of air. The loss of body heat is therefore greater in a helium atmosphere than in air. As the depth increases, the required ambient temperatures that define the upper and lower limits between which physiological adjustment can maintain thermal balance increase. These limits also become narrower with depth. Table 19-1 lists these limits as theoretically calculated to a depth of 5000 fsw.[2] These limits were calculated for a diver at rest in an appropriate helium-oxygen environment with a relative humidity of 50 percent. For the upper limit, complete peripheral vasodilation without sweating was assumed and, for the lower limit, complete peripheral vasoconstriction. As Table 19-1 shows, this range decreases from approximately 4°C at the surface to 2°C at 5000 fsw. Studies done in the ac-

Table 19-1
The Range of Ambient Temperatures in
Which a Diver at Rest ($\overset{\circ}{V}_{O_2}$ = 300 ml/min)
Can Physiologically Maintain Thermal Balance
in a Helium-Oxygen Atmosphere (relative humidity = 50%)[2].

Depth (fsw)	Minimum Temp (°C)	Maximum Temp (°C)
0	27.3	31.4
500	29.1	34.0
1000	30.2	34.6
1500	30.9	34.9
2000	31.6	35.1
2500	32.0	35.2
3000	32.4	35.3
4000	32.8	35.5
5000	33.4	35.6

tual diving situation all fall within this range to a depth of 1600 feet, beyond which this problem has not been investigated. Changes in relative humidity will raise or lower the limits shown, in an inverse relationship, but the narrowing of the range remains the same. The most comfortable range of relative humidity appears to be between 60 and 75 percent. In practical terms, this means that the saturation system must have a very good heating/cooling and humidity control system that can be maintained within very small limits. Another problem introduced by the increasing gas density is the drastic reduction of the diffusion coefficient of water; this results in the loss of evaporation of sweat as a mechanism for thermal control. As a consequence, the situation may arise in which, if a diver is required to do hard work in a chamber, the temperature may have to be lowered to maintain his thermal equilibrium. The extremely small diffusion coefficient of water probably explains the common complaint of divers in this environment of their skin feeling uncomfortably wet, although no sensible water is present. Because the water vapor cannot diffuse away from the skin as rapidly as it diffuses into it from subcutaneous tissues, the normally dry outer layers of skin become saturated with it and produce the sensation of feeling wet.

In summary, the major routes of heat loss in a dense helium-oxygen atmosphere are convective and respiratory, with the latter becoming the most important during exercise. Radiative heat loss changes very little with increas-

Table 19-2
Minimum Temperatures above Which Diver's
Breathing Gas Must Be Heated[5]

Depth (fsw)	Temperature (°C)
600	1.03
650	1.66
700	4.00
750	6.03
800	7.82
850	9.41
900	10.83
950	12.10
1000	13.25

ing density, while loss through the conductive channel may decrease moderately.

The diver's situation becomes drastically worse when he enters the water unless supplemental heating is supplied to his suit and, in many cases, his breathing gas. Several experiments have reported the consequences of breathing cold gas at depth even when the ambient environment (helium-oxygen or water) was warm. At 25 ata breathing gas at 0-2°C, there was a rapid drop in body temperature and progressively severe, incapacitating shivering, in spite of exercise and an ambient temperature of 30°C. In addition, one diver developed acute respiratory distress due to copious respiratory tract secretions. The same results occurred at 31 ata, with an inspired gas temperature of 7°C.[3] Similar results were obtained in a dive in which the divers were provided external thermal protection and were breathing gas at 3°C at 27 ata.[4] Table 19-2 lists the recommended minimum safe gas temperature limits at various depths, as calculated from these studies.[5] If the water temperature is below these, the breathing gas must be heated.

Ordinary neoprene wet suits offer no thermal protection in saturation diving because they become compressed to almost paper thinness on compression and reexpand to only about 50 percent of their original thickness. They would still be of little use if complete reexpansion did occur because the cellular structure would fill with helium. The two common methods of providing heat to divers at the present are the hot water suit and the electrical suit. The first is a loose fitting neoprene rubber suit. The space between the suit and the diver's skin is flooded with hot water, with a system of tubes, to direct some of the flow over the limbs to the hands and feet. This system is extremely comfortable, but has the disadvantage of requiring the pumping of hot water to the diver from the surface. Electrically heated suits and underwear have been in use for years, but can be unreliable because of the problems of "hot spots" and breakage of the fine-resistance wires. They are, however, commonly used.

To ensure the health and safety of the diver, the dangers of not providing an adequate thermal environment should never be minimized. If they are, the results will be disastrous.

RESPIRATORY FUNCTION IN SATURATION DIVING

The problem of increased gas density and its effect on ventilation is no different than that found in normal air diving. It is, however, intensified at depths over 750 feet because gas densities now become higher than those encountered in most air diving, and the diver must breathe this dense gas for long periods of time.

The restrictions on ventilation imposed by high gas density may well prove to be a major factor in limiting the depth that man may achieve. At 1 ata, the amount of work a man can do is generally limited by cardiovascular factors. At depth, this limitation appears to be respiratory, i.e., the diver may reach a depth at which his ventilation is impaired so much that it can support only the work of breathing and resting metabolism. Several studies indicate that there is a definite reduction in the amount of work a man can do as the depth increases. At 20.7 ata, there is little impairment to doing 900 kg-m/min work[6]; at 31.3 ata, hypercapnia was noted in two of three divers at a work load of 735 kg/minute.[7] One of two divers at a pressure of 46.4 ata showed a small increase in alveolar P_{CO_2} at a work load of 300 kg-m/min.[8] A recent analysis of respiratory studies at 60 ata suggests that at this depth the maximum amount of work that could be performed is in the region of 125 watts (750 kg-m/min).[9] From these studies, it appears this may be a bit generous, but may be proven correct. These studies were all done in dry chambers and do not take into account two other factors that affect ventilation and therefore work capability at depth. The first of these is the additional breathing resistance imposed by any underwater breathing apparatus that increases the work of breathing.[10, 11] The second factor is the hydrostatic pressure difference between the diver and his regulator, which depends on his position in the water. The resulting positive or negative pressure breathing he must do will also serve to further decrease his ventilatory capability.

COMPRESSION

Compression to depth in saturation diving causes two problems: the High Pressure Nervous Syndrome or HPNS and the syndrome of compression arthralgia. HPNS has been discussed in detail elsewhere; here the only additional point to be made is that this may be a practical problem for the physician or attendant who must join an injured diver in a chamber. In an emergency situation, a fast compression to depth may leave the physician completely unable to do any fine procedure for an hour or more afterward. It seems better to take a longer time in compression since, even with a slow compression rate of 1 meter/minute, most divers will have mild tremor and vertigo for a short time after reaching 250 meters.

The syndrome of compression arthralgia consists of ill-defined discomfort or frank pain in joints on motion associated in many cases with clicking or popping noises. The diver's ability to work is usually minimally limited, but the problem is very annoying. It has been found that by using slow compression rates the onset of these symptoms occurs at deeper depths and the severity is lessened.[12] The joints affected most often are the knees, wrists, and hips. In many cases, the symptoms will gradually disappear over a certain period of time at depth, but this also increases with depth (8 hours at 200 fsw; 41.5 hours at 850 fsw). The etiology and existence of any long-term effects of this syndrome are unknown. Because the possibility of trauma to the joints does exist, it is recommended that slow rates of compression (1 meter/minute or less) be used for deep dives, both saturation and nonsaturation.

DECOMPRESSION

Decompression from saturation diving presents the same problems that decompression from standard dives does: decompression sickness and pulmonary barotrauma. The latter is virtually unknown in saturation decompression because of the slow ascent rates, but it could occur on decompressions from excursions to a depth deeper than saturation depth and, therefore, should not be ignored in this context. The type of decompression sickness encountered is usually of the pain only type and, in contrast to standard diving, occurs almost always around the knees. In a series of saturation dives recently carried out by the Royal Navy, of 48 cases of decompression sickness, all were of the pain only variety and 46 were located around the knees. Experience of others has been similar. The cause of this great predilection for the knees to be involved is unknown. This type of decompression sickness is usually mild and is easily treated with minimal recompression. A much more serious and fortunately uncommon form of decompression sickness encountered is that involving the inner ear producing deafness and/or vertigo. Treatment of this form generally requires much deeper recompression than the pain only type. The absence of cases of decompression sickness consisting of pain and neurological signs is probably explained by the slow rate of decompression and the immediate reporting of problems by the divers, so that treatment is instituted prior to the development of other symptoms. The clearing of the pain after only a meter or two or recompression is also probably due to early treatment.

A common complaint of saturation divers during and following decompression is that of feeling "bubbles moving in their knees" and vague discomfort in the knees and anterior thighs. This latter symptom may also be described as feeling like bruising, or the aches one has after very hard exercise. These symtoms, particularly the feeling that something is moving around, lasts for only a few minutes and disappears without treatment. The aching may last for hours and may develop into the classical pain of decompression sickness, but most times does not. These symptoms simply should be observed. Treatment is necessary if other manifestations develop.

The basis for the treatment of decompression sickness occurring during or after a saturation dive is recompression. If it occurs after completion of decompression, standard treatment schedules can be used, but helium-oxygen should be substituted for air if an oxygen treatment schedule cannot be used or is unsuccessful. The reason for this is that a significant number of cases of decompression sickness will become worse on recompression using air. The usual rules of treatment that govern the use of these tables occur during decompression, recompression is begun in stages (10 fsw, U.S. Navy; 5 msw, Royal Navy) and continues until relief is noted by the diver. This depth is maintained for at least 2 hours and as long as 6 hours. During this period, the patient can be put on intermittent high oxygen mixes (1.5-2.5 bar) by mask if available. If shallower than 18 meters, pure oxygen may be used. At the end of time at treatment depth, the standard decompression schedule is resumed from that depth. If the pain is not alleviated by recompression to 20 meters (66 feet) beyond the depth at which it occurred, further recompression is not recommended. Experience has shown in cases of this type that if the pain is not relieved with this increase it is probably not decompression sickness, and other reasons for the pain should be investigated.

Saturation decompression schedules per se will not be discussed here. There are probably as many of these as there are groups doing this type of diving. There are some general points, however, with which the physician should be familiar. In general, commercial decompression schedules are shorter than navy schedules, since decompression time is expensive. This is accomplished basically by using higher oxygen partial pressures than found in more conservative schedules. In some cases, the oxygen partial pressure has been high enough to produce symptoms and laboratory evidence of pulmonary oxygen toxicity. Again, in contrast to navy schedules that use helium-oxygen mixes with a constant oxygen partial pressures, other schedules use other inert gases such as neon or nitrogen along with helium, either throughout the dive or during different portions of the decompression. Because of logistic problems, some involve the substitution of air during the shallow portions of decompression. At the present time, hydrogen is not being used, but there is research in progress to determine its usefulness in saturation diving. Finally, there are variations in the method of decompression; some schedules proceed on a constant bleed decompression, and others on the step-decompression method common to nonsaturation diving. The incidence of decompression sickness is not known on most commercial schedules because of the proprietary interest in them.

HEMATOLOGICAL AND BIOCHEMICAL CHANGES

There is some conflict in the results of hematological studies done during helium-oxygen studies, but there seems to be little argument that hematrocrit, hemoglobin, or red blood cell counts change little; if they do, it is to slightly lower values because of the hyperoxic environment. Leukocytosis has been found in some divers, but not in others. Monocytes and eosinophils have been found to be specifically increased with other leukocytes remaining in normal numbers.[1] These changes have never adequately been explained. Conflicting results on two different dives leave the question of platelet changes in doubt—in one, they remained normal, in the other they decreased sharply during decompression. Although clinical bleeding and clotting times have remained normal during helium-oxygen saturation dives, there is evidence indicating that a state of hypercoaguability does exist.

In a large series of saturation dives to 600 fsw, no changes were noted in the following serum chemistries: sodium, potassium, chloride, carbon dioxide, total protein, albumin, calcium, total bilirubin, alkaline phosphotase, or blood urea nitrogen.[13] A drop in glucose was reported, but this was thought later to be an artifact due to glucose consumption in the samples during the decompression of the blood. The results of other investigators are in agreement.

Several investigators have studied changes in enzymes (CPK, LDH, SGPT, SGOT), and it appears that in safe decompressions there is no change in these to suggest tissue damage.

Although all these studies show very little change in the constituents of blood, it cannot be assumed that deeper or longer exposures will be harmless. It may be that the stress placed on these physiological systems to date has not been enough to cause changes detectable by the methods available. A good deal more research is required in this area. For those interested, an excellent view of changes in blood during all types of diving has been published recently by Philp.[14]

WHAT IS MAN'S DEPTH LIMIT IN THE OCEAN?

This is an impossible question to answer at this time. Ten years ago diving to 500 feet appeared to be impossible, yet today, it is not uncommon to find divers working at this depth. Although the limit cannot be stated in feet, we have an idea of what factors may set the limit.

First of all is the problem of dysfunction of the central nervous system. Again, this problem has been discussed in Chapter 12 and thus will not be discussed here. However, from the investigations completed to date, it appears that unless some method of circumventing this is found (drugs and the addition of some other inert gas as nitrogen are being investigated), it may prove to be an impossible barrier.

Inadequate respiration also may be the limiting factor. As discussed earlier in this chapter, the limit for doing a moderate amount of work may be in the region of 60 ata. This is based on studies of the mechanics of breathing at depth. There are, however, other problems in respiration that also may contribute to a depth limitation. Some recent work (Winsborough, unpublished) showed that the pulmonary tissue capacitance for CO_2 increased at 250 meters, and there was evidence of an increase in the $\dot{V}_A/\dot{Q}$ maldistribution at this depth, particularly during heavy exercise. There was also a large total increase in oxygen consumption, which could not be completely related to the increased density. These changes were reversed on decompression, but what the outcome would be on longer deeper dives from both the acute affects or possible chronic affects is completely unknown.

There may also be a problem with the transfer of oxygen to the tissues. Chouteau[15] has done some experiments in which animals appeared to be hypoxic between 1280 and 1820 fsw, even though breathing normoxic helium-oxygen mixtures. Increasing the oxygen partial pressure relieved all their symptoms. He attributed the hypoxic symptoms to a disturbance of the alveolar-capillary exchange, but some recent work by Kiesow[16] has shown in vitro changes in hemoglobin which may be the reason. Pressure and inert gas shift the hemoglobin-dissociation curve to the left (nitrogen more so than helium). This means that oxygen will not transfer to the tissues normally, with resultant tissue hypoxia. It has been a personal experience that uneventful decompression from deeper than 150 meters cannot be obtained using normoxic mixtures: the oxygen partial pressure must be raised to accomplish this. If this is the case, the depth limit may be set by the oxygen partial pressures that man can breathe without inducing oxygen toxicity.

If this change in oxygen-hemoglobin dissociation does indeed take place in vivo at depths now reached, it is the earliest and shallowest evidence of pressure effects on living systems, which were not expected until much deeper depths. These effects include protein coagulation, enzyme inactivation, and disintegration of red blood cells.[17] Such changes would appear to be the ultimate barrier to diving if, in fact, the others just mentioned can be overcome.

REFERENCES

1. Vorosmarti J, Bradley ME, Linaweaver PG, et al: Helium-oxygen saturation diving I. Hematologic, lactic acid dehydrogenase and carbon monoxide-carboxyhemoglobin studies. Aerosp Med 41:1347-1353, 1970
2. Flynn ET, Vorosmarti J, Modell HI: Temperature requirements for the maintenance of thermal balance in high pressure helium-oxygen environments. USN EDU Research Report 21-73, June, 1974
3. Hoke B, Jackson D, Alexander J, et al: Respiratory heat loss from breathing cold gas to high pressures. Summary of USN EDU/NMRI studies, Feb, 1971
4. Goodman M, Colston J, Smith E, et al: Hyperbaric respiratory heat loss study Final Report on ONR Contract N00014-71-C-0099. Westinghouse Electric Corp, 1971
5. Braithwaite WR: The calculation of minimum safe inspired gas temperature limits for deep diving. USN EDU/NMRI Research Report 12-72, July 1972
6. Bradley ME, Anthonisen NR, Vorosmarti J, et al: Respiratory and cardiac responses to exercise in subjects breathing helium-oxygen mixtures at pressures from sea-level to 19.2 atmospheres, in Lambertsen CJ (ed): Proceedings of the Fourth Symposium on Underwater Physiology. New York, Academic Press, 1971
7. Salzano J, Rausch DC, Saltzman HA: Cardio-respiratory responses to exercise at a simulated seawater depth of 1000 feet. J Appl Physiol 28:34-41, 1970
8. Morrison JB, Florio JT: Respiratory function during a simulated saturation dive to 1500 feet. J Appl Physiol 30:724-732, 1971
9. Varene P, Viellefond H, LeMaire C, et al: Expiratory flow-volume curves and ventilatory limitation of muscular exercise at depth. Aerosp Med 45:161-166, 1974
10. Bradley ME, Vorosmarti J, Merz J, et al: Breathing impedance of the Mark VIII and Mark XI semi-closed underwater breathing apparatus. Submarine Development Group One Research Report 1-70, San Diego, Aug 1970
11. Sterk W: Respiratory mechanics of divers and diving apparatus. Utrecht, Drukkerij Elinkwijk, 1973
12. Bradley ME, Vorosmarti J: Hyperbaric arthralgia during helium-oxygen dives from 100 to 850 fsw. Undersea Biomed Res 1:151-167, 1974
13. Vorosmarti J, Bradley ME, Linaweaver PG, et al: Helium-oxygen saturation diving II. Serum chemistries and urinalyses. Aerosp Med 42:13-16, 1971
14. Philp RB: A review of blood changes associated with compression-decompression: relationship to decompression sickness. Undersea Biomed Res 1:117-150, 1974

15. Chouteau J: Saturation diving: The conshelf experiments, in Bennett P and Elliott D (eds): The Physiology and Medicine of Diving and Compressed Air Work. London, Bailliere, Tindall and Cassell, 1969, pp 491-504

16. Kiesow LA: Hyperbaric inert gases and the hemoglobin-oxygen equilibrium in red blood cells. Undersea Biomed Res 1:29-43, 1974

17. Fenn WO: Possible role of hydrostatic pressure in diving, in Lambertsen CJ (ed): Proceedings of Third Symposium on Underwater Physiology. Baltimore, Williams & Wilkins, 1967

STUDY QUESTIONS

1. Why is saturation diving becoming more and more common as a technique for underwater construction?

2. Although the production of 8-10 cc per day per man of carbon monoxide is only a very small percentage of the total volume of a chamber complex with a volume of 27,000 liters, this is an important atmospheric contaminant; why?

3. For a diver at rest in a chamber complex at 1000 fsw, what is the temperature range in which he can remain in thermal balance? If he makes a dive at this depth with a water temperature of 4°C, does he require heated breathing gas in addition to suit heating?

4. There is an important distinction between the factors which limit the work that can be done at 1 ata and at depth. What is the difference?

5. A diver at 850 fsw pressure is seriously injured and requires medical attention. Should a physician be locked in and rapidly compressed to this depth to give aid?

6. A diver decompressing from a saturation depth of 450 fsw complains of severe pain in his right shoulder on reaching 375 feet. He is recompressed to saturation depth without improvement. Should compression continue?

7. A diver with bilateral knee pain during decompression from a saturation dive was recompressed from 25 meters to 30 meters with complete relief. He had been intermittently breathing a helium-oxygen mixture containing 1.6 bars of oxygen for 2 hours. This was followed by a 2-hour period at 30 meter breathing chamber atmosphere. May he continue decompression and if so what schedule should be used?

Glen H. Egstrom

20
Diving Accidents

The investigation and evaluation of diving accidents has received increasing attention in the literature since 1965 when Webster published the first United States review of skin and scuba diving fatalities. The various statistical summaries of fatalities have been developed independent of data describing the growth of participation in the sport. To date, there is no coherent picture of the number of man-hours of diving in the various environments that divers enjoy. This lack of comparative baseline information has made it difficult to assess the impact of diving safety measures which have been promoted by the instructional agencies and underwater safety committees.

Each diving accident is the result of a series of complex interactions involving specific environmental conditions and other variables such as fitness, training, equipment, the ability to handle stressful situations, and the recognition of personal limits for exertion.

These interactions rarely come into consideration during the accident evaluation process as it is currently practiced. Drowning is usually listed as the cause of death without regard to the events leading to the fatality. Unfortunately, this does little to aid in understanding the nature of the accident.

A typical diving accident occurs at a site remote to immediate qualified emergency aid. It takes place during the weekend, late in the afternoon, frequently on a second or third dive. During the events preceding the accident, the victim engages in an exhausting struggle on the surface and does not ditch his weight belt, inflate personal flotation equipment, utilize the remaining air in the tank, or receive appropriate assistance from his "buddy."

These seeming contradictions to the training of the basic diver can

303

perhaps be related to conditions of state-dependent learning which may not transfer to the ocean environment. It appears that critical skills for ocean performance should be learned and practiced under conditions as similar as possible to those which might actually occur. These skills should be overlearned and reinforced at reasonable intervals to ensure prompt, accurate execution of the emergency procedures.

ACCIDENT EVALUATION

Diving accident statistics have been developed by several agencies and a summary of their findings indicates that, while the trained diving population in the United States has increased by over 100 percent during the years 1970-1974, the accident rate involving fatalities has only increased by approximately 5 percent during the same period. In essence, this points out that the diving safety programs across the country have been effective in reducing the per capita accident rate. Unfortunately, statistics relative to the exposure rate are not currently available to provide an accurate appraisal of the number of accidents versus the number of exposures. Such data might very well indicate an even more impressive safety record.

The evaluation of diving accidents, whether or not they result in a fatality, can be a valuable service for the improvement of diving safety. This evaluation should consider the specifics of the environmental conditions. Details of factors including time of day, weather conditions, and water conditions such as depth, surge, waves, visibility, vegetation, current, and temperature provide perspective when reviewing the events of the accident. Consideration should also be given to the mechanical factors of the accidents. These include specifics of the location, bottom topography, and duration of the dive, as well as the condition and behavior of the victim during the incident.

A review of 75 beach reports from 1973-1974 revealed that over 97 percent of the rescues of scuba divers involved excessive fatigue and an overestimation of the individual's abilities. Other observations were related to panic in the face of a minor emergency with struggling on the surface. These findings indicate that individuals who dive from the beach must be alert and trained to cope with the vigorous nature of this particular environment. Strength, endurance, and basic watermanship skills are fundamental to success in diving.

It is also important to know how many and what kinds of other diving activities preceded the accident. This should be specific to the date under review, as well as the past diving history. It becomes increasingly apparent that different diving environments can present substantially different kinds of demands and problems.

The assumption that a diver trained in the Florida caves will be safe and effective in California surf and kelp, or vice versa, is a tempting, but potentially dangerous, view. Unfortunately, every year there are significant numbers of individuals who are reluctant to avail themselves of "orientation"-type dives when faced with a new or unusual diving situation. Thus, they become involved in a diving mishap of varying severity, due to a lack of appropriate knowledge upon which to base their calculated risk.

Details relating to the rescue or recovery of accident victims should include (a) information on the state of all the equipment; (b) any evidence of injury or panic; (c) description of the scene at the time of rescue or recovery; and (d) a description of the situation immediately following the rescue or recovery. These details will become lost if they are not collected systematically and early. Many areas in the country have forms specifically designed for the diving circumstances of the region. Many underwater instructors and rescue personnel carry copies with their emergency equipment.

BUDDY SYSTEM FAILURE

The use of the buddy system in sport scuba dving has been an important factor in the survival of a pair in significant numbers of accidents. Unfortunately, there are no statistics that demonstrate the effectiveness of the buddy system under such circumstances. There is, however, considerable evidence of the system's failure in a number of fatal accidents and in a number of reports of rescues by lifeguards.

Much of the difficulty appears to develop as a result of lack of training and discipline in the operation of the buddy system. Common failure modes are

1. Poor visibility and separation with little or no attempt to reestablish the system.
2. Leader-follower breakdown with an excessive time period elapsing before the recognition of the problem.
3. Frustration due to dissimilar diving patterns with a subsequent reversion to solo diving with or without the partner's consent.
4. Inability to provide assistance to a buddy due to lack of knowledge of proper procedures.

It is necessary to keep the "buddy" pair close enough to permit visual or tactile contact at all times. A contact on every second or third breath is easily accomplished if the buddies are diving "shoulder to shoulder" and working as a team rather than using the "follow the leader" pattern, which frequently results in the follower stopping to check on some point of interest with the immediate dissolution of team contact. It is a common practice for trained divers to follow a simple protocol for finding a separated buddy. This protocol requires a "listen and look" behavior while rotating 360° and looking up and, if necessary, down to check for the buddy's presence. If the buddy is not immediately in sight after this check, the diver goes directly to the surface and looks for exhaust bubbles. Obviously, if both buddies follow this practice, they will meet on the surface and can resume their dive together. Effective buddy diving is dependent upon a constant awareness of the partner's behavior and is a skill which requires a common understanding of the rules of behavior between the pair. The failure to clarify and implement the rules with a diving partner is a major step in breaking the system down. The buddy system saves lives and prevents the minor emergency from becoming a catastrophe, when it is practiced as a well-learned skill in which both partners are aware and relaxed during the dive.

SURF ENTRIES AND EXITS

In an evaluation of surf entries and exits conducted at U.C.L.A., it was determined that most of the problems in the surf resulted from failure to correctly judge the surf conditions as they develop. This poor judgment is usually followed by an excessively energetic effort to recover control, and frequently leads to an avalanching of small problems into a total loss of control. Videotape analysis of over 100 entry and exit combinations resulted in the observation that 48 out of 104 trials contained multiple errors in technique, which resulted in a potentially dangerous loss of control. It was interesting that the majority of these multiple errors began with either stopping or markedly slowing down in the "drop zone," that portion of the surf zone where the waves are breaking. The failure to dive under the wave, or to otherwise reduce the surface area of the body presented to the force of the wave, results in floundering and second-order errors involving masks, snorkels, regulators, and buddy separation, to name a few. Thus, it appears that many accidents grow in severity and follow a progressive pattern with recognizable characteristics. The amount of training and reinforcement necessary to ensure safe, effective behavior under the various diving circumstances then becomes a paramount factor in accident prevention. The safe diver must be capable of appropriate, nearly reflexive, responses to specific demands of his diving environment as they change during the dive.

ACCIDENT ETIOLOGY

There is very limited information related to the etiology of diving accidents and particularly the early contributors to the ultimate problem. "Death due to drowning while scuba diving" is a common statement found in reports of diving accidents; causative information related to the state of fitness or health, poor judgment, mechanical failures, etc., is unavailable.

References to terms such as exhaustion and panic, while also common, are specifically uninformative. Accident report forms such as those used in Los Angles County and at the University of Rhode Island, while valuable, are not able to elicit adequate information on the details of the accident. This type of information is probably best gained by an on-site investigator who has knowledge of the local diving circumstances.

An example of a pattern commonly witnessed in Southern California waters begins with panic or loss of control in a minor emergency (entanglement, fatigue, struggling in current or surge, etc.). The victim then exerts additional energy in an effort to keep his head above water. The victim fails to appreciate that supporting the head, regulator, etc., out of the water requires the same amount of force as swimming to the surface 18-20 pounds negatively bouyant. This excessive work load can quickly exhaust the diver's energy reserves and leave him without adequate endurance to cope with the situation. During this struggle, one rarely witnesses a weight belt ditch or flotation device inflation, even though these are critical maneuvers in the effort to gain positive buoyancy.

The achievement of a comfortable state of positive buoyancy in advance of any need for struggling would appear to be an obvious step in accident prevention. Waiting too long to take this step can result in *unnecessary* complication of the dive and an avalanche of additional stress leading to an incapacitated diver.

REFERENCES

1. Denny M, Read R: Scuba Diving Deaths in Michigan. JAMA 192: April 19, 1965
2. De Sautels D: Cave Diving Drowning Statistics—A Twelve Year Study (1960-1972). Gainesville, Fla, personally distributed by the author, 1972
3. Kindwall E, et al: Non fatal, pressure related scuba accidents, identification and emergency treatment, in: Scuba Safety Report Series, No. 3 University of Rhode Island, 1971
4. Schenck H, et al: Skin and scuba diving fatalities involving U.S. citizens, in: Scuba Safety Report Series, No. 3. University of Rhode Island, 1971
5. Schenck H, et al: Diving accident survey, 1946-1970, including 503 known fatalities, in: Scuba Safety Report Series, No. 5. University of Rhode Island, January 1972
6. Schenck H, Mc Aniff J: Mortality rates for skin and scuba divers, in: Scuba Safety Report Series, No. 7. University of Rhode Island, April, 1972
7. Schenck H, Mc Aniff J: United States Underwater Fatality Statistics-1973. Washington, D.C., NOAA Grant Number 4-3-158-31 US Department of Commerce/US Department of Transportation, May 1975

8. Singer R: A study of southern California's scuba and free diving fatalities (1965-1970), in: Los Angeles County Underwater Instructor's Project Report. Los Angeles, March 13, 1971
9. Underwater Safety Committee, Los Angeles County: 1971 Committee Proceedings. Los Angeles, Los Angeles County Parks and Recreation Department
10. Underwater Safety Committee, Los Angeles County: Volume II-Committee Report, Los Angeles Department of Parks and Recreation, September 1974
11. Webster D: Skin and Scuba Diving Fatalities in the United States. Public Health Report 81, No. 8, August 1966

STUDY QUESTIONS

1. The cause of a diving accident is easy to determine because the majority of accidents occur where official investigators can get to the scene very quickly.
   a. True
   b. False

2. Diver training programs appear to be effective in developing a safe diving population.
   a. True
   b. False

3. Diving equipment problems rank high as a cause of diving accidents.
   a. True
   b. False

4. A separated buddy requires an immediate ascent to the surface.
   a. True
   b. False

5. Accidents generally have a progressive pattern of failure to effectively initiate an early solution to a minor problem.
   a. True
   b. False

Carl Edmonds

21

First Aid and Emergency Medical Treatment

PREVENTION

The most satisfactory way of dealing with diving morbidity and mortality is to prevent it. Initially, the potential diver should have demonstrated his ability to pass a medical examination performed by a physician knowledgeable in the field of diving medicine.[1, 3] This will ensure that the diver has reached a satisfactory state of physical fitness and has no medical diseases that are likely to prejudice his safety in an aquatic and hyperbaric environment. The second major factor in prevention is to ensure adequate diver training, including a knowledge of the medical aspects of diving. The third factor is the use of reliable equipment, appropriate to the environmental conditions and the training of the diver. Important safety equipment includes such items as communication lines, buoyancy vests, diver's buoy with flag, depth and air-tank gauges, thermal protection, underwater watch, and knife. A diver's medical kit is described later.

FIRST AID AT THE TIME OF THE ACCIDENT

No matter how much effort is put into prevention, accidents will occur in diving situations. There are two aspects of first aid; one is the rescue attempts performed following a serious accident; the other, the specific treatment given to minor injuries.

Rescue[2]

Note that in 70 percent of the diving fatalities, there is a period in excess of 15 minutes between the accident and the rescue. This is an unacceptable duration for any patient to remain underwater without functioning breathing equipment. Thus, in many cases, there is a progression from unconsciousness to death, which could have been prevented by the institution of the three basic requirements for first aid in diving, viz:

1. Immediate assistance from a companion diver, and a method of requesting this.
2. Assistance in returning to the surface or to a habitable environment.
3. The use of first aid techniques to ensure maintenance of life until professional medical treatment is obtained.

In practice the common methods of obtaining the above three requirements are

1. A lifeline to a buddy (companion diver).
2. A buoyancy vest or direct contact with surface support.
3. Mouth-to-mouth respiration and external cardiac massage.

The practice of buddy diving is the single most important factor in first aid. It requires that each diver is personally responsible for the welfare and safety of his companion. It infers a reliable method of communication between the divers, a rescue technique, and a basic knowledge of resuscitation.

Specific Treatment at the Site

Many injuries sustained by divers require a rapid assessment, diagnosis, and management. Others are of such a minor nature that expert medical assistance is not sought, although some form of treatment is indicated. The first aid is usually supplied by the diver's associates and includes the following:

1. General resuscitation, including mouth-to-mouth respiration and/or external cardiac massage in cases of unconsciousness.
2. The use of oxygen inhalation for drowning.
3. A knowledge of the management of trauma, including the use of tourniquets, e.g., with shark attack, propellor injuries, underwater explosions, etc.
4. Warming techniques for hypothermia.
5. Methods of reducing the toxicity of marine animal venoms and of obtaining symptomatic relief.
6. The general care and specific treatment of various infections ranging from otitis externa to coral cuts.

7. An ability to prevent and treat disorders environmentally associated with diving, e.g., seasickness, sunburn, fishing poisoning, etc.

It is important that the diving associates realize their limitations in treating such disorders as decompression sickness, barotrauma and hearing loss associated with diving.

LOCAL MEDICAL TREATMENT

This is usually an extension of the first aid, with the local physician augmenting the treatments with his knowledge of cardiopulmonary physiology, electrolyte disturbances, surgical techniques, the use of antitoxins, antibiotics, steroids, analgesia, and if necessary anaesthesia.

In many cases the local physician can work as a liaison officer between the divers and a specialist in the field of diving medicine, especially when recompression therapy is required. The local physician will also be important in integrating the transport and medical evacuation needs, if these are required. It is axiomatic that the local physician should have available to him direct communication with a specialist in diving medicine, so that the treatments just described and the techniques about to be described, can be instituted appropriately.

RECOMPRESSION FACILITIES

In cases of decompression sickness and pulmonary barotrauma, recompression therapy is often mandatory. In many instances, the facilities may not be available for this, and a decision has to be made as to whether the patient is to be recompressed by descent in the water, transferred to a recompression chamber, or have a recompression chamber transported to him.

Water Recompression

This technique may be of value by decreasing the size of the gas bubble, as the diver descends. It is a particularly hazardous procedure, but has been needed many times in the past as an emergency. Both mechanical and physiological problems are encountered. Requirements for diver support include a sufficient supply of gas or compressed air, tolerable weather conditions, a full face mask or helmet to prevent aspiration or water, adequate thermal protection, and an attendant to be with the diver at all times. The problems often encountered in water recompression therapy include seasickness, drowning, hypothermia, panic, and finally the aggravation of the illness by subjecting the patient to a further increase of inert gas within his tissues, compounding the problem on subsequent ascent. In many cases of water recompression therapy, the requirement has to be terminated prematurely because of adverse weather conditions, equipment failure, sharks, physiological, and, finally, psychological difficulties. When the treatment does give relief, it often needs to be supplemented with the conventional recompression therapy carried out in a chamber, soon after the patient has left the water.

A much more effective water recompression therapy uses 100 percent oxygen, at a maximum of 9 meters, and is relatively short in duration. This table has been particularly valuable in remote localities. It involves a 30-120 minute stay at 9 meters, and ascent at the rate of 12 minutes per meter. It has the advantages of not aggravating the disease by adding more inert gas, being of short duration, avoiding any problem of nitrogen narcosis, and being suited for shallow bays, protected from the open sea environment.

Recompression Chamber Therapy

General. A recompression chamber can virtually eliminate mortality from decompression sickness. It also considerably reduces the dangers associated with air embolism. A recompression chamber should be available on site if free ascents are being practiced. The armed services and regulating bodies lay down conditions in which a recompression chamber must be available for commercial operations.[1, 4-6] The British and Australian regulations require a submersible decompression chamber for dives to a depth greater than 50 meters. Amateur divers tend to a more liberal attitude to safe diving practices and the mode of treatment depends on the chamber, personnel available, and the nature of the diver's ailment. If air embolism is diagnosed or suspected, then rapid recompression to 50 meters is required. Time should not be wasted, as the diver's life may depend on the speed of compression. After the patient is at 50 meters, it is time to evaluate the situation; the diagnosis can be confirmed and further treatment instituted. Once the patient is under pressure, and no longer in immediate danger, time is available to read the appropriate book or diving manual.

After recompression has been achieved, decompression sickness can be regarded with less urgency, except when the patient is still suffering from the pulmonary, neurological, or cardiac manifestations of decompression sickness. Both the morbidity and mortality of the disease is reduced by rapid recompression.

Transport. Diving is frequently carried out in localities remote from recompression chambers. Transportation of the sick patient requiring recompression therapy then becomes a major problem. Air transport may result in a deterioration in the clinical state of the patient due to a reduction in atmospheric pressure and an associated expansion of the bubble. As most aircraft are pressurized to approximately 2000 meters above sea level (0.8 atm), ascent will increase the size of the gas bubble. If the aircraft cannot be pressurized to 1 atm, as can the C130 Hercules, then the patient should not be transported at altitude unless there is no other alternative. Even a lofty mountain range can impose a threat if the diver is being moved by road. All these factors must be evaluated before deciding on the best means of transport of the patient to the chamber, or vice versa.

The problem of treatment for the diver in a remote location can be overcome if an efficient transportation and treatment system has been established. There are two possibilities:

1. Transport the diver without compression direct to the major treatment chamber.
2. Maintain the diver in situ, breathing 100 percent oxygen, and bringing a portable recompression chamber to him. Once under pressure, his danger may be diminished, but it still remains to treat him in the best chamber available. This portable recompression chamber should have compatible transfer-under-pressure facilities with other recompression chambers, for the transfer of both patient and attendants. It may be moved to a more suitable site where a major treatment chamber can be mated to the smaller unit and the patient transferred.

The choice of system depends on the seriousness of the injury, the availability and type of recompression chambers, gas supplies, transport availability, and time and distance relationships. The initial treatment carried out by other divers on site will influence subsequent management. It is important that a central experienced authority is responsible for decisions regarding treatment and transportation. This authority is best situated where the major definitive treatment chambers are located. The capability to transfer experienced staff and equipment to remote localities will prove of great value in the decision as to whether to treat on site or transport.

Equipment. An ideal system has yet to be designed where divers in all localities can be adequately treated at all times. The following is a suggested scheme for a country where medical knowledge is available in certain centers and where transport is available from most diving localities.

Major Center. Large multicompartment recompression chamber with transfer-under-pressure facilities located within a hospital complex;

Portable recompression chamber with gas supplies and compatible transfer-under-pressure capability. These chambers should be large enough to accommodate both the patient and an attendant, but should also be capable of transport by air to remote localities.

Regional Center. Portable recompression chamber as just described with compatible transfer-under-pressure facilities, which can be transported if necessary.

It is imperative in this system that all transfer-under-pressure facilities within the one geographical area are compatible. An injured diver can be placed in a portable recompression chamber and treated at the regional center or transported to the major center in the smaller portable unit. This system, by enabling rapid recompression of the diver, would save a great deal of morbidity. Divers injured at localities remote from the regional or major center could be transported to whichever unit was most appropriate.

DIVING MEDICAL KIT

Each diving tender should be equipped for the accidents it is likely to encounter. No list of requirements will cover the range of diving activities from a shallow inspection of a coral ledge off the Hawaiian coast to a saturation exposure in the North Sea.

A basic medical kit for all diving tenders will include

Airways for mouth to mouth respiration
Respirator with an oxygen supply (for use in drowning, pulmonary barotrauma, decompression sickness)
Tropical antibiotic or antiseptic for skin injuries
Motion sickness tablets
Dressings

If diving is carried out in waters where marine animal injuries are possible

Tourniquet (sharks, barracuda, etc.) and ligature (sea snake, blue-ringed octopus, stonefish)
Alcohol, local anaesthetic ointment or spray (jellyfish)
Local anaesthetic injection, without adrenalin (scorpion fish, stonefish, stingray, catfish)
Relevant antivenins—sea snake, sea wasp, stonefish, etc.

If decompression sickness is possible

Large oxygen cylinder, for surface supply to helmet or full face mask (with an adaptor to supply the onboard respirator if needed)

A 9-meter line, marked at 1-meter intervals, and a water oxygen recompression table

Intravenous infusion system (e.g., low molecular weight dextran) and urinary catheter

Adequate compressor or air bank to support the diving attendants

A portable 2-man recompression chamber, if possible

Special circumstances will require supplementation to these medical kits. Thus, with diving in remote localities, diagnostic and therapeutic equipment varying from a thermometer to a thoracotomy set may be appropriate. The use of these in remote localities will depend to some degree on the clinical training of the attendants. It is important that these diving tenders do have available simple medication and eardrops, antibiotics, and analgesics. This diving would also require a communication link to obtain expert medical advice on the use of these drugs and equipment.

REFERENCES

1. Australian Standards CZ18 and Z67: Underwater air breathing, appendix A, in: Medical Standards for Divers. North Sydney, Standards Association of Australia, 1972
2. Scuba Safety Report Series Nos. 2, 5 and 6. Kingston, R.I., Department of Ocean Engineering, University of Rhode Island
3. Edmonds C, Lowry C, Pennefather J, Diving and Subaquatic Medicine. Mosman, NSW Australia, Diving Medical Centre, 1976
4. US Navy Diving Manual: Washington, D.C., US Government Printing Office, 1973
5. Royal Navy Diving Manual. BR 2806 London, Her Majesty's Stationary Officer, 1972
6. Royal Australian Navy Diving Manual. ABR 155

STUDY QUESTIONS

1. While examining the interior of a large submerged transport plane, a diver noted difficulty in obtaining sufficient air from his scuba cylinders. His companion diver was at a distance of only 12 feet; but, as he swam toward the companion, the latter was coincidentally swimming in the same direction, i.e., away from the diver in difficulty. An extra burst of speed was required to catch the companion diver and this, in turn, needed an air supply that was no longer available. Thus, in desperation, the diver attempted to retrace his path to the plane door. He then managed to extricate himself from the plane, triggered his carbon dioxide vest, and as-

cended the 50 feet to the surface. At that stage, he had retained all his respiratory air bursting his lungs *en route*. List the three major faults performed in this dive:

2. A diver has been swimming in the tropical Pacific and sustained a severe single tenticle contact with a jellyfish of some type. The pain was excrutiating and required the diver to ascend immediately and obtain assistance from the diving tender. On examination there was a single strip of raised erythema with small beadlike structures along it. The tenticle was not present. What form of treatment would be effective and should have been available on the tender?

3. On a small Pacific island, without airport facilities and approximately 4000 miles from the nearest recompression chamber, a diver developed severe joint decompression sickness and started developing signs suggestive of a spinal cord lesion. The island had excellent hospital facilities, with oxygen available. The harbor was sheltered and had a depth of approximately 10 meters. An experienced diving group was available, together with compressor and surface supply equipment. What instructions would you give regarding the treatment of this man.

4. If you are consulted regarding the acquisition of a hyperbaric system suitable for a specific geographical area, what recommendations would you make regarding the use of

   a. One-man chambers
   b. Connections between chambers
   c. Chamber requirements for training purposes

Mark E. Bradley

22

Near-Drowning: Pathophysiology and Treatment*

The physical nature of the water environment is intolerant of mistakes, and any incident can become a near fatal incident. In most diving accidents where death is the outcome, it is the result of drowning.[1] There may be as many as 8 million skin divers and 2 million recreational scuba divers in the United States. How many episodes of near-drowning occur in this population is unknown; but, on the basis of the large number of participants, near-drowning is probably a frequent accompaniment to many nonfatal diving accidents.

Drowning, by definition, is death from acute asphyxia while submerged, whether or not the liquid has entered the lungs. The term near-drowning has been applied by Modell[2] to those individuals who survive submersion. Near-drowning victims may or may not aspirate fluid into their lungs. These patients may survive a near-drowning episode, but may die some hours or days later.

Noble and Sharpe[3] have described a sequence of events that occurs in drowning victims. Initially the subject struggles violently and apnea or breath-holding occurs. The individual swallows large quantities of fluid. This, in turn, leads to vomiting, which is followed by gasping and the aspiration of fluid.

Drowning and near-drowning without aspiration of liquid is an interesting phenomenon, and it is often difficult to determine if aspiration has occurred even at postmortem examination. The incidence reported for drown-

*From the Bureau of Medicine and Surgery, Navy Department, Research Task MP10.01.8011. The opinions in this paper are those of the author and do not necessarily reflect the views of the Navy Department or the Naval service at large.

ing and near-drowning without aspiration varies between 10 and 20 percent.[2,4] It is thought that in these subjects there is severe reflex glottic spasm leading to asphyxia. Nonetheless, most near-drowning patients do aspirate water, and along with it, diatoms, sand, and other impurities such as chlorine, which irritate the lung.

PATHOPHYSIOLOGY AND CLINICAL FEATURES

Prior to 1960, much emphasis was on determining the type of water in which the submersion accident occurred, since it was believed that specific clinical sequelae and treatment depended on this. This belief was in large part based on the experimental work of Swann,[5] who observed that when dogs were submerged in freshwater death often resulted from ventricular fibrillation. The mechanism responsible for the fibrillation was thought to be the combination of hemodilution (secondary to aspiration of a hypo-osmolar solution), hyponatremia, and hypoxia. Swann noted that submergence of dogs in seawater caused increases in plasma sodium and chloride with hemoconcentration and development of a fulminating pulmonary edema.

There is now considerable clinical and experimental evidence that the sequelae of near-drowning are virtually identical, irrespective of whether the immersion was in fresh- or saltwater. Fuller[6] reviewed the records of 77 near-drowning victims, 20 of whom later died. He reported that, in the postimmersion period, the signs and symptoms could be ascribed to hypoxia, pulmonary edema, and aspiration injury to the lung and that, in these patients, electrolyte imbalances were not severe. Subsequently, Modell et al.[7] in a study of 12 near-drowning patients reported that pulmonary edema together with hypoxemia and metabolic acidosis were the most prominent and life-threatening complications.

Experimentally, following installation of 1 ml/kg of body weight of fresh- or seawater into the trachea of sheep, hypoxemia develops.[8, 9] With aspiration of larger quantities (3 ml/kg), there is a more profound hypoxemia, which is persistent. The functional abnormality appears to be an alteration of pulmonary ventilation/perfusion relationships with some areas of complete shunting of blood through nonventilated portions of lung.[8, 10] Pulmonary compliance decreases (the lungs become stiffer) and pulmonary hypertension develops.[8, 4] Colebatch and Halmagyi[11] have demonstrated closure of the smaller airways following aspiration of small quantities of fluid, which appears to be partly reflex in origin.

Modell[2] has proposed the following pulmonary reactions following aspiration of freshwater or seawater. The underlying mechanism for nonventilation of alveoli after aspiration of freshwater results from an alteration in the surface-active material lining the lung—the pulmonary surfactant. The surface tension of fluid extracted from the lungs of animals that aspirate fresh-water is abnormally high.[12] This high surface tension also acts in the Starling Equilibrium to pull fluid from pulmonary capillaries into alveoli and cause pulmonary edema.

Conversely, following aspiration of seawater, more fluid can be drained from the lungs than was initially instilled.[13, 14] Aspiration of seawater does not appear to alter the characteristics of pulmonary surfactant.[12] However, because of its hyperosmolar characteristics, seawater does draw fluid across the alveolar capillary membrane and causes pulmonary edema.

The changes in blood gas and acid-base status are by far the most impor-tant feature of the near-drowning situation. Modell et al.[15] studied in dogs the effects of aspiration of 22 ml/kg of various fluids: normal saline, distilled water, and chlorinated distilled water. Arterial P_{CO_2} rose to about 50-60 mm Hg and the pH fell to a minimum, at approximately the 5- to 6-minute mark. Thereafter, these parameters tended to return to normal. There was a steady fall in base excess, reflecting a general metabolic acidosis, and this plateaued after about 10 minutes. After the administration of any of these substances, arterial oxygen tension fell to 40 mm Hg and remained at that level for the duration of the experiment, which was 1 hour. This hypoxemia was more marked and prolonged in seawater aspiration.

In general, the information that has been published on human near-drowning victims is quite similar. Severe hypoxemia and the development of metabolic acidosis have been consistently noted in human victims of near drowning with aspiration.[6, 7, 14, 16, 17] The hypoxemia persists even after ar-terial carbon dioxide tensions have returned to normal.

The effects on serum electrolyte levels of aspiration of various types of fluids and in various volumes have been the subject of much experimental work. It is now clear that these animal experiments bear little relation to what happens in the drowning or near-drowning human. However, this experimen-tal work does indicate the extremes that can be achieved and is therefore of interest. In general, with increasing amounts of seawater aspiration, there are progressive rises in serum sodium, chloride, and calcium concentrations. Serum magnesium levels may also increase.[18] There is an opposite trend in freshwater drowning and near-drowning, except that serum potassium may be increased, which in part results from the hemolysis of red cells.[15, 19]

When one examines the reported data for patients who have drowned in freshwater, however, serum sodium, chloride, and potassium levels are almost in the normal range.[20] A few seawater drowning victims have been noted to have high serum sodium levels; but, in most victims, serum sodium as well as serum chloride and potassium levels fall within a normal range. The same ob-servations have been made of serum electrolyte concentrations of patients who had experienced freshwater or seawater near-drowning (Table 22-1).

Experimentally, after aspiration of 11 ml/kg of freshwater, there are

Table 22-1
Serum Electrolyte Levels of Human Near-Drowning Patients*

Type of Water	Sodium (meq/liter)			Chloride (meq/liter)			Potassium (meq/liter)		
	Patients	Mean	Range	Patients	Mean	Range	Patients	Mean	Range
Fresh water	22	137	126-146	25	101	88-116	21	4.4	3.0-6.3
Seawater	26	147	132-160	28	111	91-127	25	4.2	3.2-5.4

*Data from Modell,[2] pp. 45, 49.

detectable increases in blood volume. With aspiration of 44 ml/kg or more, blood volume increases level off.[15, 21] The influx of hypotonic fluid into the circulation causes a reduction in the osmolality and viscosity of blood and a rise in central venous pressure. The hypervolemia that occurs after freshwater aspiration is transient and central venous pressure returns to normal in about 15 minutes.

After aspiration of 11 ml/kg of seawater, there is a significant decrease in blood volume, primarily as the result of loss of plasma into the lungs.[22] This hypovolemia can persist for as long as 48 hours and is accompanied by increases in blood osmolality and viscosity. Following aspiration of quantities of seawater greater than 11 ml/kg, the changes in blood volume are inversely proportional to the quantity of seawater aspirated.

The changes in blood volume in human near-drowning patients are extremely variable. Since the duration of submersion, quantity of water aspirated, and time of study after submersion differ widely, no general predictions of blood volume changes can be made when evaluating near-drowning patients.[2]

On the basis of his animal experiments,[20, 22] Modell has been able to estimate the volumes of water aspirated by victims of drowning or near-drowning. It appears that approximately 85 percent of the humans who drown, and presumably most of all who survive, aspirate less than 22 ml/kg of water. Changes in serum electrolyte levels appear minor. In only a few patients who have experienced freshwater near-drowning, did hemolysis appear to be of any significance.[2] There is no evidence of hemolysis in subjects exposed to seawater near-drowning episodes. The most likely explanation for the human near-drowning situation is that very small volumes of fluid are aspirated and that the volume and electrolyte disturbances are seldom life-threatening or of primary importance in therapy.

The effects on cardiovascular function of a near-drowning episode are extremely variable.[2] With the outpouring of protein-rich exudate into aveoli, the patient may be hypotensive. On the other hand, patients have been reported to be either normotensive or hypertensive following a near-drowning episode. Bradycardia is a common feature initially and is frequently followed by tachycardia. The most common cardiac picture seen in the near-drowning patient is directly related to myocardial hypoxia and acidosis. The electrocardiogram may show QRS changes, P-wave changes, A-V dissociation, or depression of the ST segment in both fresh- and seawater near-drowning.[6, 16] These changes are usually transient and respond well to improved myocardial oxygenation. In the past, there has been considerable emphasis on the development of ventricular fibrillation in human drowning and near-drowning victims. In fact, this appears to be an extremely uncommon phenomena.

After a severe asphyxic episode, there are likely to be neurological symptoms and signs. The most severely ill patients may have trismus, motor hyperactivity, convulsions, and headaches. Fuller[6] noted that in the 14 of his 77 near-drowning cases in which coma returned, the outcome was uniformly fatal.

The other clinical fetures of near-drowning are varied. About half of the patients will develop pyrexia—sometimes as high as 105-106°F; most will have an associated neutrophil leukocytosis. Albuminuria, hemoglobinuria and anuria all can occur, but are usually not severe.[2]

TREATMENT

Immediate Therapy

The emergency care of the near-drowning victim should be airway clearance and mouth-to-mouth or mouth-to-nose ventilation.[23] Artificial ventilation always should be started as soon as possible—if feasible, even before the victim is moved out of the water. When removed from the water, the patient should have standard artificial ventilation and, if pulseless, should receive external cardiac compression.

Drowning victims often swallow large volumes of water and their stomachs usually become distended. This impairs ventilation and circulation and should be alleviated as soon as possible. To relieve this distension, the patient may be turned on his side and his upper abdomen compressed to force the water out.

There should be no delay in moving the patient to a hospital emergency room where advanced life-support facilities are available. During transportation to the emergency room, high-inspired oxygen concentrations should be administered, ideally by positive end-expiratory pressure respirators. Every near-drowning patient, even one who requires minimal resuscitation, should be admitted to a hospital for a 24-hour observation.

Emergency Room Therapy

At the emergency room level, the immediate objective should be to normalize arterial blood gas and acid-base levels by effective ventilation, by oxygenation, and by buffers or bicarbonate.[2] Mechanical ventilation with positive end-expiratory pressure using 100 percent oxygen is the treatment of choice. This form of therapy has been demonstrated both experimentally[24, 25] and clinically [14, 17] to give significantly higher levels of oxygenation and to enhance the near-drowning victim's chances of survival. Obviously, tracheal intubation will usually be necessary in most patients to provide a suitable airway for providing prolonged mechanical ventilation.

Since the majority of near-drowning victims have some degree of metabolic acidosis, it is reasonable to give all near-drowning patients 50 meq of sodium bicarbonate intravenously immediately upon arrival at the emergency room. As soon as possible, arterial blood should be obtained for determination of pH, P_{O_2}, P_{CO_2}, and bicarbonate. Further, bicarbonate therapy and the extent of ventilatory support will depend upon the results of these values. Isoproternol may be helpful in reducing bronchospasm secondary to aspiration of fluid. Gastric decompression with a Levin tube will withdraw swallowed water, which prevents vomiting and aspiration.

Obviously, if circulatory arrest is present, closed chest cardiac massage should be conducted along with pulmonary support, and an electrocardiogram obtained to determine if the heart is arrested in asystole or in ventricular fibrillation. Electrical defibrillation should be attempted immediately if ventricular fibrillation is present. Epinephrine, calcium chloride, atropine sulfate, and lidocaine may be administered as adjuvants to cardiac resuscitation, as appropriate.

With the outpouring of protein-rich exudate into the alveoli, the patient may be hypovolemic. Here, the correct intravenous infusion is plasma, or if this is not available, blood. There is certainly no place for giving hypotonic or hypertonic solutions to correct electrolyte imbalances expected on the basis of animal experiments where the lungs were flooded with fresh- or seawater.[5, 18, 26] In all severe near-drowning cases, a plasma infusion should be started on arrival at the emergency room.

Hospital Therapy

Continued close observation and treatment of the near-downing patient is essential and should ideally be done in a respiratory intensive-care unit. Vital signs (e.g., pulse, respiration, blood pressure, and temperature) should be regularly monitored.

Serial determinations of arterial P_{O_2}, P_{CO_2}, pH, and bicarbonate obtained via an indwelling arterial catheter will serve as an evaluation and guide to the efficiency of positive end-expiratory pressure ventilation and the adequacy of inspired O_2 levels.[2] Although 100 percent oxygen can initially be administered, it is best to decrease inspired oxygen tensions as soon as possible to avoid pulmonary oxygen toxicity. Arterial P_{O_2} should be maintained at the range of 60-90 mm Hg; measurement of arterial oxygen tension will provide a reliable guide to therapy.

Determinations of serum electrolytes, hematocrit, and hemoglobin should be obtained on the patient's admission to the hospital. These measurements should be repeated 12-24 hours thereafter. Central venous pressure monitoring will assist in assessing the extent of blood volume changes and in guiding intravenous therapy.[2] If abnormal serum electrolyte concentrations or signs of hypovolemia are present, specific correction by the appropriate intravenous solutions is indicated.

An early chest x-ray is valuable. Follow-up chest x-rays should be obtained to determine the development or resolution of atelectasis, pulmonary edema, or pneumonia.

The reactive alveolitis in near-drowning has been likened to the syndrome after aspiration of acid gastric contents. In this situation, there is some evidence that steriod therapy is beneficial. The place of steroids in near drowning remains to be determined, but Sladen and Zauder[27] have provided evidence that intravenous Methylprednisolone (5 mg/kg of body weight per 24 hours in 6 divided doses) may favorably influence the outcome. If the near-drowning has occurred in particularly foul water, then antibiotic therapy may be instituted on admission to the hospital. Otherwise, antibiotics should be given only if an infection becomes apparent.

Most patients who survive the initial 24 hours will recover; if pneumonia does not occur, 3 to 5 days will bring full recovery. Prolonged hospitalization is usually due to hypoxic brain damage. Fortunately, reports of severe neurological deficits following near drowning are quite rare. One has only to look at the case of a chilled child who with vigorous therapy survived 40 minutes of submersion with no residual neurological deficit.[14] This case, in particular, emphasizes the importance of attempting resuscitation even in cases of lengthy submersion.

Supportive psychotherapy might be needed for the survivor to cope with various phobias and anxieties associated with his experience. A mild-to-moderate depression is common 3 to 6 weeks following the incident.[16]

SUMMARY

Near-drowning, whether from submersion in freshwater or seawater, presents the same clinical picture. Hypoxia, pulmonary edema, acidosis, and aspiration are the main considerations in treatment. Therapy should begin at the time of rescue and should be pursued vigorously. The fundamentals of therapy are (a) immediate mouth-to-mouth resuscitation; (b) closed-chest cardiac massage if pulse is absent; (c) tracheal intubation; (d) PEEP with 100 percent oxygen; (e) cardiac defibrillation if indicated; (f) sodium bicarbonate, 1-2 ampules immediately; (g) plasma and intravenous fluids; (h) steriod therapy; and (i) reassessment of oxygenation.

ACKNOWLEDGMENT

The author gratefully acknowledges the assistance of Mrs. Elizabeth Grunewald and Mrs. Peggy Matzen in the preparation of this manuscript.

REFERENCES

1. Webster VP: Skin and scuba diving fatalities in the United States. Public Health Rep 81(8):703-711, 1966
2. Modell JH: The pathophysiology and treatment of drowning and near-drowning. Springfield, Charles C Thomas, 1971, pp 8, 17, 48, 58, 61-64, 72, 92, 105, 107, 119
3. Noble CS, Sharpe N: Drowning—its mechanism and treatment. Can Med Assoc J 89:402-405, 1963
4. Fuller RH: Drowning and the postimmersion syndrome: A clinicopathologic study. Milit Med 128:22-36, 1963
5. Swann HG: Mechanism of circulatory failure in fresh and seawater drowning. Circ Res 4(3):241-244, 1956
6. Fuller RH: The clinical pathology of human near-drowning. Proc R Soc Med 56:33-38, 1963
7. Model JH, Davis JH, Giammona ST, et al: Blood gas and electrolyte changes in human near-drowning victims. 203(5):337-343, 1968
8. Colebatch JHJ, Halamgyi DFJ: Lung mechanics and resuscitation after fluid aspiration. J Appl Physiol 16(4):684-696, 1961
9. Halmagyi DFJ, Colebatch HJH: Ventilation and circulation after fluid aspiration. J Appl Physiol 16(1):35-40, 1961
10. Halmagyi DFJ, Colebatch HJH: The Drowned Lung: A physiological approach to its mechanism and management. Aust Ann Med 10(1):68-77, 1961
11. Colebatch HJH, Halmagyi DFJ: Reflex airway reaction to fluid aspiration. J Appl Physiol 17(5):787-794, 1962
12. Giammona ST, Modell JH: Drowning by total immersion. Effects on pulmonary surfactant of distilled water, isotonic saline and sea-water. Am J Dis Child 114:612-616, 1967
13. Halmagyi DFJ: Lung changes and incidence of respiratory arrest in rats after aspiration of sea and fresh-water. J Appl Physiol 16(1):41-441, 1961
14. Siebke H, Breivik H, Rod T, et al: Survival after 40 minutes' submersion without cerebral sequelae. Lancet 1:1275-1277, 1975
15. Modell JH, Gaub M, Moya F, et al: Phsiologic effects of near-drowning with chlorinated fresh-water, distilled water and isotonic saline. Anesthesiology 27(1):33-41, 1961
16. Griffin GE: Near-Drowning: Its pathophysiology and treatment in man. Milit Med 131(1):12-21, 1966
17. Rutledge RR, Flor RJ: The use of mechanical ventilation with positive end-expiratory pressure in the treatment of near-drowning. Anesthesiology 38(2):194-196, 1973
18. Swann HG, Spafford NR: Body salt and water changes during fresh and sea-water drowning. Tex Rep Biol Med 9:356-382, 1951
19. Modell JH, Weibley TC, Ruiz BC, et al: Serum electrolyte concentrations after fresh-water aspiration: A comparison of species. Anesthesiology 30(4):421-425, 1969
20. Modell JH, Davis JH: Electrolyte changes in human drowning victims. Anesthesiology 30(4):414-420, 1969

21. Modell JH, Moya F: Effects of volume of aspirated fluid during chlorinated fresh-water drowning. Anesthesiology 27:662-672, 1966
22. Modell JH, Moya F, Newby EJ, et al: The effects of fluid volume in sea-water drowning. Ann Intern Med 67(1):68-80, 1967
23. Standards for Cardiopulmonary Resusciation (CPR) and Emergency Cardiac Care (ECC) JAMA 227(7):833-888, 1974
24. Modell JH, Calderwood HWC, Ruiz BC, et al: Effects of ventilatory patterns on arterial oxygenation after near-drowning in sea-water. Anesthesiology 40(4):376-384, 1974
25. Ruiz BC, Calderwood HW, Modell JH, et al: Effect of ventilatory patterns on arterial oxygenation after near-drowning with fresh-water: A comparative study in dogs. Anesth Analg 52(4):571-577, 1973
26. Swann HG, Brucer M, Moore C, et al: Fresh-water and Sea-Water Drowning: A study of the terminal cardiac and biochemical events. Tex Rep Biol Med 5:423-437, 1947
27. Sladen A, Zauder HL: Methylprednisolone therapy for pulmonary edema following near-drowning. JAMA 215(11):1793-1796, 1971

STUDY QUESTIONS

1. In near-drowning, all of the following factors are frequently important *except*
   a. Hypoxia
   b. Acidosis
   c. Serum electrolyte abnormalities
   d. Pulmonary edema

2. The emergency treatment of severe near-drowning includes
   a. Ventilation with positive end-expiratory pressure using 100 percent oxygen
   b. Determination of arterial blood gases
   c. Infusion of intravenous bicarbonate solution
   d. Plasma infusion
   e. All of the above

3. Antibiotics should always be given following near-drowning in order to prevent pneumonia.
   a. True
   b. False

4. A swimmer was brought to the emergency room following an undetermined period underwater. He is cold, blue, and without signs of cardiorespiratory activity. The physician should
   a. Begin resuscitation and therapy
   b. Not attempt resuscitation because permanent brain damage has already occurred

5. A near-drowning victim who revives quickly
   a. Can be sent home
   b. Should be admitted to a hospital for observation.

Carl Edmonds

23

Investigation of Diving Accidents

In the investigation of diving accidents, there are five separate areas which may require assessment. These are

Personal and past medical history
Environmental conditions
Dive profile and history
Diving equipment
Autopsy investigation

Only the last of these will be discussed in detail in this chapter, the others being more relevant to investigation by diving authorities. A knowledge of the predisposing factors and clinical sequelae of the specific medical conditions is detailed elsewhere in other chapters.

PERSONAL AND PAST MEDICAL HISTORY

There is certain personal data that may be relevant in assessing the diving accident. First and foremost is the presence of diseases likely to predispose to the diving accident and reference should be made to Chapter 24, Medical Standards for Diving. Other information that may be very pertinent is the degree of experience of the diver and his companions. The incidence of accidents is far greater with the inexperienced diver, especially during his first "open water" sea dive. The history of previous diving accidents should be taken into consideration. Many disorders experienced by divers in the past are likely to be repeated under similar conditions. These comprise a wide range of accidents and include such potentially dangerous conditions underwater as breath-hold following hyperventilation, panic with hyperventilation, saltwater aspiration, alternobaric vertigo, barotrauma and especially pulmonary barotrauma, nitrogen narcosis, syncope of ascent, decompression sickness, oxygen toxicity, and carbon dioxide toxicity.

ENVIRONMENTAL CONDITIONS

Note should be made of the weather and environmental conditions prevailing at the time of the accident. Over one-quarter of the fatalities are associated with adverse environmental conditons of this nature. Not only may the diver be exposed to an increased risk of injury during entry into or exit from the water, but also, during the dive, there may be exceptional stress in the form of impaired visibility, seasickness, tidal currents, rips, etc. A diver who has to battle a 1 knot current is exerting himself to a considerable degree, probably consuming 2 liters or more of oxygen/minute and ventilating 40 liters of gas/minute/atm., surface equivalent. It is virtually impossible for an unassisted diver to make significant headway against a current of 2 knots or more; thus, not only is the speed of the current important, but also the direction. If the diver initially swims with a strong current, his removal from his site of entry will be rapid, and his return much more difficult. Also, surface currents do not necessarily reflect those at depth. The temperature of the water will influence his susceptibility to hypothermia and also the functioning of various pieces of diving equipment. Carbon dioxide absorbents are less effective under cold conditions, and with the temperature approaching the freezing point, regulators may cease to function. Environmental hazards include exposure to explosives, dangerous marine animals, inability to surface (e.g., in caves, under ledges, in kelp, etc.) and many others.

DIVE PROFILE AND HISTORY

In the assessment of predisposition to decompression sickness, a history of recent dives is of importance. It may be equally relevant in cases of undisclosed pulmonary barotrauma, saltwater aspiration, hypothermia, etc. In cases of breath-hold diving, the estimated depth and duration are very relevant to the possibility of hypoxia, as is the practice of preceding hyperventilation. With the use of diving equipment, the depth and duration parameters of each dive are germane to the development of decompression sickness, especially if there are recommended stoppages that have been omitted, or if the dive is in excess of that suggested in the tables, e.g., beyond the "limiting line" in the Royal Navy tables, or in the exceptional exposure tables of the United States Navy. The depth is of paramount importance in the assessment of nitrogen narcosis and its influence on the behavior of the diver, and also in other gas toxicity disorders such as with carbon dioxide and oxygen. The speed of ascent is relevant, especially if it is excessive, since it can be correlated with pulmonary barotrauma, decompression sickness, or syncope of ascent. It is of note that the Blackpool Tables prepared in 1969 recommend a maximum rate of ascent of 50 feet/minute to the first stop and 10 feet/minute between stops. Some civilian amateur divers have been timed to exceed 200 feet/minute in their routine daily practice.

The amount of exercise performed during the dive is of considerable importance when assessing the medical disorders associated with rebreathing equipment. With strenuous exercise, there is an increased oxygen requirement which may be in excess of that supplied by the flow rate for the particular gas mixture chosen. With the increased oxygen consumption, there is also an increased carbon dioxide production, which places an added load on the absorbent system. Thus, the dangers of both hypoxia and carbon dioxide toxicity are increased. Exercise also increases the incidence of oxygen toxicity with susceptible partial pressures of oxygen. Even with open circuit scuba, there are problems to be encountered with increased exercise. Firstly, there is an increased consumption of gas, and this may not be allowed for by the diver who is not wearing a tank pressure gauge to indicate this consumption. Second, there is a problem in the production of an increased resistance to breathing with a resultant dyspnea and physical exhaustion. Panic is then a common complication.

Following one of the hazards mentioned above, or associated with underwater rescue attempts, there is likely to be a panic and rapid ascent. Inadequate training will then become manifest. The practice of buddy breathing is a particular hazard, often resulting in one of the companions making a desperate dash to the surface. Probably the most neglected information relevant to any accident, and also to the interpretation of the autopsy findings, is that involving the first aid and resuscitation methods employed.

The information regarding the symptoms of each specific disorder can be found by reference to the respective chapters of this book.

DIVING EQUIPMENT

It is necessary to ensure that there is little or no interference after the accident with the diving equipment that has been used by all the divers, until a detailed written report has been completed and photographs taken. The cause of the accident, or factors likely to aggravate it, is often ascertained from the examination of this equipment. The information may vary from such obvious faults as the absence of protective clothing in a diver exposed to cold water, to the complex analysis techniques for oxygen, carbon dioxide, carbon monoxide, inert gases, and hydrocarbons of the remaining contents of the gas cylinders. Functioning of the equipment also requires assessment, e.g., demand valve performance, determining the flow rate through the reducer, the efficiency of the carbon dioxide absorbent system, etc.

The equipment may have been affected by the accident, as can be seen when there is loss or displacement of movable items or damage to the protective clothing, diving set, or accessories. Gas spaces, such as the face mask, buoyancy vest, or counterlung may be flooded. The lugs of the mouthpiece may be bitten during a convulsion. Vomitus may be present on the equipment or on the mouthpiece, and this could either be a cause of the accident or one of the events in the sequence, which may have aggravated the situation.

Other observations on the equipment may reflect both on the diver and on the rescue procedure. The ease with which the weight belt can be released, or whether this was actually done, is of obvious importance. A depth gauge, watch, pressure gauge on the gas cylinder, decompression meter, etc., will be worn by the diver who takes precautions against accidents. A knife is important to overcome entanglements in ropes, kelp, etc. The use of a buoyancy vest and its ease of operation are very relevant to the first aid capability. Similarly, a buddy line or direct contact with the surface support is often necessary for a rapid rescue.

Note, that in 70 percent of the diving fatalities, there is a period in excess of 15 minutes between the accident and rescue. This is an unacceptable duration for any patient to remain without functioning breathing equipment. Thus, in many cases, there is a progression from unconsciousness to death, which could have been prevented by the institution of the three basic requirements for first aid in diving, viz:

1. Immediate assistance from a companion diver, and a method of requesting this
2. Assistance in returning to the surface or to a habitable environment
3. The use of first aid techniques to ensure maintenance of life until professional medical treatment is obtained

In practice, the common methods of obtaining the above 3 requirements are

1. A lifeline to a buddy (companion diver)
2. A buoyancy vest or direct contact with the surface support
3. Mouth-to-mouth respiration and external cardiac massage.

AUTOPSY PROCEDURE

Site and Time of the Autopsy

To overcome the generalized and disruptive effects of the liberation of gas from the deceased diver who is brought to the surface, i.e., postmortem decompression sickness, it is often advantageous to perform the autopsy prior to decompression. This is possible when the death has occurred in a recompression facility, and where the pathologist can be transferred to the same pressure, and can perform the autopsy under those conditions. This is very relevant in saturation diving, where the environment is such as to sustain life for an indefinite time. It is much more difficult under operational diving conditions where the pathologist himself may be exposed to the hazards of nitrogen narcosis and decompression sickness. The former is likely to influence his ability to perform the autopsy and the latter, his enthusiasm.

The results of the autopsy must always be assessed in relation to the time between the diving accident and the diver's death, and also between the death and the time of autopsy. If there has been a substantial period of time between the accident, injury, drowning, or decompression sickness and the time of death, then many of the pathological changes will have time to be corrected, even though the disease progresses to a fatal termination. Thus the electrolyte changes of drowning and the gas changes associated with decompression sickness may well be totally corrected. The pathological lesions demonstrated hours or days later may reflect only the previous existence of the disease. A prolonged time between death and autopsy will nullify any electrolyte changes, and putrefaction influences both gas and alcohol production. The widespread disruptive influence of postmortem decompression sickness has already been mentioned.

The results of bacteriological investigations will also be greatly influenced by these factors. A time delay between the dive and death from encephalitis due to *Naegleria* is expected in divers who have exposed themselves to contaminated freshwater areas. A paracolon growth from shark wounds is also possible for some days following the injury. Unfortunately, many bacteriologically positive results may reflect contamination as opposed to actual aquatic infection. This is so with organisms such as *Clostridium tetani* and *C. welchii*. Nematocyst identification may remain possible for many days, even though the actual lesion may decrease in its florid appearance, not only between the injury and the time of death, but also postmortem.

General

An investigation of the cause of death following diving is often poorly understood by the average pathologist. Once death has been certified, it is important that no further interference is caused with either the body, its clothing, or the equipment, except for sealing the equipment and the closure of any valves associated with it.

The observations will commence with an examination of the deceased prior to cleaning or removal of foreign bodies or clothing. This examination may demonstrate damage from either the cause of the accident, e.g., shark attack; or injuries from the search and recovery, e.g., damage from a grappling hook or line.

An examination of the integument of the diver may also reveal important information. Trauma to the skin from marine animals may either be caused after death or be instrumental in the death. If there are marine animal lesions, these are usually easy to diagnose. Shark "bumping" produces parallel lacerations, whereas multiple crescentic teeth marks and tearing wounds illustrate the direction of the attack and the size of the animal. Teeth particles are very commonly found in the wound, and will assist in identifying the species of shark. Barracuda bites are clean-cut incisions. Coelenterate injuries will be recognizable by the number and distribution of the whiplike marks, which commonly fade after death. An accurate identification of the type of coelenterate or jellyfish is possible by taking a skin scraping for examination of the nematocysts by a marine biologist. Cone shell and blue-ringed octopus bites appear as single hemorrhagic blebs, whereas a sea snake bite will show two or more fang marks with surrounding teeth impressions. Where a large octopus has held a victim, multiple bruising from round sucker marks is seen along the extent of the tentacle contact.

External evidence of barotrauma is important in ascertaining the sequence of events. An unconscious diver, or one who has not been able to equalize his physiological or equipment gas spaces during submergence, will have evidence of barotrauma as described in previous chapters. Thus, there must always be an examination for evidence of mask or face squeeze with hemorrhage into the conjunctiva, ear squeeze with hemorrhage or perforation of the tympanic membrane, and suit squeeze with long whiplike marks underneath the folds of the protective clothing. Total body squeeze may occur when a standard diving rig is being used.

Pulmonary barotrauma of ascent may be inferred by evidence of surgical (subcutaneous) emphysema localized to the supraclavicular areas. If this finding is generalized over most of the body, then it is more likely to be due to the liberation of gas following death, i.e., postmortem decompression sickness. This should not be confused with putrefactive changes. Where the diver has suffered from decompression sickness, there is often a reddish or cyanotic distension of the tissues of the head, arms, and upper trunk. The body will therefore have an appearance not unlike that seen in clinical cases of the superior vena cava syndrome.

The skin of the fingers may show the effects of immersion, i.e., pale and wrinkled with the so-called washerwoman's skin. There may be lacerations from where the diver has attempted to clutch barnacles, coral, etc. Injury inflicted by aquatic animals in the early postmortem period is normally restricted to the fingers, nose, lips, eyelids, etc.

There is often evidence of vomitus, which may be either causative or an integral part of the sequence of events. In cases in which seawater has been aspirated, there may be white, pink, or blood-stained foam from the nose and mouth. Where the patient has been brought to the surface following a significant exposure at depth, there may also be distension of the gas spaces within the body resulting in a distended abdomen, fecal extrusions, etc.

Radiology

Prior to any invasive technique, total body radiology should be performed for evidence of gas within the tissues, pneumothorax, abdominal gas, and gas occupying the vessels and heart. The interpretation of this must include consideration of pulmonary barotrauma, decompression sickness, and postmortem decompression sickness. X-rays should also be performed for bone lesions and dysbaric osteonecrosis. In the case of marine animal injuries, there may also be evidence of bone damage and foreign bodies, such as shark teeth.

Air Embolism

Some technique to demonstrate air emboli is of paramount importance in the investigation of diving accidents. Although in most general medicine situations information is sought regarding gas in the venous system or on the right side of the heart, in cases of diving accidents the important emboli are arterial. There are two methods of detecting this, and neither is particularly well-known among general pathologists. In each case, the presence of a few cubic centimeters of air is very significant; whereas, in general medicine, one requires more than 1 cc of air per kg body weight rapidly infused into the venous system to cause death. The first technique[4] is for the incision to be made in the scalp initially, and the calvarium removed. This may introduce artefactual "air emboli" into the superficial cerebral veins and venous sinuses, but these are not of diagnostic importance. The circle of Willis and its related arteries are the areas to be examined meticulously for evidence of the significant air bubbles. Before any arteries are cut, the frontal lobes are reflected and the optic nerves severed. The circle is then carefully inspected, including the anterior cerebral and vertebral arteries. The middle cerebral arteries may be inspected by spreading the insula very carefully. If bubbles are found, they should be photographed in situ, or after clamping the carotids and cutting proximal to the clamp, in order to obtain a better exposure.

The other technique of demonstrating cerebral air emboli is to make a

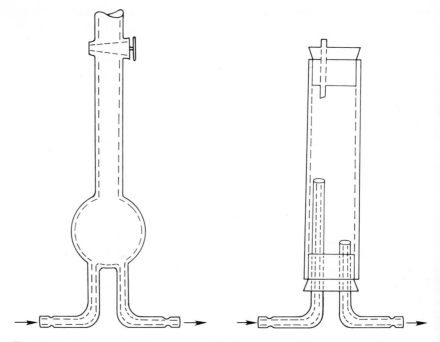

Fig. 23-1. Examples of air traps used during autopsy. The trap is initially filled with water and sealed at the top before blood is passed through.

midline or Y incision in the neck and expose, by careful dissection at as low a level as convenient, all vessels on both sides including the vertebral arteries and veins. All these vessels are then ligated and the trachea is clamped. The esophagus should also be ligated. Two air traps are set up as shown in Fig. 23-1, one on each side of the head and each one connected to a cannula tied in the jugular vein above the ligature. Care is taken to ensure that the air trap system is free of air bubbles beforehand. The cannuli are then perfused from the common carotid, and , if possible, the vertebral artery on each side, with a 3.8 percent sodium citrate solution. This will force air out of the cerebral circulation into the respective air traps. For a satisfactory perfusion of the brain, the vertebral artery should be injected as well as the common carotid. If this is particularly difficult to do, the pathologist may complete the ligation at that stage and then wait until the lungs and heart have been removed from the thorax in order to use the right innominate artery.

Cardiothoracic Investigation

Prior to the opening of the thorax, it is recommended that the body be totally immersed in slowly flowing water, so that any air escape can be easily detected. The concept of an underwater autopsy has received considerable lip service, although practical experience seems very limited. A Y-shaped incision can then be performed, noting the presence or absence of foaming blood or gross bubbles in the vessels and subcutaneous tissue. Intapleural pressure can be measured using a water manometer, and the presence of air in the intrapleural space can be verified at the same time by aspiration through a needle inserted via an intercostal space. The sternum, costal cartilage, and the inner two-thirds of each clavicle are removed, after dividing the pectoral fascia and the sternomastoid. The costal cartilages are divided by using a guillotine type of shears and not a knife to prevent damaging the visceral pleura. The sternoclavicular joints are not dissected, but each clavicle is divided at the outer third in order not to damage the underlying suclavian vessels. Any fluid or air is observed in the pleural cavities. The appearance of the lungs is noted, and an inspection is made for mediastinal emphysema. The heart is also inspected for distension, as both sides may contain air. In cases of possible drowning, a specimen of blood should be taken with a needle and syringe from each ventricle. It is important not to palpate or disturb any air bubbles at this time. The diaphragm is freed from below by cutting along the attached border and reflecting it downward, in order to cut between the ligatures or clamps on the inferior vena cava, aorta, and esophagus. Any injury to the pleura, either recent or in the form of old adhesions, is recorded. The trachea is divided above a clamp, with the tongue and larynx left in situ, and the lungs and heart are removed *en bloc.* This will entail the cutting between the ligatures of the following vessels: right and left innominate veins; right and left internal mammary veins if possible; right innominate artery; left common carotid; left subclavian artery. The heart and lungs can then be x-rayed independently of the remainder of the body. The lungs can be partly inflated by blowing a small quantity of air into the trachea, and this may be performed underwater in order to detect either small blebs or bullae (these are often difficult to find without this test), and the site of rupture in cases of pneumothorax. Each hilum is then clamped at the lungs and cut away distal to the clamp. The pericardial sac is opened underwater and any air bubbles noted. An attempt must be made at this stage to observe the coronary vessels and to ascertain whether they also contain any bubbles. The chambers of the heart are also opened underwater to test for the presence of air bubbles. Frothy blood may be found in the left ventricle, aorta, aortic arch, or in the right heart.

Most of this procedure can be performed, without the necessity of having the full body immersed, by immersing only the heart and lungs underwater. This is achieved by performing a neck incision extending down the midline from the sternal notch to the midpoint between the xiphisternum and umbilicus, and then to each of the anterosuperior iliac spines. The skin and the muscles over the chest and the skin over the abdomen are then widely reflected by undercutting, and the trough between the body and the skin filled with water. The body cavities can then be opened, and the presence of any abnormal gas collection noted.

Abdomen

Apart from these observations, it is necessary to inspect the inferior vena cava and descending aorta for gas bubbles and to examine the gastrointestinal tact for hemorrhages and infarcts, which may be related to either emboli or decompression sickness. In cases of underwater blast, most of the hemorrhages occur between a gas and fluid interface, and the abdomen and gastrointestinal tract are expecially involved. under these conditions, there are seldom any external sings of violence on the skin or subcutaneous tissue despite severe hemorrhages within the bowel itself.

Bone Lesions

It is important for biopsies to be performed on all potential dysbaric osteonecrotic lesions.

Temporal Bones

In diving accidents, in diving pathology, the temporal bone and its associated middle ear and mastoid air cell cavities are of special importance. Not only will hemorrhage occur within this area in situations leading to barotrauma of descent, but also there are specific disorders related to disorientation which may be instrumental in the diving accident. These include such injuries as tympanic membrane perforation, middle ear barotrauma of descent, and inner ear disturbances, either from hemorrhage or round window rupture. It is thus important to record the appearance of the tympanic membrane on otoscopy, the presence of any fluid within the middle ear cavity, and, finally, a histological examination of the temporal bones performed by an experienced laboratory.

Other Laboratory Examinations

It is necessary to record the presence of alcohol and drugs as contributions to the diver's death. The alcohol level must be correlated with the postmortem interval to assess the putrefactive neoformation of this substance. Other biochemical investigations that may be relevant include serum electrolytes, performed on both the right and left side of the heart, serum hemoglobin and haptoglobin levels, and carboxyhemoglobin estimation. Histological examination of the blood, the tissues, and the bone marrow, as well as the material in the respiratory and gastrointestinal tracts, is necessary for the identification of diatoms and aquatic organisms. This information should be compared with similar investigation on a sample of water taken from the areas in which the diver could have died.

CONCLUSION

There needs to be close cooperation between the investigations performed by the diving supervisors, the diving physician, and the pathologist to obtain data and then to assess it. There is little available systematized work perfomed on the pathology and autopsy techniques associated with diving accidents. In most countries there are no analogous units to those investigating aircraft accidents; thus, the usual practice is for the investigation of the dive to be performed by a police inspector moderately ignorant in the technical aspects of diving equipment, a local clinician who has no training in diving medicine, and a pathologist who is overworked and not amenable to varying his standardization and venerable techniques. The result is often either a mistaken diagnosis of decompression sickness or drowning, without an explanation as to the sequence of events leading to this.

There is thus a regrettable tendency to lose valuable information and not to learn from the mistakes of the past.

REFERENCES

1. Royal Austrialian Navy Medical Technical Instruction No. 110.
2. Scuba Safety Report Series, Nos. 3, 5, 7. University of Rhode Island 1972
3. Edmonds C, Lowry C, Pennefather J, Diving and Subaquatic Medicine. Sidney, A Diving Medical Centre Publication, 1976
4. Goldhahn RT: Scuba deaths in the military: an approach for pathologists, Annual Meeting, American Academy of Forensic Sciences, Las Vegas, Nevada, February 20, 1973

STUDY QUESTIONS

1. A diver, who had been collecting abalone near San Diego, was brought aboard with severe hemorrhages from lacerations of the left leg. Because a tourniquet was not applied, he bled to death. On examination of the body, it was noted that the lacerations were in four groups. The two major ones were on the lateral and the medial aspect of the leg, and there were minor ones on the opposite sides of the ankle. In each case, there was a series of concentric curved lacerations. Because of the variety of explanations offered by local divers and medicos, a definitive diagnosis was required. What was this diagnosis, and how could it be verified?

2. X-rays performed postmortem at sea level on a diver who had died while in a habitat at a depth of 200 feet revealed gas in all the subcutaneous areas and in the lumen of the vessels. He had previously performed some excursion diving from the habitat at a depth of 300 feet.

What is the pathological diagnosis of the injury described, and explain its relevance to the remainder of the autopsy.

3. Of what relevance is an examination of the temporal bone, both morbid and histological, in a postmortem on a diver.

4. Of what importance is the demonstration of dysbaric osteonecrotic lesions in divers when detected during the postmortem radiological examinations?

5. A diver ascended very rapidly from a depth of 60 feet, reached the surface, and immediately lost consciousness. Bloody froth issued from the mouth, and the diver died within minutes of being rescued from the water.

During the autopsy, the skull was opened through a horizontal saw cut and the calvarium reflected. On examination, there was seen to be gas in the cortical veins. Based on this finding what is the pathological diagnosis?

Eric P. Kindwall

24

Medical Examination of the Diver*

Depending upon what kind of diver one is examining, and what sort of work he intends to do, different physical standards are observed. Navy divers, commercial divers, caisson workers, and sport scuba divers all have different physical requirements.

Navy divers must initially pass a very rigid standard Navy physical examination which has no direct relevance to diving. Then, additional requirements are made. With commercial divers, there is more leeway, but it is incumbent on the examining physician to be sure that the diving applicant is physically capable of doing the kind of work he may be called upon to do. Some commercial divers may saturate for days at a time, where medical help cannot reach them. Others may be flown to a foreign country at a moment's notice. These men should not have any physical illness that might give them trouble if they were to be isolated from immediate emergency medical aid.

Caisson workers also experience an environment of increased ambient pressure. However, they are not surrounded by water and, in some respects, the stringent physical requirements for divers are somewhat relaxed for these men. However, caisson workers usually experience very long exposure times to compressed air and, therefore, often suffer from decompression sickness when working at pressure greater than 12 psig. For this reason, those factors that could contribute to an increased susceptibility to decompression sickness are especially important to notice in caisson workers. Economically, the most important single item in commercial divers and caisson workers is to rule out

---

*The physical standards for sport scuba divers used in this chapter have been adapted from "Physical Standards for Sport Scuba Diving," approved by the Undersea Medical Society, 9650 Rockville Pike, Bethesda, Maryland 20014, February, 1974.

the presence of aseptic necrosis of the bone before the applicant is employed by any given company. Skeletal surveys should be done at regular yearly intervals thereafter. This is not only for the protection of the worker, but because workmen's compensation can create tremendous insurance losses should aseptic necrosis be discovered. This is the single, most important, factor in performing physical examinations on the commerical diver or caisson worker.

Sport scuba divers are the most varied group of underwater mammals the doctor is asked to examine. Scuba divers may range from young children to grandmothers. This chapter will be devoted to the examination of the sport scuba diver. It must be borne in mind that there are no laws preventing anyone from engaging in sport diving at the present time, and insurance company regulations do not apply in the same way to sport scuba divers as they do to commercial workers. Therefore, the physician's recommendations will, at best, be taken as "a direct order" and at worst, completely ignored. The examining physician should, however, be able to advise the sport scuba diver intelligently when it comes to the peculiar requirements of diving.

ABSOLUTE CONTRAINDICATIONS TO DIVING

1. Persons subject to spontaneous pneumothorax.
2. Persons subject to epileptic seizures or syncopal attacks.
3. Lung cysts or definite air-trapping lesions seen on a chest x-ray.
4. Perforated eardrum.
5. Active asthma.
6. Drug addiction.
7. Brittle diabetes, or individuals subject to insulin shock or diabetic coma.
8. Ear surgery with placement of plastic strut in air conduction chain.

Persons subject to repeated pneumothorax must be disqualified from diving. Should a pneumothorax occur while the diver is submerged, it would be life threatening for him to return to the surface with the subsequent expansion of the intrathoracic air. A person with a history of one spontaneous pneumothorax may be subject to more attacks. It is up to the physician to make the determination whether or not the would-be diver is subject to further pneumothoraces.

The same applies to patients subject to epileptic seizures or syncopal attacks. Having an epileptic seizure underwater would probably be fatal. In addition, it would endanger a diving buddy.

Lung cysts or definite air-trapping lesions, as seen on a chest x-ray, raise the question of adequate ventilation of the lungs. In a free ascent situation, a person with marginal patency of his pulmonary air passages might conceivably trap air if he buoyantly ascended from 50 feet to the surface in 7 or 8 seconds. For this reason, close attention should be paid to the chest x-ray. Pulmonary function tests may be indicated if there is any question.

Perforated eardrum is usually considered disqualifying. However, the author has seen divers with perforated eardrum who have been diving for years without difficulty, and apparently never suffer from vertigo or nystagmus when cold water enters the middle ear. If a diver has been successfully diving with a perforated eardrum and continues to dive in the same waters, there is no reason to disqualify him if he has proven his ability. Unless the applicant has proven ability as a diver, perforated eardrum is absolutely disqualifying as cold water entering the middle ear can cause sudden and catastrophic vertigo and disorientation. Infection of the middle ear is also a potential complication.

Active asthma, in which airway obstruction occurs, is disqualifying because of the occasional necessity to make very rapid ascents. Drug addiction needs no comment, nor does the question of insulin shock or diabetic coma.

Certain types of ear surgery involve the insertion of a plastic or metal strut in place of the bony ossicles of the ear. The trauma of equalizing pressure in the middle ear or performing a Valsalva maneuver might very well disrupt this kind of surgery, and the patient should not engage in diving.

RELATIVE CONTRAINDICATIONS

Decrease of pulmonary reserve from any cause is a relative contraindication. The work of breathing is many times greater as one descends deeper underwater and the breathing gas becomes more dense. The prospective diver should be warned that if he undertakes deep or strenuous diving, or if he finds himself suddenly in an emergency situation even in shallow water where he must work hard, he may endanger his life. This is a very real hazard and cannot be overstressed.

Pregnant women often ask if scuba diving is safe. The safety of scuba diving during pregnancy has not been established. Little is known about inert gas transport across the placenta. Until more information is available, decompression diving or any diving deeper than 30 feet should be discouraged during pregnancy, especially during the first trimester. The results of a nitrogen bubble developing in an embryonic central nervous system or a limb bud can only be surmised. Also, the effects of an increased partial pressure of oxygen on the foetus (84% effective at 99 ft) must be considered. The prospective diver should be apprised of this. After all, it is not a great hardship to wait a few months until the pregnancy is over to begin diving once again.

Obesity is a problem for the diver only when he intends to do decompression diving. Otherwise, fat can be helpful because of its insulating properties in cold water. A correlation has been established between an increased bends incidence, body weight 20 percent greater than that allowed in actuarial height-weight charts, and excessive skin-fold fat thickness over the triceps area of the arm and the area below the scapula on the back. Other fat areas of the body, such as the skin-fold thickness on the legs or the size of the abdominal panniculus, oddly enough do not correlate with the incidence of decompression sickness. Obesity is particularly dangerous in divers requiring decompression due to long bottom times, even at moderate depths. The prospective diver should be apprised of this if obesity is present.

History of thoracotomy may rule out diving for a prospective scuba enthusiast. The reason for the thoracotomy may be determining in this case. In such a case, pulmonary function studies should be carried out to detect air trapping, as well as the usual chest film. Even if these are normal, the patient should preferably have a pressurization-depressurization test in a dry chamber at a medical facility under controlled conditions before diving. The chamber tests should be conducted in a chamber with 165-foot capability. Decompression should be from a minimum of 60 feet at a rate approaching, but not exceeding, 60 feet/minute.

The physician must be very careful with the patient who has a history of myocardial infarction. The prospective diver, having had an infarct, should be over 1 year postcoronary. He must have no angina, arrythmia, or demonstrable heart failure and must have a normal exercise tolerance capability even to be considered for diving. A stress EKG should be normal. If such an individual is approved for diving, he should be informed that a myocardial infarction occurring underwater may well prove fatal. Additionally, it is advisable that anyone who has had a myocardial infarction have a stress test EKG done at 6-month intervals, plus other medical followup if he intends to dive. Interestingly, a recent article implied that pilots who had suffered a myocardial infarction may be safer in the air than their peers of the same age who had not suffered a similar episode. This is because in such a case the cardiovascular system has been thoroughly investigated, and is kept under much better medical surveillance than the cardiovascular system of someone of equal age who has not had previous cardiac difficulty.

CONDITIONS NECESSITATING TEMPORARY
DISQUALIFICATION FROM DIVING

1. Severe hay fever or other allergy that causes sinus and middle ear blockage.

2. Upper and lower respiratory infection causing sinus or middle ear blockage or chest congestion.
3. Alcoholic intoxication.
4. Medication that might interfere with normal diving.

These conditions need no further explanation as their relation to diving is obvious. On very rare occasions, patients have suffered severe pain in sinuses during decompression, especially if clearing the sinus has been difficult on the way down. Normally, however, congestion presents problems only during descent. It is perfectly acceptable to use a decongestant to overcome these difficulties if they are not too severe.

THE PHYSICAL EXAMINATION*

An otherwise standard history and physical examination must be carried out keeping the previously noted points in mind. The examining physician should interpret any physical findings strictly on the basis of what kind of diving a prospective diver intends to do. By using this frame of reference, the applicant's cardiovascular, gastrointestinal, genitourinary, neuromuscular, and central nervous systems can be assessed to determine if the *physical exertion* necessitated by the type of diving planned will be harmful to the organ system in question. It should also be determined if the organ system's status would make it difficult, impossible, or dangerous for the prospective diver to carry out the planned dives or exertion.

As much information as possible about the type of diving planned should be elicited. If the diver simply states, "I will never dive deeper than 10 feet," this is not adequate information. In one case, it might mean cleaning the family swimming pool, and in another, it could conceivably mean open sea, night diving in heavy current and cold water with a long swim from the beach to the dive site. The maximum sustained speed a good swimmer in top condition can maintain is only 0.6 knot (without fins).

The diving physician should try to familiarize himself with the underwater conditions likely to be encountered (visibility, temperature, thermoclines, current, depth, etc.) in his diving area, so he can better appraise prospective divers. This can be done by diving himself or by questioning experienced local divers. The prospective diver must be informed of any possible physical limitations detected by the physician and how they might exclude him from certain kinds of diving.

*Examples of history and physical examination forms are found in Appendix 4.

MISCELLANEOUS FACTORS TO KEEP IN MIND WHEN
ADVISING PROSPECTIVE DIVERS OR THEIR PARENTS

In regard to the extremes of age, a youngster must obviously be physically of sufficient size to be able to handle his heavy diving equipment. Very young children may swim and dive well, but they have not yet had the chronologic opportunity to develop experience and judgment in emergency situations. Any youngster must be old enough to understand the basic physics involved in diving and to pass written and oral tests on these subjects.

In older age groups, arteriosclerosis will tend to predispose to decompression sickness. Individuals over 50 should be informed of this and must be cautious in undertaking dives approaching no-decompression limits or decompression diving.

The physician should also consider the individual's personality profile if possible. The applicant must be personally motivated to dive. When asked why he wants to dive, he should give an appropriate answer. Always ask the prospective diver *himself,* and this should be done in private. Often, a spouse or child takes up diving because of pressure from the husband, wife or parents. If the individual is forced into diving and is psychologically unmotivated, there is a distinct risk of accident.

Another thing to remember is that people with a history of multiple serious fractures, automobile or motorcycle accidents, chronic alcoholism, or impulsive behavior are more prone to have serious scuba diving accidents.

STUDY QUESTIONS

1. Persons subject to epileptic seizures or syncopal attacks should never dive.
   a. True
   b. False
2. Which of the following organ systems is least important with regard to diving:
   a. central nervous system
   b. pulmonary system
   c. genitourinary system
   d. Ears and sinuses
   e. musculoskeletal system
4. A perforated ear drum is disqualifying because it can cause severe external ear squeeze.
   a. True
   b. False

5. Pregnant women may dive with perfect safety as long as they follow standard air decompression tables or use a decompression meter.
   a. True
   b. False
6. The size of the abdominal panniculus correlates well with susceptibility to decompression sickness.
   a. True
   b. False
7. A history of myocardial infarction is an absolute contraindication to sport diving.
   a. True
   b. False
8. A young child who can swim and dive well has what is required to be an excellent scuba diver.
   a. True
   b. False

Appendix 1

Pressure Conversion Table

Pressure Units Found in Articles

	kg/cm^2	at*	atm†	bar
kg/cm^2	1	1.000	1.033	1.020
at*	1.000	1	1.033	1.020
atm†	9.678× 10^{-1}	9.678× 10^{-1}	1	9.869× 10^{-1}
bar	9.807× 10^{-1}	9.807× 10^{-1}	1.013	1
torr mm Hg	735.5	735.5	760	750.1
lbs/in^2	1.422× 10^1	1.422× 10^1	1.470× 10^1	1.450× 10^1
meters sea water (msw)	1.000× 10^1	1.000× 10^1	1.033× 10^1	1.020× 10^1
feet sea water (fsw)	3.198× 10^1	3.198× 10^1	3.305× 10^1	3.261× 10^1

Pressure units of the reader (row label, left of table)

*Technical atmosphere, equal to 1 kg/cm^2.

†Standard atmosphere, equal to pressure exerted by a column of mercury 760 mm high at a temperature where the density of mercury is 13.5951 g/cm^3.

Courtesy *Undersea Biomedical Research,* 9650 Rockville Pike, Bethesda, Maryland, 20014, 1974.

torr mm Hg	lbs/in^2	meters sea water (msw)	feet sea water (fsw)
1.360×10^{-3}	7.031×10^{-2}	1.026×10^{-1}	3.127×10^{-2}
1.360×10^{-3}	7.031×10^{-2}	1.026×10^{-1}	3.127×10^{-2}
1.316×10^{-3}	6.805×10^{-2}	9.927×10^{-2}	3.026×10^{-2}
1.333×10^{-3}	6.8945×10^{-2}	1.0052×10^{-1}	3.067×10^{-2}
1	51.71	75.5	23.
1.934×10^{-2}	1	1.458	4.445×10^{-1}
1.360×10^{-2}	7.031×10^{-1}	1	3.048×10^{-1}
4.347×10^{-2}	2.247	3.281	1

In order to convert the pressure units presented in an article to those used by the reader, enter the table at the top with the author's units and read down to the row corresponding to the reader's units; note the number, x. Convert any pressure unit cited by the author by multiplying it with x.

> Example: author citation = 33 feet seawater (fsw)
> reader's units are atm
> so, $x = 3.026 \times 10^{-2}$.
> The reader's equivalent pressure would be
> $(3.026 \times 10^{-2}) \times (33) = 1.000$ atm.

Whenever pressures are given in absolute terms (e.g., ata), one must convert them to applicable gauge pressures by subtracting the barometric pressure cited by the author.

Appendix 2

U. S. Navy Standard Air Decompression Tables* and Treatment Tables

U. S. NAVY STANDARD AIR DECOMPRESSION TABLE

Depth (feet)	Bottom time (min)	Time first stop (min:sec)	50	40	30	20	10	Total ascent (min:sec)	Repetitive group
40	200						0	0:40	*
	210	0:30					2	2:40	N
	230	0:30					7	7:40	N
	250	0:30					11	11:40	O
	270	0:30					15	15:40	O
	300	0:30					19	19:40	Z
	360	0:30					23	23:40	**
	480	0:30					41	41:40	**
	720	0:30					69	69:40	**
50	100						0	0:50	*
	110	0:40					3	3:50	L
	120	0:40					5	5:50	M
	140	0:40					10	10:50	M
	160	0:40					21	21:50	N
	180	0:40					29	29:50	O
	200	0:40					35	35:50	O
	220	0:40					40	40:50	Z
	240	0:40					47	47:50	Z
60	60						0	1:00	*
	70	0:50					2	3:00	K
	80	0:50					7	8:00	L
	100	0:50					14	15:00	M
	120	0:50					26	27:00	N
	140	0:50					39	40:00	O
	160	0:50					48	49:00	Z
	180	0:50					56	57:00	Z
	200	0:40				1	69	71:00	Z
	240	0:40				2	79	82:00	**
	360	0:40				20	119	140:00	**
	480	0:40				44	148	193:00	**
	720	0:40				78	187	266:00	**
70	50						0	1:10	*
	60	1:00					8	9:10	K
	70	1:00					14	15:10	L
	80	1:00					18	19:10	M
	90	1:00					23	24:10	N
	100	1:00					33	34:10	N
	110	0:50				2	41	44:10	O
	120	0:50				4	47	52:10	O
	130	0:50				6	52	59:10	O
	140	0:50				8	56	65:10	Z
	150	0:50				9	61	71:10	Z
	160	0:50				13	72	86:10	Z
	170	0:50				19	79	99:10	Z

* See No Decompression Table for repetitive groups
**Repetitive dives may not follow exceptional exposure dives

From the U. S. Navy Diving Manual, 1973.

*Those decompression schedules that are enclosed by solid lines are for exceptional exposure dives and should not be used by sport divers because of the higher risk of decompression sickness.

U. S NAVY STANDARD AIR DECOMPRESSION TABLE

Depth (feet)	Bottom time (min)	Time first stop (min:sec)	50	40	30	20	10	Total ascent (min:sec)	Repeti-tive group
80	40						0	1:20	*
	50	1:10					10	11:20	K
	60	1:10					17	18:20	L
	70	1:10					23	24:20	M
	80	1:00				2	31	34:20	N
	90	1:00				7	39	47:20	N
	100	1:00				11	46	58:20	O
	110	1:00				13	53	67:20	O
	120	1:00				17	56	74:20	Z
	130	1:00				19	63	83:20	Z
	140	1:00				26	69	96:20	Z
	150	1:00				32	77	110:20	Z
	180	1:00				35	85	121:20	**
	240	0:50			6	52	120	179:20	**
	360	0:50			29	90	160	280:20	**
	480	0:50			59	107	187	354:20	**
	720	0:40		17	108	142	187	455:20	**
90	30						0	1:30	*
	40	1:20					7	8:30	J
	50	1:20					18	19:30	L
	60	1:20					25	26:30	M
	70	1:10				7	30	38:30	N
	80	1:10				13	40	54:30	N
	90	1:10				18	48	67:30	O
	100	1:10				21	54	76:30	Z
	110	1:10				24	61	86:30	Z
	120	1:10				32	68	101:30	Z
	130	1:00			5	36	74	116:30	Z
100	25						0	1:40	*
	30	1:30					3	4:40	I
	40	1:30					15	16:40	K
	50	1:20				2	24	27:40	L
	60	1:20				9	28	38:40	N
	70	1:20				17	39	57:40	O
	80	1:20				23	48	72:40	O
	90	1:10			3	23	57	84:40	Z
	100	1:10			7	23	66	97:40	Z
	110	1:10			10	34	72	117:40	Z
	120	1:10			12	41	78	132:40	Z
	180	1:00		1	29	53	118	202:40	**
	240	1:00		14	42	84	142	283:40	**
	360	0:50	2	42	73	111	187	416:40	**
	480	0:50	21	61	91	142	187	503:40	**
	720	0:50	55	106	122	142	187	613:40	**
110	20						0	1:50	*
	25	1:40					3	4:50	H
	30	1:40					7	8:50	J
	40	1:30				2	21	24:50	L
	50	1:30				8	26	35:50	M
	60	1:30				18	36	55:50	N
	70	1:20			1	23	48	73:50	O
	80	1:20			7	23	57	88:50	Z
	90	1:20			12	30	64	107:50	Z
	100	1:20			15	37	72	125:50	Z

* See No Decompression Table for repetitive groups
**Repetitive dives may not follow exceptional exposure dives

U. S. NAVY STANDARD AIR DECOMPRESSION TABLE

Depth 120

Bottom time (min)	Time to first stop (min:sec)	70	60	50	40	30	20	10	Total ascent (min:sec)	Repetitive group
15								0	2:00	*
20	1:50							2	4:00	H
25	1:50							6	8:00	I
30	1:50							14	16:00	J
40	1:40						5	25	32:00	L
50	1:40						15	31	48:00	N
60	1:30					2	22	45	71:00	O
70	1:30					9	23	55	89:00	O
80	1:30					15	27	63	107:00	Z
90	1:30					19	37	74	132:00	Z
100	1:30					23	45	80	150:00	Z
120	1:20				10	19	47	98	176:00	**
180	1:10			5	27	37	76	137	284:00	**
240	1:10			23	35	60	97	179	396:00	**
360	1:00		18	45	64	93	142	187	551:00	**
480	0:50	3	41	64	93	122	142	187	654:00	**
720	0:50	32	74	100	114	122	142	187	773:00	**

Depth 130

Bottom time (min)	Time to first stop (min:sec)	70	60	50	40	30	20	10	Total ascent (min:sec)	Repetitive group
10								0	2:10	*
15	2:00							1	3:10	F
20	2:00							4	6:10	H
25	2:00							10	12:10	J
30	1:50						3	18	23:10	M
40	1:50						10	25	37:10	N
50	1:40					3	21	37	63:10	O
60	1:40					9	23	52	86:10	Z
70	1:40					16	24	61	103:10	Z
80	1:30				3	19	35	72	131:10	Z
90	1:30				8	19	45	80	154:10	Z

Depth 140

Bottom time (min)	Time to first stop (min:sec)	90	80	70	60	50	40	30	20	10	Total ascent (min:sec)	Repetitive group
10										0	2:20	*
15	2:10									2	4:20	G
20	2:10									6	8:20	I
25	2:00								2	14	18:20	J
30	2:00								5	21	28:20	K
40	1:50							2	16	26	46:20	N
50	1:50							6	24	44	76:20	O
60	1:50							16	23	56	97:20	Z
70	1:40						4	19	32	68	125:20	Z
80	1:40						10	23	41	79	155:20	Z
90	1:30					2	14	18	42	88	166:20	**
120	1:30					12	14	36	56	120	240:20	**
180	1:20				10	26	32	54	94	168	386:20	**
240	1:10			8	28	34	50	78	124	187	511:20	**
360	1:00		9	32	42	64	84	122	142	187	684:20	**
480	1:00		31	44	59	100	114	122	142	187	801:20	**
720	0:50	16	56	88	97	100	114	122	142	187	924:20	**

* See No Decompression Table for repetitive groups
**Repetitive dives may not follow exceptional exposure dives

U. S. NAVY STANDARD AIR DECOMPRESSION TABLE

Depth (feet)	Bottom time (min)	Time to first stop (min:sec)	90	80	70	60	50	40	30	20	10	Total ascent (min:sec)	Repetitive group
150	5										0	2:30	C
	10	2:20									1	3:30	E
	15	2:20									3	5:30	G
	20	2:10								2	7	11:30	H
	25	2:10								4	17	23:30	K
	30	2:10								8	24	34:30	L
	40	2:00							5	19	33	59:30	N
	50	2:00							12	23	51	88:30	O
	60	1:50						3	19	26	62	112:30	Z
	70	1:50						11	19	39	75	146:30	Z
	80	1:40					1	17	19	50	84	173:30	Z
160	5										0	2:40	D
	10	2:30									1	3:40	F
	15	2:20								1	4	7:40	H
	20	2:20								3	11	16:40	J
	25	2:20								7	20	29:40	K
	30	2:10							2	11	25	40:40	M
	40	2:10							7	23	39	71:40	N
	50	2:00						2	16	23	55	98:40	Z
	60	2:00						9	19	33	69	132:40	Z
	70	1:50					1	17	22	44	80	166:40	Z

Depth (feet)	Bottom time (min)	Time to first stop (min:sec)	110	100	90	80	70	60	50	40	30	20	10	Total ascent (min:sec)	Repetitive group
170	5												0	2:50	D
	10	2:40											2	4:50	F
	15	2:30										2	5	9:50	H
	20	2:30										4	15	21:50	J
	25	2:20									2	7	23	34:50	L
	30	2:20									4	13	26	45:50	M
	40	2:10								1	10	23	45	81:50	O
	50	2:10								5	18	23	61	109:50	Z
	60	2:00							2	15	22	37	74	152:50	Z
	70	2:00							8	17	19	51	86	183:50	Z
	90	1:50						12	12	14	34	52	120	246:50	**
	120	1:30				2	10	12	18	32	42	82	156	356:50	**
	180	1:20			4	10	22	28	34	50	78	120	187	535:50	**
	240	1:20			18	24	30	42	50	70	116	142	187	681:50	**
	360	1:10		22	34	40	52	60	98	114	122	142	187	873:50	**
	480	1:00	14	40	42	56	91	97	100	114	122	142	187	1007:50	**
180	5												0	3:00	D
	10	2:50											3	6:00	F
	15	2:40										3	6	12:00	I
	20	2:30									1	5	17	26:00	K
	25	2:30									3	10	24	40:00	L
	30	2:30									6	17	27	53:00	N
	40	2:20								3	14	23	50	93:00	O
	50	2:10								2	9	19	30	65	128:00	Z
	60	2:10								5	16	19	44	81	168:00	Z

* See No Decompression Table for repetitive groups
**Repetitive dives may not follow exceptional exposure dives

U. S NAVY STANDARD AIR DECOMPRESSION TABLE

Depth (feet)	Bottom time (min)	Time to first stop (min:sec)	110	100	90	80	70	60	50	40	30	20	10	Total ascent (min:sec)	Repetitive group
190	5												0	3:10	D
	10	2:50										1	3	7:10	G
	15	2:50										4	7	14:10	I
	20	2:40									2	6	20	31:10	K
	25	2:40									5	11	25	44:10	M
	30	2:30								1	8	19	43	63:10	N
	40	2:30								8	14	23	55	103:10	O
	50	2:20							4	13	22	33	72	147:10	Z
	60	2:20							10	17	19	50	84	183:10	Z

NO-DECOMPRESSION LIMITS AND REPETITIVE GROUP DESIGNATION TABLE FOR NO-DECOMPRESSION AIR DIVES

Depth (feet)	No-decompression limits (min)	A	B	C	D	E	F	G	H	I	J	K	L	M	N	O
10		60	120	210	300											
15		35	70	110	160	225	350									
20		25	50	75	100	135	180	240	325							
25		20	35	55	75	100	125	160	195	245	315					
30		15	30	45	60	75	95	120	145	170	205	250	310			
35	310	5	15	25	40	50	60	80	100	120	140	160	190	220	270	310
40	200	5	15	25	30	40	50	70	80	100	110	130	150	170	200	
50	100		10	15	25	30	40	50	60	70	80	90	100			
60	60		10	15	20	25	30	40	50	55	60					
70	50			5	10	15	20	30	35	40	45	50				
80	40			5	10	15	20	25	30	35	40					
90	30				5	10	12	15	20	25	30					
100	25				5	7	10	15	20	22	25					
110	20					5	10	13	15	20						
120	15					5	10	12	15							
130	10						5	8	10							
140	10						5	7	10							
150	5							5								
160	5								5							
170	5								5							
180	5								5							
190	5								5							

RESIDUAL NITROGEN TIMETABLE FOR REPETITIVE AIR DIVES

*Dives following surface intervals of more than 12 hours are not repetitive dives. Use actual bottom times in the Standard Air Decompression Tables to compute decompression for such dives.

Repetitive group at the beginning of the surface interval

A	0:10 / 12:00*
B	0:10 / 2:10	2:11 / 12:00*
C	0:10 / 1:39	1:40 / 2:49	2:50 / 12:00*
D	0:10 / 1:09	1:10 / 2:38	2:39 / 5:48	5:49 / 12:00*
E	0:10 / 0:54	0:55 / 1:57	1:58 / 3:22	3:23 / 6:32	6:33 / 12:00*
F	0:10 / 0:45	0:46 / 1:29	1:30 / 2:28	2:29 / 3:57	3:58 / 7:05	7:06 / 12:00*
G	0:10 / 0:40	0:41 / 1:15	1:16 / 1:59	2:00 / 2:58	2:59 / 4:25	4:26 / 7:35	7:36 / 12:00*
H	0:10 / 0:36	0:37 / 1:06	1:07 / 1:41	1:42 / 2:23	2:24 / 3:20	3:21 / 4:49	4:50 / 7:59	8:00 / 12:00*
I	0:10 / 0:33	0:34 / 0:59	1:00 / 1:29	1:30 / 2:02	2:03 / 2:44	2:45 / 3:43	3:44 / 5:12	5:13 / 8:21	8:22 / 12:00*
J	0:10 / 0:31	0:32 / 0:54	0:55 / 1:19	1:20 / 1:47	1:48 / 2:20	2:21 / 3:04	3:05 / 4:02	4:03 / 5:40	5:41 / 8:40	8:41 / 12:00*
K	0:10 / 0:28	0:29 / 0:49	0:50 / 1:11	1:12 / 1:35	1:36 / 2:03	2:04 / 2:38	2:39 / 3:21	3:22 / 4:19	4:20 / 5:48	5:49 / 8:58	8:59 / 12:00*
L	0:10 / 0:26	0:27 / 0:45	0:46 / 1:04	1:05 / 1:25	1:26 / 1:49	1:50 / 2:19	2:20 / 2:53	2:54 / 3:36	3:37 / 4:35	4:36 / 6:02	6:03 / 9:12	9:13 / 12:00*
M	0:10 / 0:25	0:26 / 0:42	0:43 / 0:59	1:00 / 1:18	1:19 / 1:39	1:40 / 2:05	2:06 / 2:34	2:35 / 3:08	3:09 / 3:52	3:53 / 4:49	4:50 / 6:18	6:19 / 9:28	9:29 / 12:00*
N	0:10 / 0:24	0:25 / 0:39	0:40 / 0:54	0:55 / 1:11	1:12 / 1:30	1:31 / 1:53	1:54 / 2:18	2:19 / 2:47	2:48 / 3:22	3:23 / 4:04	4:05 / 5:03	5:04 / 6:32	6:33 / 9:43	9:44 / 12:00*
O	0:10 / 0:23	0:24 / 0:36	0:37 / 0:51	0:52 / 1:07	1:08 / 1:24	1:25 / 1:43	1:44 / 2:04	2:05 / 2:29	2:30 / 2:59	3:00 / 3:33	3:34 / 4:17	4:18 / 5:16	5:17 / 6:44	6:45 / 9:54	9:55 / 12:00*
	0:10 / 0:22	0:23 / 0:34	0:35 / 0:48	0:49 / 1:02	1:03 / 1:18	1:19 / 1:36	1:37 / 1:55	1:56 / 2:17	2:18 / 2:42	2:43 / 3:10	3:11 / 3:45	3:46 / 4:29	4:30 / 5:27	5:28 / 6:56	6:57 / 10:05	10:06 / 12:00*

NEW → GROUP DESIGNATION

Z	O	N	M	L	K	J	I	H	G	F	E	D	C	B	A

REPETITIVE DIVE DEPTH

Depth	Z	O	N	M	L	K	J	I	H	G	F	E	D	C	B	A
40	257	241	213	187	161	138	116	101	87	73	61	49	37	25	17	7
50	169	160	142	124	111	99	87	76	66	56	47	38	29	21	13	6
60	122	117	107	97	88	79	70	61	52	44	36	30	24	17	11	5
70	100	96	87	80	72	64	57	50	43	37	31	26	20	15	9	4
80	84	80	73	68	61	54	48	43	38	32	28	23	18	13	8	4
90	73	70	64	58	53	47	43	38	33	29	24	20	16	11	7	3
100	64	62	57	52	48	43	38	34	30	26	22	18	14	10	7	3
110	57	55	51	47	42	38	34	31	27	24	20	16	13	10	6	3
120	52	50	46	43	39	35	32	28	25	21	18	15	12	9	6	3
130	46	44	40	38	35	31	28	25	22	19	16	13	11	8	6	3
140	42	40	38	35	32	29	26	23	20	18	15	12	10	7	5	2
150	40	38	35	32	30	27	24	22	19	17	14	12	9	7	5	2
160	37	36	33	31	28	26	23	20	18	16	13	11	9	6	4	2
170	35	34	31	29	26	24	22	19	17	15	13	10	8	6	4	2
180	32	31	29	27	25	22	20	18	16	14	12	10	8	6	4	2
190	31	30	28	26	24	21	19	17	15	13	11	10	8	6	4	2

RESIDUAL NITROGEN TIMES (MINUTES)

TABLE 5—MINIMAL RECOMPRESSION, OXYGEN BREATHING METHOD FOR TREATMENT OF DECOMPRESSION SICKNESS AND GAS EMBOLISM

1. Use—treatment of pain-only decompression sickness when oxygen can be used and symptoms are relieved within 10 minutes at 60 feet. Patient breathes oxygen from the surface.
. Descent rate—25 ft/min.
3. Ascent rate—1 ft/min. Do not compensate for slower ascent rates. Compensate for faster rates by halting the ascent.
4. Time at 60 feet begins on arrival at 60 feet.
5. If oxygen breathing must be interrupted. allow 15 minutes after the reaction has entirely subsided and resume schedule at point of interruption.
6. If oxygen breathing must be interrupted at 60 feet. switch to TABLE 6 upon arrival at the 30 foot stop.
7. Tender breathes air throughout. If treatment is a repetitive dive for the tender or tables are lengthened. tender should breathe oxygen during the last 30 minutes of ascent to the surface.

Depth (feet)	Time (minutes)	Breathing Media	Total Elapsed Time (minutes)
60	20	Oxygen	20
60	5	Air	25
60	20	Oxygen	45
60 to 30	30	Oxygen	75
30	5	Air	80
30	20	Oxygen	100
30	5	Air	105
30 to 0	30	Oxygen	135

TABLE 5 DEPTH/TIME PROFILE

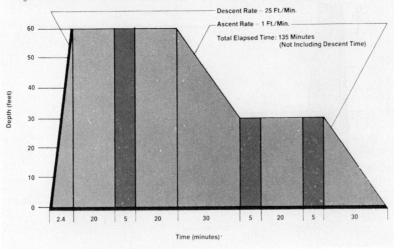

Descent Rate = 25 Ft./Min.
Ascent Rate = 1 Ft./Min.
Total Elapsed Time: 135 Minutes
(Not Including Descent Time)

Depth (feet)

Time (minutes)

TABLE 5A—MINIMAL RECOMPRESSION, OXYGEN BREATHING METHOD FOR TREATMENT OF DECOMPRESSION SICKNESS AND GAS EMBOLISM

1. Use—treatment of gas embolism when oxygen can be used and symptoms are relieved within 15 minutes at 165 feet.

2. Descent rate—as fast as possible.

3. Ascent rate—1 ft/min. Do not compensate for slower ascent rates. Compensate for faster ascent rates by halting the ascent.

4. Time at 165 feet—includes time from the surface.

5. If oxygen breathing must be interrupted, allow 15 minutes after the reaction has entirely subsided and resume schedule at point of interruption.

6. Tender breathes air throughout. If treatment is a repetitive dive for the tender or tables are lengthened, tender should breathe oxygen during the last 30 minutes of ascent to the surface.

Depth (feet)	Time (minutes)	Breathing Media	Total Elapsed Time (minutes)
165	15	Air	15
165 to 60	4	Air	19
60	20	Oxygen	39
60	5	Air	44
60	20	Oxygen	64
60 to 30	30	Oxygen	94
30	5	Air	99
30	20	Oxygen	119
30	5	Air	124
30 to 0	30	Oxygen	154

TABLE 5A DEPTH/TIME PROFILE

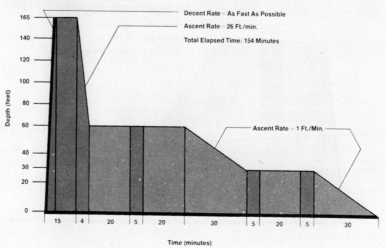

Decent Rate = As Fast As Possible

Ascent Rate = 26 Ft./min.

Total Elapsed Time: 154 Minutes

Ascent Rate = 1 Ft./Min.

Depth (feet)

165, 140, 120, 100, 80, 60, 40, 30, 20, 0

Time (minutes)

15 4 20 5 20 30 5 20 5 30

TABLE 6—MINIMAL RECOMPRESSION, OXYGEN BREATHING METHOD FOR TREATMENT OF DECOMPRESSION SICKNESS AND GAS EMBOLISM

1. Use—treatment of decompression sickness when oxygen can be used and symptoms are not relieved within 10 minutes at 60 feet. Patient breathes oxygen from the surface.

2. Descent rate—25 ft/min.

3. Ascent rate—1 ft/min. Do not compensate for slower ascent rates. Compensate for faster rates by halting the ascent.

4. Time at 60 feet—begins on arrival at 60 feet.

5. If oxygen breathing must be interrupted, allow 15 minutes after the reaction has entirely subsided and resume schedule at point of interruption.

6. Tender breathes air throughout. If treatment is a repetitive dive for the tender or tables are lengthened, tender should breathe oxygen during the last 30 minutes of ascent to the surface.

Depth (feet)	Time (minutes)	Breathing Media	Total Elapsed Time (minutes)
60	20	Oxygen	20
60	5	Air	25
60	20	Oxygen	45
60	5	Air	50
60	20	Oxygen	70
60	5	Air	75
60 to 30	30	Oxygen	105
30	15	Air	120
30	60	Oxygen	180
30	15	Air	195
30	60	Oxygen	255
30 to 0	30	Oxygen	285

TABLE 6 DEPTH/TIME PROFILE

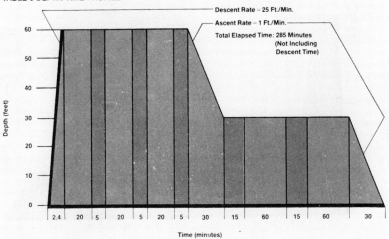

Descent Rate = 25 Ft./Min.

Ascent Rate = 1 Ft./Min.

Total Elapsed Time: 285 Minutes (Not Including Descent Time)

Depth (feet)

2.4 20 5 20 5 20 5 30 15 60 15 60 30

Time (minutes)

TABLE 6A — MINIMAL RECOMPRESSION, OXYGEN BREATHING METHOD FOR TREATMENT OF DECOMPRESSION SICKNESS AND GAS EMBOLISM

1. Use—treatment of gas embolism when oxygen can be used and symptoms moderate to a major extent within 30 minutes at 165 feet.
2. Descent rate—as fast as possible.
3. Ascent rate—1 ft/min. Do not compensate for slower ascent rates. Compensate for faster ascent rates by halting the ascent.
4. Time at 165 feet—includes time from the surface.
5. If oxygen breathing must be interrupted, allow 15 minutes after the reaction has entirely subsided and resume schedule at point of interruption.
6. Tender breathes air throughout. If treatment is a repetitive dive for the tender or tables are lengthened, tender should breathe oxygen during the last 30 minutes of ascent to the surface.

Depth (feet)	Time (minutes)	Breathing Media	Total Elapsed Time (minutes)
165	30	Air	30
165 to 60	4	Air	34
60	20	Oxygen	54
60	5	Air	50
60	20	Oxygen	79
60	5	Air	84
60	20	Oxygen	104
60	5	Air	109
60 to 30	30	Oxygen	139
30	15	Air	154
30	60	Oxygen	214
30	15	Air	229
30	60	Oxygen	289
30 to 0	30	Oxygen	319

TABLE 6A DEPTH/TIME PROFILE

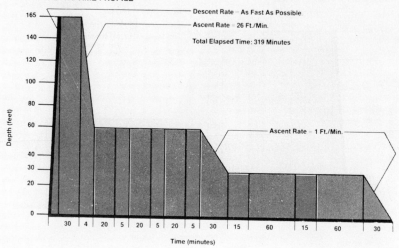

Descent Rate = As Fast As Possible

Ascent Rate = 26 Ft./Min.

Total Elapsed Time: 319 Minutes

Ascent Rate = 1 Ft./Min.

Depth (feet)

Time (minutes)

Appendix 3

Decompression Tables for Diving at Altitude*

DECOMPRESSION - TABLE 0 - 700 m ABOVE SEA LEVEL

Depth m	Bottom-time min	15	12	9	6	3	Repet. group
15	90					5	J
	120					10	K
	150					15	L
20	50					4	H
	60					6	J
	75					18	K
	90					23	K
	105				3	31	K
25	30					5	G
	40					8	H
	50					12	J
	60					20	K
	75				3	30	K
	90				10	38	L
30	25					5	G
	30					9	H
	35					12	J
	40				5	14	J
	50				5	25	K
	60			6	8	32	K
	75			7	15	42	L
	90			8	25	52	L
35	20					5	G
	25					9	H
	30					12	J
	35				5	17	J
	40				7	30	J
	50			3	10	35	K
	60			7	15	45	K
	75			10	15	62	L
40	15				2	5	G
	20				2	10	H
	25				3	12	J
	30			2	5	20	J
	35			2	10	30	K
	40			5	15	35	K
	50		2	7	20	40	K
	60		2	10	25	50	L

Depth m	Bottom-time min	18	15	12	9	6	3	Repet. group
45	10						4	F
	15					2	6	G
	20					3	11	H
	25					5	20	J
	30				3	10	30	K
	35				5	10	35	K
	40			2	5	15	45	K
	50		2	5	10	20	55	L
	60		2	5	20	25	60	-
50	10						5	F
	15					3	8	H
	20					5	17	J
	25				3	10	27	J
	30				5	10	35	K
	40		2	5	12	15	50	K
	50		2	10	15	20	60	L
	60		3	12	20	30	70	-
55	10				1	2	5	F
	15				1	4	11	F
	20			1	4	8	24	G
	25			2	7	10	32	J
	30		1	3	9	13	38	K
	40	1	5	8	17	18	58	K
60	10				2	3	5	H
	15				3	5	15	J
	20			2	6	10	29	J
	25		2	2	10	10	35	K
	30		2	4	12	15	40	L
65	10			1	2	3	6	H
	15			1	3	8	18	J
	20		1	2	6	13	33	J
	25		2	4	10	13	40	K
	30	1	2	8	14	18	46	L
70	10			2	3	4	6	H
	15			2	3	10	20	J
	20		2	3	5	15	35	J
	25	2	2	5	10	15	43	K
	30	2	3	10	15	20	50	L

Courtesy of Professor Dr. A. A. Buhlmann, Medizinische Universitatsklinik, Kantonsspital, CH-8006 Zurich, Switzerland.

*1 meter = 3 feet, 3 inches

Max. ascent rate 10m/min

		No decompression limits (0 - 700 m)							
m	9	12	15	18	20	25	30	35	40
min		200	75	50	30	25	20	15	10
	Each dive must include a decompression stop of 3 min at 3 m								

REPETITIVE SYSTEM 0 - 700 m ABOVE SEA LEVEL

SURFACE INTERVAL TABLE (min)

Repetitive group at the end of the surface interval

	K	J	H	G	F	E	D	C	B	A	"O"
L	14	30	47	68	94	127	149	174	206	255	440
K		16	34	55	80	113	135	160	194	240	426
J			18	39	65	98	119	145	180	225	409
H				22	47	80	101	127	160	206	394
G					26	59	80	106	139	186	372
F						34	55	80	113	160	346
E							22	47	80	127	312
D								26	59	106	292
C									34	80	266
B										47	233
A											186

Repetitive group at the beginning of surface interval

REPETITIVE TIMETABLE (min)

Depth m	6	9	12	15	20	25	30	35	40	45	50	55	60	65	70
L		>400	300	160	96	69	55	45	39	34	30	27	25	23	21
K		>400	250	127	80	59	47	39	34	29	26	24	22	20	18
J		400	150	101	67	50	40	33	29	25	23	21	19	17	16
H		200	113	80	55	42	34	27	25	22	19	17	16	15	14
G	>200	135	85	63	44	34	27	22	20	18	16	14	13	12	11
F	200	108	61	47	34	26	22	17	16	14	13	12	11	10	9
E	113	61	42	34	25	19	16	13	12	11	9	8	8	7	7
D	85	48	34	27	20	16	13	10	10	9	8	7	7	6	6
C	61	37	26	22	16	13	10	8	8	7	6	6	5	5	5
B	43	26	19	16	12	9	8	6	6	5	5	4	4	4	4
A	26	17	12	10	8	6	6	4	4	3	3	3	3	3	3

Repetitive - group

DECOMPRESSION - TABLE 701 - 1500 m ABOVE SEA LEVEL

Depth m	Bottom-time min	16	13	10	7	4	2	Repet group
12	120					4	4	H
15	40					5	5	F
	75					8	8	H
	90					13	13	H
	105					16	16	J
	120						19	J
20	20						4	E
	25						6	F
	30					2	8	F
	40					3	9	G
	50					5	11	H
	60					5	19	H
	75					8	25	J
	90					12	25	J
	105					15	30	-
	120					20	37	-
25	15					1	5	D
	25					4	8	F
	30				3	4	9	G
	35				4	5	13	G
	40				5	5	17	H
	50				5	7	23	H
	60				7	12	25	J
	75				10	15	30	J
	90				15	17	38	-
30	10					1	3	D
	15					3	6	E
	20					5	9	F
	25				3	5	10	G
	30				6	6	12	G
	35				7	7	18	H
	40			3	10	10	23	H
	50			5	10	15	25	J
	60			6	15	15	31	J

Depth m	Bottom-time min	16	13	10	7	4	2	Repet. group
35	10					2	3	D
	15				3	5	8	F
	20			2	5	5	11	G
	25			3	7	7	13	H
	30			4	8	8	16	H
	35			5	8	8	22	H
	40		2	5	10	10	25	J
	50		3	6	12	15	32	J
40	5					1	3	C
	10				2	2	6	E
	15			3	3	5	9	F
	20			4	5	6	12	G
	25			5	7	8	16	H
	30		3	6	8	10	20	J
	35		4	8	8	11	25	J
	40		6	8	9	17	32	J
45	5					2	3	C
	10				3	4	8	F
	15		2	3	5	5	12	G
	20		3	4	6	8	15	H
	25	1	4	6	6	10	19	H
	30	2	5	7	10	16	28	J
50	5				1	3	4	D
	10			3	4	5	10	F
	15	1	3	5	6	6	15	G
	20	3	3	6	6	10	18	H
	25	3	4	8	10	10	25	H
	30	6	6	8	13	18	35	J
55	10		2	4	5	6	12	F
	15	1	3	5	7	7	17	G
	20	4	5	6	7	10	24	H
60	10		1	3	4	6	13	G
	15	2	3	4	8	8	18	G
	20	5	6	6	8	10	30	H

Max. ascent rate 10m/min

	No decompression limits (701 - 1500 m)							
m	9	12	15	18	20	25	30	35
min	720	90	30	20	15	10	5	4
	Each dive must include a decompression stop of 3 min at 2 m							

REPETITIVE SYSTEM 701 - 1500 m ABOVE SEA LEVEL

SURFACE INTERVAL TABLE (min)

Repetitive group at the end of the surface interval

	J	H	G	F	E	D	C	B	A	"O"
J		17	35	59	87	105	125	150	183	265
H			19	42	71	89	109	134	166	250
G				23	52	69	90	115	147	230
F					29	46	67	92	124	207
E						18	39	64	96	178
D							21	46	78	161
C								25	58	141
B									33	115
A										81

Repetitive group at the beginning of the surface interval

REPETITIVE TIMETABLE (min)

Depth m	6	8	10	12	15	20	25	30	35	40	45	50	55	60
J			320	171	120	73	53	43	35	30	26	23	21	19
H		>225	190	125	93	60	44	35	30	25	22	20	18	16
G	>330	225	130	92	71	47	35	29	24	21	18	16	15	13
F	330	132	90	67	53	36	27	23	19	16	14	12	11	10
E	142	83	59	46	37	26	20	16	14	12	11	9	8	7
D	103	64	47	37	30	21	16	13	11	10	9	7	7	6
C	73	48	36	28	23	16	12	10	9	8	7	6	6	5
B	51	34	26	21	17	12	9	8	7	6	5	5	4	4
A	32	21	16	13	11	8	6	5	5	4	4	3	2	2

Repetitive - group

DECOMPRESSION - TABLE 1501 - 2000 m ABOVE SEA LEVEL

Depth m	Bottom-time min	16	13	10	7	4	2	Repet. group
12	60						4	H
	90						5	H
	120						6	H
15	30						4	E
	40						6	E
	50						7	F
	60						8	F
	75						12	G
	90						16	H
	105						20	H
20	15						5	C
	20						7	D
	25					2	7	E
	30					2	10	F
	40					3	12	G
	50					5	18	H
	60					6	24	H
25	10						5	C
	15					2	6	D
	20					4	8	E
	25					6	10	F
	30				3	6	12	F
	40				5	7	20	G
	50				7	10	25	H
	60				8	15	25	H
30	5						4	C
	10					1	4	D
	15					4	7	E
	20				2	4	10	F
	25				5	5	10	G

Depth m	Bottom-time min	16	13	10	7	4	2	Repet. group
30	30				6	8	16	G
	40			3	10	12	25	H
	50			3	12	15	30	H
	60			5	14	20	35	H
35	5						4	C
	10					2	5	E
	15				4	5	10	F
	20			1	6	6	14	F
	25			3	7	8	17	G
	30			4	8	10	20	G
	40		2	7	10	15	30	H
	50		3	8	12	20	40	H
40	5					2	4	C
	10				2	3	8	D
	15			3	5	5	11	F
	20			4	6	7	14	G
	25		3	5	8	8	20	H
	30		3	6	10	11	25	H
	40		6	6	11	18	40	H
45	5					3	4	C
	10			1	3	4	9	E
	15		2	4	5	5	14	G
	20		3	5	7	8	19	G
	25	1	4	6	8	10	25	H
	30	2	5	7	10	17	35	H
50	5				2	3	6	D
	10		1	3	4	5	12	F
	15	1	3	6	6	7	18	G
	20	3	4	6	8	10	23	H
	25	3	5	8	10	12	28	H

Max. ascent rate 10 m/min

No decompression limits (1501 - 2000 m)							
m	9	12	15	18	20	25	30
min	360	50	25	15	10	6	4

Each dive must include a decompression stop of 3 min at 2 m

REPETITIVE SYSTEM 1501 - 2000 m ABOVE SEA LEVEL

SURFACE INTERVAL TABLE (min)

	Repetitive group at the end of the surface interval							
	H	**G**	**F**	**E**	**D**	**C**	**B**	**A**	**"O"**
H	17	37	60	74	90	108	130	191
G		20	44	58	75	93	116	179
F			24	39	55	73	96	160
E				15	31	49	72	136
D					17	35	58	113
C						19	42	106
B							23	88
A								65

Repetitive group at the beginning of the surface interval

REPETITIVE TIME TABLE (min)

Depth m		6	8	10	12	15	20	25	30	35	40	45	50
Repetitive - group	H	-	-	361	168	103	63	46	37	30	25	23	20
	G	-	>224	184	119	77	50	37	30	25	21	19	17
	F	>437	224	118	83	57	39	29	23	19	17	15	13
	E	437	119	75	57	41	28	21	17	14	12	11	9
	D	194	89	58	45	33	23	17	14	12	10	9	8
	C	122	65	45	36	25	18	14	11	9	8	7	6
	B	78	45	32	25	19	13	10	8	7	6	5	5
	A	46	28	21	16	12	9	7	6	5	4	3	3

DECOMPRESSION - TABLE 2001 - 2500 m ABOVE SEA LEVEL

Depth m	Bottom-time min	DECO - stops 16	13	10	7	4	2	Repet. group
12	50						4	E
	60						6	F
	75						8	F
	90						10	F
	120						15	G
15	20						4	C
	25						5	D
	30						6	D
	40						9	E
	50						12	F
	60						14	F
	75						18	G
	90						22	G
20	10						4	B
	15						7	C
	20						10	D
	25					2	10	E
	30					3	12	E
	40					5	16	F
	50					6	20	F
	60					8	26	G
25	5						4	B
	10						6	C
	15					3	8	D
	20					5	10	E
	25				1	7	10	F
	30				3	7	18	F
	40				5	10	30	F
	50				8	15	30	G
	60				8	20	35	G

Depth m	Bottom-time min	DECO - stops 16	13	10	7	4	2	Repet. group
30	5					1	5	B
	10					3	7	C
	15					5	9	E
	20				3	7	10	F
	25				6	9	18	F
	30				8	10	25	F
	40			3	12	15	33	G
	50			5	15	20	38	G
35	5					2	4	B
	10				1	3	6	D
	15				4	5	13	E
	20			2	6	7	15	F
	25			3	8	9	24	F
	30			5	8	10	30	G
	40		3	7	10	18	45	G
40	5					3	5	B
	10				2	4	9	D
	15			3	5	6	13	F
	20			4	7	8	17	F
	25		2	5	9	10	25	G
	30		3	6	11	15	32	G
45	5				1	3	7	C
	10			1	3	6	10	E
	15		1	4	5	8	15	F
	20		3	5	8	10	25	G
	25	1	4	6	10	12	30	G
50	5				2	4	8	C
	10			3	4	6	14	E
	15	1	3	6	7	9	21	F
	20	3	4	6	9	12	28	G

Max. ascent rate 10 m/min

	No decompression limits (2001 - 2500 m)				
m	9	12	15	18	20
min	240	40	15	7	5
	Each dive must include a decompression stop of 3 min at 2 m				

REPETITIVE SYSTEM 2001 - 2500 m ABOVE SEA LEVEL

SURFACE INTERVAL TABLE (min)

Repetitive group at the end of the surface interval								
H	**G**	**F**	**E**	**D**	**C**	**B**	**A**	**"O"**
H 17	36	58	72	87	104	124	180	
G	19	42	55	70	88	108	163	
F		23	36	51	69	89	146	
E			14	29	46	66	121	
D				15	33	53	109	
C					18	38	94	
B						21	27	
A							57	

Repetitive group at the beginning of surface interval

REPETITIVE TIMETABLE (min)

Depth m		6	8	10	12	15	20	25	30	35	40	45	50
Repetitive - group	H	-	-	>206	180	106	65	47	37	31	26	23	20
	G	-	>280	206	124	80	51	38	30	25	22	19	17
	F	-	280	127	87	59	39	29	23	20	17	15	13
	E	>258	132	80	58	42	28	22	17	15	13	11	10
	D	258	97	63	46	34	23	18	14	12	10	9	8
	C	145	70	47	36	26	18	14	11	10	8	7	7
	B	89	48	34	26	19	13	10	9	7	6	6	5
	A	51	30	22	17	13	9	7	6	5	4	4	3

DECOMPRESSION - TABLE 2501 - 3200 m ABOVE SEA LEVEL

Depth m	Bottom-time min	DECO - stops m 16	13	10	7	4	2	Repet. group
12	40						5	D
	50						8	D
	60						10	E
	75						14	F
	90						18	F
15	15						4	B
	20						6	C
	25						8	D
	30						10	D
	40						14	E
	50						18	E
	60						20	F
	75					2	26	F
	90					2	32	F
20	10						4	B
	15						8	C
	20					2	10	D
	25					2	12	D
	30					3	14	E
	40				1	7	18	E
	50				1	10	24	F
	60				2	12	30	F
25	5						5	B
	10						8	C
	15					3	10	D
	20				1	5	13	D
	25				3	7	18	E
	30				4	10	23	F
	40				6	12	35	F
	50				8	15	40	F

Depth m	Bottom-time min	DECO - stops m 16	13	10	7	4	2	Repet. group
30	5					2	6	B
	10					3	9	C
	15				1	5	12	D
	20				3	8	13	E
	25			2	5	12	20	F
	30			3	9	12	30	F
	40			4	12	16	40	F
	50			6	15	22	50	F
35	5				1	3	6	B
	10				1	4	9	D
	15			1	2	6	12	E
	20			2	4	9	18	F
	25			3	9	13	25	F
	30		1	5	10	15	33	F
	40		3	7	12	22	50	F
40	5				1	3	8	B
	10				2	5	10	D
	15			2	3	8	14	E
	20		1	4	8	10	22	F
	25		3	5	11	14	30	F
	30		3	8	14	18	35	F
45	5				2	3	9	C
	10			1	3	6	12	D
	15		2	4	6	10	18	E
	20	1	2	6	10	14	32	F
	25	1	2	8	12	17	38	F
50	5			1	2	3	10	C
	10		1	2	5	8	14	E
	15	1	3	6	8	12	22	F
	20	3	4	7	11	16	34	F

Max. ascent rate 10 m/min

No decompression limits (2501 - 3200 m)			
m	9	12	15	18
min	150	30	10	5

Each dive must include a decompression stop of 3 min at 2 m

REPETITIVE SYSTEM 2501 - 3200 m ABOVE SEA LEVEL

SURFACE INTERVAL TABLE (min)

Repetitive group at the end of the surface interval						
F	**E**	**D**	**C**	**B**	**A**	**"O"**
F	22	34	47	63	80	127
	E	13	26	42	59	106
		D	14	29	47	94
			C	16	34	80
				B	18	65
					A	47

Repetitive group at the beginning of surface interval

REPETITIVE TIMETABLE (min)

Depth m		6	8	10	12	15	20	25	30	35	40	45	50
Repetitive - group	F	-	>160	145	94	63	41	30	24	20	17	15	13
	E	-	160	89	63	44	29	22	18	15	13	11	10
	D	-	113	69	50	35	24	18	15	12	11	9	8
	C	206	80	51	38	27	19	14	12	10	9	8	7
	B	113	55	36	27	20	14	11	9	7	7	6	5
	A	63	35	23	18	13	9	7	6	5	4	4	3

Example of a repetitive dive

1. - Mountain lake: 1620 meters above sea level
    → Decompression Table 1501 - 2000 meters above sea level

    - Depth 28 meters → 30 meters on the table.

    - Bottom time 17 minutes → 20 minutes on the table.

    - After the decompression you are in the repetitive group F.

2. - Second dive after 45 minutes on the surface. On the "surface interval ta-
    ble" you can determine that you are in repetitive group D after 45 min-
    utes.

    - For a second dive, to 20 meters, you see that you have to add 23 minutes
    to the bottom time because you are still in repetitive group D. Addi-
    tional decompression is therefore necessary.

Appendix 4

Medical Examination Forms*

MEDICAL HISTORY
(To be completed by applicant)

Name_____Age _____Sex _____Date_____

Address_____Phone _____

1. Have you had previous experience in diving? Yes___No___
2. When driving through mountains or flying, do you have trouble equalizing pressure in your ears or sinuses? Yes___No___
3. Have you ever been rejected for service, employment, or insurance for medical reasons? Yes___No___
   (If yes, explain under remarks or discuss with doctor.)
4. When was your last physical examination?
   Date_____Results _____
5. When was your last chest x-ray?
   Date_____Results _____
6. Have you ever had an electrocardiogram? Yes___No___
   Date_____Results _____
7. Have you ever had an electroencephalogram (brain wave study)? Yes___No___
   Date_____Results _____
8. Do you smoke? Yes___No___
   If so, how much? _____

(Check the blank if you have, or ever have had, any of the following. Explain under "remarks", giving dates and other pertinent information, or discuss with the doctor.)

9. ____ Frequent colds or sore throat.
10. ____ Hay fever or sinus trouble.
11. ____ Trouble breathing through nose (other than during colds).
12. ____ Painful or running ear, mastoid trouble, broken eardrum.
13. ____ Hardness of hearing.
14. ____ Asthma or bronchitis.
15. ____ Shortness of breath after moderate exercise.
16. ____ History of pleurisy.
17. ____ Collapsed lung (pneumothorax).
18. ____ Chest pain or persistent cough.
19. ____ Tiring easily.
20. ____ Spells of fast, irregular, or pounding heartbeat.
21. ____ High or low blood pressure.
22. ____ Any kind of "heart trouble."
23. ____ Frequent upset stomach, heartburn or indigestion, peptic ulcer.
24. ____ Frequent diarrhea or blood in stool.
25. ____ Anemia or (females) heavy menstruation.
26. ____ Belly or backache lasting more than a day or two.

*Modified from Safety Regulations for Scuba Diving, Department of Labor and Industries, State of Washington.

27. ____ Kidney or bladder disease; blood, sugar or albumin in urine.

28. ____ Broken bone, serious sprain or strain, dislocated joint.

29. ____ Rheumatism, arthritis, or other joint trouble.

30. ____ Severe or frequent headaches.

31. ____ Head injury causing unconsciousness.

32. ____ Dizzy spells, fainting spells, or fits.

33. ____ Trouble sleeping, frequent nightmares, or sleepwalking.

34. ____ Nervous breakdown or periods of marked nervousness or depression.

35. ____ A phobia for closed-in spaces, large open places, or high places.

36. ____ Any neurological or psychological condition.

37. ____ Train, sea, or air sickness or nausea.

38. ____ Alcoholism or any drug or narcotic habit (including regular use of sleeping pills, benzedrine, etc.).

39. ____ Recent gain or loss of weight or appetite.

40. ____ Jaundice or hepatitis.

41. ____ Tuberculosis.

42. ____ Diabetes.

43. ____ Rheumatic fever.

44. ____ Any serious accident, injury, or illness not mentioned above (describe under "remarks", give dates).

45. ____ Dental bridgework or plates.

46. ____ Susceptibility to panic.

47. ____ Pain from altitude or flying.

48. What sports or exercise do you regularly engage in?_____

_____

Remarks: _____

_____

_____

_____

Signature of applicant

MEDICAL EXAMINATION

(This form and the medical history form are retained by the physician for his records.)

A. NURSING STATION DATA:

Height____(in.) Weight____(pds.)

Blood Pressure____Pulse____

Vision:	Right eye	Left eye
uncorrected	_____	_____
corrected	_____	_____

B. MEDICAL HISTORY: Is there a significant past history which would disqualify the applicant from scuba diving? (See medical history form.)   Yes____No____

Remarks: _____

_____

C. EXAMINATION: (Check following items. If abnormal, give details below.)

	Normal	Abnormal		Normal	Abnormal
1. General appearance (including obesity, gross defects, postural abnormalities)			11. Inguinal rings (males)		
2. Head and neck			12. Genitalia (males)		
3. Eyes			13. Anus and rectum (if indicated)		
4. Nose and sinuses			14. Extremities		
5. Ears (including otitis, perforation)			15. Skin reactions or eruptions		
6. Mouth and throat			16. Neurologic		
7. Spine			17. Psychiatric (including apparent motivation for diving, emotional stability, claustrophobia)		
8. Lungs and chest					
9. Heart					
10. Abdomen					

Explanation of abnormals: _____

_____

_____

D. TEST RESULTS:

All applicants: As indicated:

Chest x-ray(s) _____   EKG _____   Hematocrit _____

                            V.C. and FEV$_1$ _____   Urinalysis _____

                            Audiogram _____   Other _____

E. FINAL IMPRESSION (circle one):

Approval: I find no defects that I consider incompatible with diving.

Conditional Approval: I do not consider diving in this person's best interests, but find no defects that present marked risk. I have discussed my impression with him/her.

Disapproval: This applicant has defects which, in my opinion, constitute unacceptable hazards to his/her health and safety in diving.

_____   _____

Date   Signature of physician

(The form below is completed and returned
to the examinee if he requires evidence of medical examination.)

IMPRESSION (circle one):

I have examined _____ and reached
the following conclusion concerning his/her fitness for diving:

Approval: I find no defects that I consider incompatible with diving.

Conditional Approval: I do not consider diving in this person's best interests, but find no defects that present marked risk. I have discussed my impression with him/her.

Disapproval: This applicant has defects which, in my opinion, constitute unacceptable hazards to his/her health and safety in diving.

                            Signature of Physician: _____
                            Address: _____

                                     _____

                            Date: _____

Appendix 5

Case Histories

This group of case histories has been selected to demonstrate the general problems that may confront a physician who treats divers. The treatment the patient received is included. In some cases, the immediate relief and full recovery that can be achieved by the use of recompression is demonstrated. In other cases, both oxygen and recompression failed to provide complete restitution. No claim is made that the treatment prescribed was optimal, when judged either at the time of the incident, or subsequently in the light of newer knowledge. However, the degree of medical rehabilitation afforded by the treatment would seem to be a useful criterion.

In addition to treatment, there are two things these cases were also meant to demonstrate: (1) that decompression sickness is a protean disease, which may affect many parts of the body simultaneously; and (2) that the more complete and definitive the physical examination, the more apparent the protean nature of this disease becomes.

In our experience, it has only been through the combined efforts of a multidisciplinary team of specialists that the various disparate lesions have been identified.

CASE HISTORY 1*

Type of Exposure:
Scuba Diving

History of the Present Illness

This 53-year-old man accompanied several companions in a sport dive off the coast of Kenosha, Wisconsin, to explore a wrecked vessel in August of 1974. The dive began at approximately 1215 hours and, within approx-

*Submitted by Eric P. Kindwall, M.D.

Summary of Case Histories Presented

Case History No.	Occupation	Presenting Complaints		Diagnosis
		Initial	Secondary	
1	Diver	Double vision	Pain in shoulder	Decompression sickness — Type 2
2	Caisson worker	Pain — abdomen	Pain & numbness in hip	Decompression sickness — Type 2 — CNS
3	Diver	Sudden loss of hearing — right	Dizzyness	Decompression sickness — Type 2 — vestibular, peripheral
4	Diver	Sudden onset of tinnitus	Dizzyness & nausea	Barotrauma — left inner ear — Fracture of stapes
5	Diver	Tremors	Dizzyness & nausea	High-pressure nervous syndrome
6	Diver	Mental confusion	Amnesia	Compressed air intoxication
7	Patient	Unconscious episode	L. hemiparesis L. hemianopsia	Air embolism — iatrogenic
8	Diver	Semiconscious	L. hemiparesis loss of vision	Air embolism — decompression
9	Diver	Pain — shoulder	Loss of shoulder motion	Dysbaric Osteonecrosis
10	Diver	Pain — chest	Tightness in chest — dyspnea	Decompression Pneumothorax

imately 3 minutes, the divers reached the bottom depth of 128 feet. The time spent at the bottom was approximately 18 to 20 minutes. The diver engaged in swimming and some mild work in an attempt to salvage some equipment from the wrecked vessel. He used a decompression gauge to determine bottom time and, when ascent was decided upon, he and his fellow divers noted that the anchor line by which they had planned to ascend had broken free and could not be found. The patient then began his ascent, but due to his increasing buoyancy became separated from his companions and reached the surface in approximately 2 minutes. Twenty minutes after surfacing, he noticed that the shoreline appeared double. This condition persisted. About an hour after surfacing, he noted that he had pain in both shoulders, which was followed by pain in both elbows and both wrists. Purple splotches were also noted on his abdomen and chest. His companions then brought him by auto to the hyperbaric facility (a distance of about 50 miles).

Past History

The patient denied taking a hot bath or shower after surfacing, and did not exercise or sleep in a cramped position after surfacing. He denied any injury, strains, or sprains prior to present attack. His sleep was normal the night before, but he does report having a low-grade cough for approximately 3 to 4 weeks prior to this episode. After surfacing, the patient consumed approximately 3 to 4 ounces of Scotch whiskey and 2 beers. Water recompression was not attempted.

Past History of Diving

The patient has been a sport diver, trained by the Y.M.C.A., for the past 8 years, having logged 232 dives. He has no history of exposure to compressed air in his occupation other than sport dives, as just noted.

The patient did report that he had one episode of untreated bends approximately 3 years ago following a 29-minute dive. He noted that the pain in the back of his neck occurred several hours after he surfaced, and was present for approximately 1 day, and then subsided spontaneously. The patient's past medical history is without significant illness. He has been taking Xyloprim for the past 3 months for elevated uric acid. He had no history of gout prior to this, but says that an attack of gout was precipitated shortly after the medicine was begun. The patient was a heavy smoker in the past, but quit smoking cigarettes 15 years ago.

Physical Examination

This 53-year-old, white male, height 6 feet, weight 190 pounds, was seen in the emergency room at 1700 hours, about 3-1/2 hours after finishing a sport dive. At that time, he had some numbness and tingling in his left hand, diplopia, pains in his shoulders, and clouded sensorium.

Treatment

An intravenous injection of 500 ml of Rheomacrodex was begun and the patient was recompressed on Navy Table 6. Recompression was begun at 1717 hours. Relief of shoulder pain was noted at 1736 hours. Relief of "skin bends" was noted at 1810 hours.

Factors Contributing to This Attack of Decompression Sickness:

1. Loss of anchor ascent line making a timed ascent difficult.
2. Separation of patient from his diving companions due to his increased buoyancy.

Impression

1. Decompression sickness, Type 2, with diplopia, pain in both shoulders, both elbows and both wrists, numbness and tingling of the left hand, weakness of the legs, clouded sensorium, and abdominal marbling.
2. Complete relief of all symptoms on U.S. Navy low pressure oxygen treatment Table 6 with administration of 500 ml of Rheomacrodex intravenously.

CASE HISTORY 2*

History of the Present Illness

The patient is a 34-year-old, black male caisson worker of muscular build, who weighs 162 pounds and is 5 feet 8 inches tall. He had been working in a tunnel heading which had been at a pressure of 18 pounds for several weeks. The patient entered compressed air at 1:55 PM on May 29, 1971, and worked for 7 hours, during which time he spent long periods lying on his stomach with his buttocks and legs hanging without support. This was in the process of pouring concrete. The patient states that this is the first time he has done this type of work under increased air pressure. At 9:05 PM the patient started decompression which took 1 hour and was completed at 10:05 PM.

*Submitted by Eric P. Kindwall, M.D.

The patient smoked one or two cigarettes while undergoing decompression in the lock, as did two or three others. There was no ventilation of the decompression lock during the entire decompression.

The patient left the job site shortly after decompressing. At approximately 1:00 AM, May 30, he developed abdominal pain in the periumbilical area. The pain became gradually worse and by 6:00 AM, the patient became nauseated and vomited, and had a bout of diarrhea as well. The pain continued to get worse during the day, and began to migrate downward to the lower part of the stomach. By 3:00 PM the pain in the stomach had become very severe, and he had also developed pain in his hip. Approximately 1-1/2 hours after the development of hip pain, he noted a patch of numbness over the anterior aspect of his left hip and a "pins and needles" feeling in this area. By evening, the patient decided that he ought to get some sort of treatment for his symptoms and reported to the hyperbaric facility that served his company at approximately 7:40 PM. When the patient arrived at the hospital admitting room, he stated that he had abdominal pain. He was asked to wait. In due course, he was seen and gave this recent history.

The patient denied any exercise during decompression, and he also denied sitting in a cramped position during decompression. The patient denied postdecompression exercise. He denied any history of strains or sprains prior to his attack, and he had 8 hours of sleep prior to going on shift. There was no alcoholic intake in the immediate history before pressurization, and he denied having a severe cold. He denied that he had been chilled in the tunnel, or that there had been any smoke or fumes while he was working.

Past History

The patient first worked under compressed air in 1955 when he was employed by a construction company at a maximum pressure of 15 pounds, on a job which lasted for 3 years. In 1961, he worked for another construction company for 3-1/2 years at a maximum pressure of 32 pounds. The patient later went to work for another construction company in 1967 for a 2-1/2-year period at a maximum pressure of 29 pounds.

Previous Attacks of Decompression Sickness

In 1961, the patient developed pains in his legs, arms, and knees after working 3 hours at 31 pounds and spending 1 hour in decompression. The patient recompressed himself back to 31 pounds on the job and remained there for 2 hours after which he slowly bled off the air. The patient denies having frequent untreated air pains, and he also denies a history of trauma to his bones or joints. The patient had x-rays 1 month ago, which showed no evidence of aseptic necrosis.

Physical Findings

On admission, the patient's hematocrit was 49.4 percent with a hemoglobin of 16.3 and a white count of 6100. The patient demonstrated no pathologic reflexes and his physical examination did not differ from his preemployment physical, which had been performed exactly 1 month previously, with the exception of the findings related to the present illness. His hematocrit was 3 points higher, however.

Treatment

The patient was recompressed at 9:11 PM. Because of the nature of his symptoms and because they took some time to resolve, the patient was committed to U.S. Navy Table 6, which requires 285 minutes. When the patient got to pressure, he stated that his abdominal symptoms were much better, but some soreness persisted. After 17 minutes on oxygen at 60 feet, the patient said that the "pins and needles" feeling in his hip had disappeared. After a total of 88 minutes of recompression, the patient stated that all of his symptoms had disappeared. While at pressure, the patient was given 500 ml of Rheomacrodex intravenously. The patient completed Table 6 with no further difficulty, and was sent home with no residual symptoms.

When seen the following day, the patient complained of a stiff neck and still had an occasional queasiness in his stomach.

Factors Which Contributed to This Attack of Decompression Sickness

1. This patient demonstrates no facts from his history that would tend to materially increase his chances for getting decompression sickness. However, the following observations should be made:
    a. Smoking was permitted during decompression. This practice is forbidden by state law.
    b. Albeit the combination lock is large in terms of cubic capacity, there was no ventilation of this lock for a 1-hour period of decompression.
    c. This patient very possibly was victim of some sort of vital illness which would have lowered his resistance to getting decompression sickness, but this can be only conjecture. The only evidence we have for this hypothesis is that he developed stiffness in the neck and questionable gastrointestinal symptoms unrelated to decompression sickness, even after treatment.
2. *The patient waited for a period of 19 hours before asking for recompression treatment.* This is excessive. Had he been treated early, it is quite probable that a short treatment table could have been used with a resulting

economy in time, air, oxygen, money, and pain. I think it is imperative that a statement be posted in the decompression lock saying that if a workman experiences "niggles" or "air pains" that persist for more than 1/2 hour, he is to immediately notify the cognizant hyperbaric treatment facility.

Impression

1. Decompression sickness, Type 2, with spinal cord symptoms (sensory and possibly visceromotor involvement).
2. Nineteen hour delay in treatment.
3. Possible concomitant viral enteritis.

CASE HISTORIES 3 AND 4*

The following two cases are presented to illustrate several ways in which the auditory and vestibular systems can be severely damaged under hyperbaric conditions, and how the primary symptoms may be similar. While vestibular involvement is frequently seen in diffuse central nervous system decompression sickness, peripheral injury may also occur without evidence of other CNS involvement. Labyrinthine fistula must also be considered in the differential diagnosis. We recommend surgical exploration in all cases where the history and physical examination exclude decompression sickness or air embolism as the likely etiology; in those cases that fail to respond at all to recompression therapy; and where vertigo and hearing loss are the only complaints.

We also feel that a thorough otoneurological examination and routine audiometric studies should be prerequisites for all who work under hyperbaric conditions.

On the basis of history, physical examination, and test results, case 3 represents peripheral decompression sickness and case 4 represents inner ear barotrauma.

CASE HISTORY 3

In November 1973, this 46-year-old veteran commercial diver descended to 246 feet on air for 12 minutes. Decompression proceeded uneventfully until he was told that he was being brought up to his 10-foot stop.

*Submitted by Paul Winkleman, M.D. Department of Otolaryngology, University of Texas Medical Branch

Instead, he found himself on the surface due to a 10-foot error in the pneumofathomer.** He then descended 10 feet on a weighted line and completed his last stop. Approximately 1 hour after leaving the water, he was sitting in the mess hall when he noted the sudden onset of decreased hearing and high-pitched tinnitus in the right ear and whirling vertigo that rendered him unable to walk unassisted. He was then recompressed and treated on Treatment Table 5. After 15 minutes of recompression and breathing on 100 percent oxygen, the vertigo subsided and his hearing improved. Following treatment, he noted some decrease in hearing on the right, but complained mainly of tinnitus. He continued to dive until August 1974, when he sought medical attention for persistent tinnitus, hearing loss, and episodic vertigo. Otoneurologic examination at that time was normal. Audiometries revealed a right sensorineural hearing loss and initial ENG (electronystagmogram) showed a right beating spontaneous nystagmus with eyes closed, a direction changing positional nystagmus, an asymetrical torsion test, and a decreased response in the right ear to caloric stimulation.

Otoneurologic examination in April 1975 was again normal. Audiometric testing showed a mild to moderate low-frequency and severe high-frequency sensorineural hearing loss in the right ear, of cochlear origin. Central auditory tests were normal. The vestibular test battery at this time was within normal limits.

Diagnosis

Vestibular decompression sickness—peripheral lesion with central compensation.

CASE HISTORY 4

This 25-year-old policeman was sport diving in March 1975. He had made repeated descents to a depth of about 25 feet and noted no difficulty clearing his ears, though he customarily employed the Valsalva maneuver to clear. Almost immediately following his final ascent, he noted tinnitus and the sensation of fullness in his left ear. On the way home, he began experiencing whirling vertigo associated with nausea and vomiting which was precipitated by any head movement. He presented 24 hours later with persistent tinnitus and vertigo, and stated that he could stop the vertigo only by lying down with his head slightly elevated and turned to the right.

Examination revealed a pale, dehydrated caucasian male in his midtwen-

---

**The pneumofathometer (NEMO in diver language) is an air pressure gauge mounted on the dive barge and connected to a long tube, the other end of which is attached to the diver to give the pressure at the depth of the diver.

ties. Otoscopic exam showed an air fluid level on the left, but the Weber was midline and the Rinne was positive at 256 and 512 Hz. The neurological examination was normal except for cerebellar tests, which could not be done because the patient experienced severe vertigo when he closed his eyes. The audiogram revealed a bilateral high-frequency loss, which was worse on the left. The VTB (Vestibular Test Battery) showed an 18.8° right-beating spontaneous nystagmus. In addition, he had a 20 percent left unilateral weakness and 28 percent right-beating directional preponderance on caloric stimulation.

A labyrinthine fistula was suspected, and an exploratory left tympanotomy was performed the night of his admission. The stapes footplate was found to be fractured and subluxed into the vestibule with complete disruption of the annular ligament. The stapes footplate was returned to its normal position, and the fistula was closed with a fat graft taken from the lobule. The patient felt almost completely better immediately postoperatively, and all vertigo and imbalance were gone by the third postoperative day. He returned to light duty at work 2 weeks later.

Two months later, the VTB remained abnormal with persistence of an 11°/second spontaneous right-beating nystagmus. However, the patient has remained asymptomatic, and there has been a 20 decibel improvement in the pure tone threshold at 600 Hz and 8000 Hz. This case illustrates inner ear barotrauma, probably from autoinflation.

Diagnosis

Barotrauma, inner ear, left, with fracture and subluxation of footplate of stapes.

CASE HISTORY 5*

Experimental Simulated Dive—He/O$_2$
Compression to 1000 feet in 33 minutes

"During compression, the chamber became quite hot—although not nearly as bad as the previous dive. I began to notice distinct tremors long before reaching the bottom. I was not aware of much dizziness or nausea during most of the descent although this developed strongly near the bottom. On arrival at the depth the tremors became very severe and I became extremely dizzy and nauseated. I was only able to put in a couple of pegs in the Peg

*Submitted by Peter B. Bennett, Ph. D.

Board during the first battery and writing was virtually impossible. The arithmetic and matching scores were down largely due to tremor and to a lesser extent from an unclear head. I noticed that there was a very definite feeling of loss of mental acuity, almost like narcosis. Perhaps the pressure itself causes this? I found the ball bearing test impossible to do and, on one occasion, had to abandon it completely because I was feeling so sick. I did not manage to get in one single ball. The nausea and dizziness improved slightly during the second battery, 40 minutes later, and I was able to do the peg board, although I still felt pretty ill. This general condition persisted through the ascent to 850 feet and transfer to the other chamber, and did not fully wear off until this evening at about 2000 hours. During most of this time, I felt very unsteady on my feet and had to move slowly. During the ascent to 850 feet, I noticed a mild pain in my upper right thigh and occasional sensation in the knees. Occasional mild sensation in lower back and shoulders persists." (Duke University Medical Center Experiments described by Bennett, Blenkarn, Roby, and Youngblood. Undersea Biomed Res 3: 221, 1974.)

Comment

Even at a relatively slow rate of compression such as 1 hour to 650 feet (commercial divers often compress at 100 feet/minute), HPNS signs and symptoms can be quite debilitating. Fast compression to depths greater than 500 feet or so will produce signs and symptoms of HPNS, especially tremors, nausea, dizziness, sometimes visual effects such as "sparkling" of lights. Arthralgia is common in such deep dives and can be very painful in some divers. There is considerable variation in sensitivity to HPNS.

Treatment

These signs and symptoms can be controlled by adding 10 percent nitrogen to the oxygen-helium breathing mixture. This works well at 1000 ft. A slightly higher amount of 12-15 percent may be used at depths between 400-700 feet. Alternatively, it may be possible to choose individuals who are less sensitive. In general, the signs and symptoms will abate after about 1 1/2 hours. A further alternative is to compress slowly over approximately 24 hours, for example, to 1000 feet and saturate. Then rapid excursions may be made some 200-300 feet deeper without inducing HPNS. With increasing depths greater than 1000 feet this tends to be less successful.

CASE HISTORY 6*

Compressed Air Intoxication

When exposed to compressed air at pressures of 4 ata (100 feet) or greater, compressed air intoxication occurs with euphoria, dizziness, impaired neuromuscular and intellectual function, and alterations of behavior similar to that of alcoholic intoxication or the early stages of anesthesia.

Simulated Chamber Dive on Compressed Air at 275 feet (Wearing Standard Hard Hat and Suit)

Condition previous 24 hours: Normal except for loss of sleep due to 2 AM to 6 AM watch. The physical examination revealed no defects, and the Schneider score was 13.

Required suit-dive task

Remove nut from spill pipe attached to iron workbench, hand nut to diving partner, take hose from partner, attach hose to spill pipe, tighten loose fitting with wrench, open spill pipe valve, close spill pipe valve, take hose off, put nut on and tighten nut with wrench. Subject started task as usual without being told, but dropped the nut after removing it; he picked it up (should have let partner do this), and put it on the pipe instead of putting on the hose. Next, he opened the spill pipe valve as if the hose had been attached, but did not close the valve. Then he took the wrench and tightened the nut as if the job was completed.

The instructor told him to repeat the job and he responded, "Stand by to come up." As further instructions failed to elicit any response, his partner was asked to take his turn on the same job. His partner removed the nut and tried to hand it to him, but he would not take it, so his partner placed the nut on the workbench. Instead of handing his partner the hose, as he should have done, he tied the hose around the spill pipe.

At this point, it seemed wise to terminate the run and reduce the pressure. The instructors kept in communication with him during the decompression, but at 120 feet, he suddenly left his tank air-control valve and picked up the nut from the bench and started to put it back on the pipe. They did not succeed in getting him back to his valve until the first stop (110 feet) in the decompression had been reached. In response to phoned questions during the remaining decompression, he repeatedly stated he was all right and that he had completed his job correctly.

*Submitted by Peter B. Bennett, Ph. D.

Upon reaching the surface and being questioned, he at first stated that he had attached the hose and completed the job; but upon further questioning, he admitted he could only remember the following incidents: Taking off the nut, turning on the valve, seeing his partner with him by the workbench, and being told to stand by to come up. He has no memory of the other happenings until he saw the nut on the workbench. He not only knew that he should not pick up the nut when he was doing the job, but he also knew it should be on the pipe for a finished job; consequently, this started a debate in his mind that seemed to last for a long time, and to be a thing apart from him. He further stated, "these two ideas were coming from two directions like, and they seemed to bounce back and forth in my mind until the idea to pick up the nut became so strong I had to do it, and so I made a dive for it and put it on." At this point, although he thought he was still on the bottom, he was actually at 120 feet. He said that during the dive he knew vaguely that something was wrong, but could not tell what, and cannot now explain. However, when his partner, at the 110-foot stop, punched him in order to get him back to his valve and away from the nut, "everything became clear and plain, like something had been rubbed out." (From Shilling and Willgrube, US Naval Med Bull 35: 373, 1937.)

CASE HISTORY 7

The patient is a 21-year-old female with Eisenmenger's complex (ventricular septal defect, overriding aorta and right ventricular hypertrophy). A recent cardiac evaluation revealed her not to be a surgical candidate because of pulmonary hypertension with a right to left shunt. She was being treated at a local hospital with occasional phlebotomies for her polycythemia secondary to her cardiac disease. While undergoing a routine phlebotomy, difficulty was encountered which resulted in air being introduced into her right antecubital vein. She immediately became apprehensive, followed by loss of consciousness for approximately 15 minutes. She was subsequently noted to have a left hemiparesis, left central VII paralysis, and a left homonymous hemianopsia. There was no evidence of a peripheral phlebitis or an endocarditis. It was felt that she had had iatrogenic air embolism secondary to the phlebotomy accident. She was started on treatment with intravenous steroids.

A telephone consultation was held with a representative of the Hyperbaric Facility of the University Hospital who recommended immediate transfer and treatment by recompression and with hyperbaric oxygen therapy. Instead, *watchful* expectancy was instituted. When this therapy was found to have been unsuccessful after 24 hours, the patient was transferred.

Hospital Admission

Upon admission, the patient was examined, both by the cardiologist and neurologist, and found to be semicomatose in addition to having the other neurological deficits that had been demonstrated immediately after the phlebotomy.

Hyperbaric Treatment

The treatment of the patient was begun 29 hours after the initial insult, and the U.S. Navy Minimal Recompression Oxygen Breathing method for treatment of air embolism Table 6A was followed.

The patient had an ear squeeze at 1.5 ata and a bilateral myringotomy was performed. She was then taken to 6 ata for 30 minutes breathing compressed air. While at 6 ata, the patient became more alert, and her headache resolved. She had a remarkable improvement in her neurologic function: the left central facial nerve lesion cleared; she was able to move her left lower extremity; and her Babinski reflex resolved. She was also noted to have an improvement in her left homonymous hemianopsia and to have regained minimal movement in her left hand. The patient was then brought to 2.8 ata and then to 1.9 ata and ventilated with 100 percent oxygen. She showed no signs of oxygen toxicity. The patient was given 4 mg of Decadron at 1.9 ata to prevent rebound of her suspected cerebral edema. The patient's neurologic functions continued to improve with increase in strength in her left lower extremity and left upper extremity. She still had marked weakness in her left shoulder and her left biceps at the completion of the hyperbaric therapy. The treatment time was 5 hours and 35 minutes.

The patient continued to improve during the hospital stay. Her laboratory values such as CBC, chest x-ray, and EKG were compatible with her Eisenmenger's complex. All other lab values, including a brain scan, were within normal limits. She was treated with Decadron 2 mg q6h IM, ASA 10 grains qd, and Persantin 25 mg qid. The Decadron was discontinued after 2 days. The patient regained full use of her left leg and could again walk well. She had no left facial weakness. She had no defect in her visual fields to gross confrontation. She was discharged ambulatory after a 6-day hospital stay with only minimal weakness in the fourth and fifth fingers of the left hand and of her left shoulder.

CASE HISTORY 8

History of Present Illness

This 22-year-old, white female R.N. was in good health until 24 hours prior to admission, when she became confused, developed blindness, and lost the use of her left arm and leg following a short dive to 30 feet. The patient had been on a charter dive boat for the previous 2 days and had been diving at the Flower Garden Reef 100 miles southwest of Galveston. Her scuba dives from the boat had been as follows:

5-25-75 #1 1430-1500 hours 110 fsw x 30 minutes
        #2 1845-1910 hours 80 fsw x 25 minutes
        #3 Night dive—aborted shortly after entering the water because
           of fatigue and muscle pains in both upper extremities.
5-26-75 #1 0935-1005 hours 80 fsw x 30 minutes
        #2 1321-1331 hours 30 fsw x 10 minutes

During her last dive, a 2 - 2.5 knot current was running and she was trying to swim from the dive station at the stern of the vessel forward to the anchor line, which was being used as a descending line. She became tired swimming against the current. She accidentally dislodged her mask and while trying to replace and clear her mask, she dislodged her regulator. Before she realized what was happening, she was on the surface. She denies breath-holding, but recalls aspirating seawater on the way to the surface. Her dive buddy then helped her back to the boat. On deck, she told him that she felt okay except for a tightness in her chest and some pain in her right chest on inspiration. She complained of feeling tired and wanted to go to her bunk to rest, which she did. She was checked again 45 minutes later by the skipper of the boat who found her to be confused, lethargic, and complaining that she could not see. She complained of tingling sensations all over her body, but worse over her left face and arm. She was also unable to move her left arm. She was unable to help herself and had to be carried to the recompression chamber.

She was recompressed to 165 fsw. She became reoriented during descent, but did not regain the use of her left arm until after 25 minutes under pressure. Treatment was then continued on a U.S. Navy Treatment Table 6A which was completed at about 8:30 PM.

After treatment, she felt tired, but had no headache. Her ears were "stopped up," and she felt slightly unsteady. She was able to walk and use her arms, although she noticed that the left side of her face and body still felt slightly numb. As soon as the boat was able to get back to port, she was brought to the hyperbaric facility for evaluation and treatment.

Previous Medical History

Appendectomy, age 16; cholecystectomy following abdominal trauma in motorcycle accident, age 20.

Patient denied any visual disturbances since previous chamber treatment. She had no localizing neurological complaints other than imbalance. Her ears felt stopped up, and she thought her hearing was diminished. She denied tinnitus or whirling vertigo. She had no G.I. or G.U. complaints.

Diving History

Patient had had only a basic diving course, and had received her first open-water diving experience during the dives prior to the present incident.

Admission Physical Examination

The general physical examination was essentially negative, except for bilateral serous otitis media and lateralization of the Weber test to the right. The Rinne test was positive bilaterally.

The neurological examination disclosed that the patient was cooperative and intelligent. Memory was intact in all spheres.

The patient had decreased sensation to pinprick over the entire left upper extremity. Muscle strength to gross testing was weaker on the left than would be expected for her age and physical condition. Examination of cranial nerves disclosed normal corneal reflex bilaterally, but decreased sensation to pinprick on the left side of her face. Otherwise, central nervous function was intact.

Testing for cerebellar function disclosed that she did well on all tests with her eyes open, but fell to the right with her eyes closed.

She had no pathological reflexes, and deep tendon reflexes were normoactive and symmetrical.

Impression

Air embolism due to diving, with sensory defect of left upper extremity and fifth cranial nerve.

Treatment

Patient was admitted to hospital for observation and treatment. She was given a repeat treatment on the U.S. Navy Air Embolism Treatment Table 6A, with the initial depth increased to 200 fsw (the maximum allowed in that chamber). The time at 200 fsw was 15 minutes, with the remainder of the treatment schedule according to the standard Table 6A.

Following the treatment, the patient felt a subjective improvement of the sensation both of her left face and left upper extremity. Her imbalance had disappeared.

Hospital Notes

Examination by consultant neurologist on the following day was summarized as follows:

Impression: "Air embolism with evidence of resolving, mild left hemiparesis, and central brain stem defect of cranial nerves V & VII connections. I believe no further specific treatment required and that patient will improve and likely escape any significant neurologic defect."

CASE HISTORY 9

History of Present Illness

This young, civilian, commercial diver was brought by helicopter to the U.S. Navy Dispensary at Ismalia, Egypt, in August 1974. His complaint was of severe pain in his right shoulder which had been continuous since its onset 4 hours previously at the time of surfacing after a repetitive working dive to 65 feet in the Suez Canal.

The patient reported that he was one of the divers under civilian contract who had come to Egypt to assist the Navy in clearing the Suez Canal. He had worked daily since his arrival in May. He was one of the divers who was working in the south end of the Canal; he lived in a hotel in Port Said and had been referred by the Navy corpsman who was stationed there.

This diver had been working at this part of the canal since his arrival. The water here was 65 feet deep. They had been diving on the U.S. Navy Standard Air Decompression Tables and took their stops in the water as they did not have a chamber on their diving barge. The divers wore light-weight surface supply gear, and they rotated dives, beginning at 7:00 AM and working until early evening. They made either one or two dives, depending on the work to be done. This diver's work included hand jetting under the wrecks, burning (i.e., cutting with an electric arc cutting torch), and then rigging for the cranes to lift out the pieces of scrap.

The patient stated that he had not been bent on this job, but that there had been both ordinary bends and CNS hits from the type of diving that they were doing.

The diver stated that he had been feeling okay. He was finishing his second dive and had just completed his water stops and was climbing up the dive ladder onto the deck of the barge when he felt a sharp pain in his right shoulder that radiated down his arm. It was so severe that he could not pull off the jacket of his wet suit and had to be helped. He denied any trauma to his shoulder either during the dive or in the immediate past. He did acknowledge that his shoulder had felt sore after diving for the previous several days.

The diver had reported this pain to the diving supervisor, who decided that he should be sent back to see the Navy corpsman at their hotel. This was done and this corpsman gave him a shot of morphine and had him transferred to the main dispensary at Ismalia.

Past History

The patient had the usual diseases between the ages of 6 and 8 without sequellae and had infectious mononucleosis without jaundice or sequellae at age 18. He had a successful surgical repair of a right inguinal hernia as a child and had a fracture of his third metacarpal of the right hand at age 12, which was satisfactorily treated.

He had a predeployment diving physical before leaving for Egypt which qualified him for diving. It did not include either a chest or long bone study, but he had had a contusion to his right shoulder in February while diving, and the treating physician had taken an x-ray which was negative.

Since he had been in Egypt, he had lost 10-15 pounds, which he blamed partly on the food and partly on the fact that he, like all of the divers, had a continual case of "Gippy Tummy."

Diving History

He had received his basic training by taking the Commercial Diving Center Course for Commercial Diving in 1971. Since that time, he had worked when possible as a diver, first in California and then in the Gulf of Mexico. He had not had a regular diving job until he took the job in Egypt.

Physical Examination

The patient was a well-developed, white male who looked his age of 25 years. He was ambulatory and was in no great pain when examined. He complained of soreness of his right shoulder and tenderness on palpation of the head of the humerus. Passive movement of the arm was possible, but evinced moderate additional discomfort. The physical findings were otherwise normal. (This dispensary did not have an x-ray machine or physician.)

Treatment No. 1:

The patient was given:

1. pills for pain
2. pills for sleep
3. a sling for his arm
4. 7 days sick leave
5. a helicopter ride back to Port Said

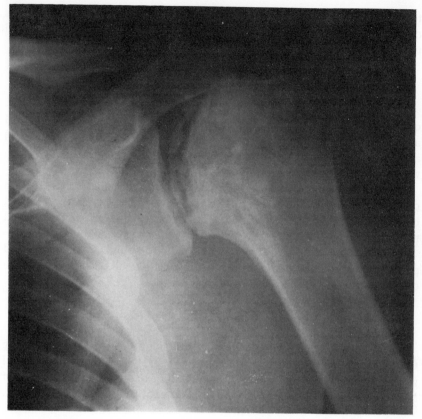

Fig. 1. Roentgenogram of right shoulder of diver taken seven months after onset of pain.

Progress Notes

1. The leave was found to be more beneficial than the pills, inasmuch as his wife came over to keep him company during his illness.
2. After 7 days, he reported back to the dispensary. They were so pleased with his improvement that they sent him back to work.
3. Diver stated that his shoulder continued to bother him and was very uncomfortable at night when he tried to sleep on it. He nevertheless continued to dive, and did the best job that he could, although he could not lift much with his right arm.
4. Diver's 6-month contract was completed in November 1974 and he returned to the States.

5. Since he was still having much trouble with his right shoulder, he sought the advice of an orthopedic surgeon who made a diagnosis of dysbaric osteonecrosis of the head of the right humerus. The surgeon treated the lesion with intracapsular injections of cortisone at intervals over a 2-month period, without relief.

Diver was referred to the Marine Medicine Clinic, U.T.M.B., in April 1975. The diagnosis of dysbaric osteonecrosis of the right humeral head was confirmed. The lesion had progressed, and there was now a multiple sequestra of the articular surface of the head of the humerus with fracture lines easily visible.

Diagnosis

Dysbaric osteonecrosis, right humerus, A-4 lesion. (See Fig. 1, roentgenogram of right shoulder.)

Treatment Advised

1. Prohibited from further diving.
2. Limited load bearing of right arm.
3. Regular examination to observe progress of disease.
4. Consider prosthetic replacement of joint if pain or loss of mobility indicate.

CASE HISTORY 10

Report On Diving Incident Leading to Death of Diver in Decompression Chamber

This is the account of a diving accident that occurred during the course of regular diving operations in the North Sea. The dive was carried out from a drilling platform. The diving support equipment consisted of a chamber complex including a deck decompression chamber (DDC) and a submersible decompression chamber (SDC) which could be mated together mechanically. This permitted the transfer of the diver into and back out of the SDC or bell. In this case, the diver entered the bell, or SDC, at the start of the "dive," and was transported into the water and to the dive site in the SDC. The bell was opened at the work site, the work accomplished, and the diver then reentered the bell. The bottom hatch was closed, and the bell brought back up to the surface (still under pressure). The bell was then mated to the decompression chamber, which had been pressurized to an equal pressure. The diver could then transfer from the small SDC into the larger more comfortable DDC for decompression.

The log of the dive is given, representing the company's report, and the medical officer's report is interspersed as appropriate to represent the medical developments.

DIVING LOG

Pressure/depth (feet)   Date

Sunday, 30 June 1974

02.24	Start pressurizing up for the dive.
02.43/492	Dive complete start decompression.
04.23/90	First symptoms occur (shortness of breath, chest pain).
04.53/100	Atmosphere changed and recompressed to 100 feet where relief was complete. Diving Superintendent (on shore) informed by radiophone.
07.53/85	Symptoms present again at 85 feet.
09.53/185	Recompress to 185 feet on saturation schedule.

Monday, 1 July 1974

02.53/105	Symptoms recur at 105 feet. This is technically the firs recurrence of symptoms.
12.03/85	Symptoms recur for the second time, this time at 85 feet. Recompressed to 185 feet to get complete relief of symptoms.
14.33/185	Leave 185 feet on saturation schedule.

Tuesday, 2 July 1974

13.00/75	Restricted breathing reported at 75 feet. Recompress to 125 feet. Complete relief. Third recurrence.
23.25/83	Difficulty breathing at 83 feet. Recompress to 135 feet. Complete relief. Fourth recurrence. Diving Superintendent and physician called for.

Wednesday, 3 July 1974

10.49/90	Superintendent and physician arrive. Diver now at 90 feet.

Report of Physician

History and Examination July 3, 1974

"No previous diving incident. History of having had pain in left chest wall posteriorly, attributed by himself to a "pulled muscle" while using chest expanders on day preceding dive, i.e. on Saturday June 29. Asked for and obtained "embrocation cream" ("Deep Heat") from Rig medic, and had got relief from its use. No other diving personnel had been informed and he had not mentioned symptoms himself until day of examination. He said the pain had been worse on deep breathing and coughing, but he had not had any symptoms of a florid "cold." Had found dive to be uneventful and without symptoms, as was first decompression to 90 feet when he had experienced symptoms similar to those he had at time of examination, i.e., pleuritic-type pain left chest posteriorly over midthoracic region, and a generalized chest tightness, felt worse over front of chest across line level with nipples.

("Most recent diving medical was at 231 Union Street, "3 to 4 months ago" passed as "fit for deep sea diving.")

"On examination—there was no cyanosis, respiratory rate was increased to approximately 30 per minute, blood pressure 118/74, pulse rate 108/minute. Temperature at this point was not taken, but was read every 4 hours afterward and found to be normal, then below normal by 1°.

"Detailed examination of the chest revealed a pleural "friction rub" at the left apex, decreased air entry over the whole lung field, but breath sounds still heard, decreased percussion note, vocal resonance, and tactile vocal fremitus over the entire left lung field as compared with the right. The trachea was central, and the apex beat of the heart was not displaced. Examination of the abdomen was normal.

"My diagnosis therefore in view of the history, the presence of a pleural friction rub at the left apex, the nondisplacement of the apex beat or trachea was that of an untreated pneumonia at the stage of consolidation. Treatment was prescribed by me as follows:

"Penicillin, 1 million units 6 hourly, reduce rate of ascent, observe closely, and possibility of adding injections of an analgesic if pain became too intolerable, or recompress if this not feasible.

"At this point, diving superintendent asked if it might be prudent to obtain a second opinion, to which I replied that I was sufficiently sure of my diagnosis for me to be able to leave the rig noontime, to return at a moments notice, but if he still thought it necessary after further ascent, I would welcome a second opinion and give any help required to a second doctor. Finally agreed that we should see how further ascent progressed.

"After obtaining extra supplies of penicillin from nearby rig, I returned to Aberdeen. Phoned Rig in evening to find that ascent to 59 feet has been made, but increase in chest pain led to recompression to 70 feet and held there for 1 hour. As diver had only had one injection of penicillin at that time, I asked that when ascent was resumed that it be slowed further, until more injections had been given and drug had had time to take effect."

DIVING LOG (cont)

13.49/80	Doctor diagnosis says pneumonia and pleurisy and no pneumothorax. Doctor instructs to bring patient to surface at 3 feet per hour. Depth is 80 feet.
16.40/70	Diver breathing reported improving all the time.
17.30/67	First penicillin injection.
21.00/70	Recompress to 70 feet.
21.45/70	Pain killing injection (first).

Thursday, 4 July 1974

06.00/60	Diver reports shortness of breath held at 60 feet.
08.40/60	New tender reports diver sleeping at 60 feet. Diving superintendent (on Rig) requests opinion of second doctor.
12.30/50	Diver condition getting worse again at 50 feet.

12.41/53	Diver got some relief at 53 feet given pain killer injection.
15.24/48	Diver breathing okay, rate of ascent increased.
16.00/47.5	Diver feeling bad but breathing O.K. at 47.5 feet.
17.11/48	Recompressed to 48 feet from 46 feet. Chest pains and swelling (not certain) over left pectoral muscle. Pain killing injection.

Physician's Report

"*July 4.* Kept in touch with Rig by radiotelephone. Treatment continued as on the 3rd with the addition at midday of intramuscular injections of Pethidine and a further slowing of rate of ascent. Conditions apparently satisfactory up to 1600-1700 hrs when it was reported that Rig medic, while giving injection, had noticed swelling at front of chest on left, below the left clavicle region. Instructions given for him to re-enter chamber to find out nature of swelling (whether any sign that swelling could be air), the position of the apex beat of the heart to see if there was any displacement to the right, and to check that the trachea was not displaced. While this was being done, I phoned the Royal Naval Physiological Laboratory at Alverstoke to seek further advice. Immediately before the appearance of the swelling as described, Diving Superviser, on my advice and at his request, tried to get a doctor to go to the Rig and give a second opinion. However, no other physicians were available. The Senior Medical Officer I spoke to in Alverstoke could only agree that in the cirumstances I should return to the Rig earlier than originally planned and make a reappraisal of the situation. I phoned the Rig to be told that the swelling was no longer evident on the chest wall and that apex beat and trachea appeared to be in their normal positions. Informed them that I would be traveling to the Rig once I had all the necessary equipment, not only for the immediate condition, but also for the planned helicopter trip at low altitude late Saturday or early Sunday, the ascent having been stopped."

DIVING LOG (cont)

19.11/46	Diver held at 46 feet examined by medic. Diver sleeping. Temperature 96.6. pulse 104.
19.22/44	No swelling of pectoral muscle noted by medic at 44 feet.
20.50/43	Diver feeling very bad at 43 feet.
21.00/43	Diver vomits after drinking orange juice.
22.50/43	Pain killer and penicillin injection.

Friday, 5 July 1974

01.30/41	Diver condition worse, wretching, 41 feet. Medic administers tranquilizer.
03.30/40	Diver received Valium injection at 40 feet.
03.40/39	Physician makes examination. Claims diver condition is improving with pneumonia disappearing. At 39 feet orders decompression rate increased.

Physician's Report (cont)

"Examination—again could find no evidence of a mediastinal shift, the apex beat being in the 5th interspace just outside the midclavicular line, the trachea central, and adequate oxygenation on comparing the color of the nail beds of both the diver and my own. Auscultation with the stethescope showed a disappearance of the pleural friction rub at the apex but now audible in the midaxillary line in the midlung zone. Breath sounds were more easily audible over the apex and the upper lobe than had been the case before, but were still less than on the right side. The breath sounds lower down in the midaxillary line I thought were faintly amphoric, which I took to indicate the beginnings of a pleural effusion, and the whole picture to be one of the stages of resolution of a lobar pneumonia. There was some disorientation and a degree of distress and restlessness in relation to that caused by the pain, which I attributed to the effects of Pethidine. These were alleviated to a large extent by an intramuscular injection of Valium 10 mg at 0400. At 0400 the Rig medic gave injection of penicillin and 75 mg of Pethidine intramuscularly, while awaiting delivery of Physopiton injections with equal analgesic effect, but less disorientation accompanying its use.

"Last spoke to diver at 0645 when he appeared to be settling down to sleep, though still with a rapid respiratory rate (pulse on examination had been 100/min while blood pressure was still maintained at 110/70)."

DIVING LOG (cont)

05.30/30	Medic administers penicillin and sleeping pill at 30 feet.
06.20/33	Tender administers 75 mg Mettradin at 33 feet. Diver sleeping.
09.00/32	Tender reports no pulse or breathing. Administers mouth-to-mouth resuscitation at 32 feet.

Physician's Report (cont)

"At 0910 was informed by Diving Superintendent that diver's pulse had stopped—after quick compression to 35 feet entered inner chamber where examination of diver showed absence of pulse and respiration, pupils dilated and unresponsive to light, with the retinal vessels and retina itself showing pallor suggesting that death had probably occurred at least 20 minutes earlier. I certified death at 0920 on Friday, July 5, 1974.

"Postmortem examination performed by Police Surgeon, on July 6 showed cause of death to be a left pneumothorax."

Appendix 6

Answers to Study Questions

Chapter 2. The Physics of Gases

1. 304 mm Hg
2. 12 liters
3. 3.16 atm or 2402 mm Hg
4. a
5. b

Chapter 3. Diving Equipment

1. d
2. False
3. True
4. False
5. False
6. True

Chapter 4. Respiratory System

1. a and d are correct
2. During lung rupture by expanding gas, the gas pressures are probably high enough to block the pulmonary circulation by squeezing the capillaries. On reaching surface, the diver breathes, lung gas pressure drops, blood flow begins again, and gas emboli are on their way.
3. 265 feet = 9 ata. The maximum voluntary ventilation should be about one-third that measured on the surface.
4. No. Pressure (pleural) around intrathoracic extrapulmonary airways is very negative during forced inspiration.
5. a. Divers tend to ventilate less than most other people in response to CO_2 and exercise.
   b. Divers breathe slowly, depressing CO_2 response.
   c. Increased gas density depresses CO_2 response.
   d. High O_2 depresses CO_2 response.

6. a. They have very high O_2 solubility—they contain enough O_2 for metabolic needs when equilibrated with O_2 at 1 ata.

   b. They do not mix with water and they have low surface tension so some surface tension lung recoil is preserved; and they do not wash out surfactant.

Chapter 5. Barotrauma

1. Blood vessels
2. a
3. Air embolism, mediastinal emphysema, subcutaneous emphysema, dyspnea, hemoptysis, and pneumothorax
4. Air embolism
5. Immediate recompression

Chapter 6. Decompression Sickness

1. c
2. b
3. a
4. e
5. b
6. a
7. Obesity, exertion, poor physical conditioning, aging, cold, dehydration, injury
8. b
9. 2 hours
10. b
11. a
12. a
13. a

Chapter 7. Hyperbaric and Ancillary Treatment

1. True
2. False
3. True
4. True
5. False
6. True
7. e
8. False
9. a
10. False

11. True
12. False
13. False
14. True
15. False
16. False
17. True
18. False

Chapter 8. Aseptic Necrosis of Bone

1. a. At least 3 months must elapse from the causal incident until radiological signs can be expected.
   b. A single radiograph gives no indication of the prognosis.
   c. Radiographs do not indicate the true extent of the lesion.
2. The head of the humerus
3. 6 months
4. Any five of the following:
   steroid therapy
   sickle cell anemia
   diabetes
   chronic alcoholism
   cirrhosis of the liver
   hepatitis
   pancreatitis
   Gaucher's disease
   trauma
   rheumatoid arthritis
   gout
   ionizing radiation
   syphilis
   alcaptonuria
   arteriosclerosis
   hyperlipidemia
5. Yes: in order to exclude the possibility of neoplastic change in a shaft lesion.

Chapter 9. Ear and Sinus Problems in Diving

1. a. Inner ear barotrauma with probable round window fistula.
   b. Bedrest with head elevation. Avoid any maneuvers that can increase CSF or middle ear pressure. If no improvement of hearing or vertigo occurs in 48 hours, a left exploratory tympanotomy for a possible round window fistula should be undertaken. Recompression treat-

ment in this situation is contraindicated, since decompression sickness is extremely unlikely with this dive profile and further compression might result in a relatively negative middle ear pressure when compared to inner ear pressure. This would worsen a round window tear or fistula.

2. a. Otologic decompression sickness.
    b. Immediate return to the presymptom helium-oxygen atm; immediate recompression to at least 220 feet (3 ata above symptom depth), or to the deepest dive depth or depth of relief if conditions will allow; use of oxygen treatment tables and low molecular weight dextran; use of parenteral Valium for symptomatic relief; complete otologic evaluation after surfacing.
3. Alternobaric vertigo; ascent.
4. a. bubble
    b. inert gases
5. a. Diving helmets

Chapter 10. Eyes, Vision, and Diving

1. In the submerged state, the cornea has no air interface. The refractive properties of the cornea depend on the air-cornea interface which comprises the largest single portion of the refractive power of the eye. Without this component, the human eye is highly hyperopic.
2. The upper bound of the size of the visual field is determined by the critical angle of reflection, not the size of the faceplate.
3. Retinal blood vessels, particularly the retinal arterioles, are very sensitive to high partial pressures of oxygen.
4. Light is attenuated during its passage through water by absorption as well as by scatter.
5. The content of both mineral and biological matter varies in different bodies of water. Hence, the particular absorption pattern in terms of wavelengths varies from body of water to body of water, as does color appreciation.

Chapter 11. Diving Gases

1. 20 parts per million (0.002 percent)
2. a. Carbon monoxide from the compressor's engine or from traffic
    b. Oil vapor from oil lubricated compressors
    c. Solvents used to clean hoses
3. To have the patient breathe 100 percent oxygen at 1 atm, or in a hyperbaric chamber if available.
4. a. True. In open-circuit scuba, however, buildup of CO_2 to such levels does not occur.

5. a. True
6. a. True

Chapter 12. The Physiology of Nitrogen Narcosis

1. b
2. c
3. a
4. a
5. d
6. Tremors, dizziness, nausea, theta increase of EEG, alpha decrease of EEG microsleep, convulsions in animals.
7. c
8. a. Exponential compression rate
    b. Stages plus slow compression
    c. Rest for the first 2-3 hours on bottom
    d. Excursions from a saturation mode
    e. Addition of narcotic or anesthetic agents
9. b
10. d

Chapter 13. Human Performance Underwater

1. Panic is implicated in most sport diving accidents. A major means of preventing panic is to make sure that the diver first obtains as much information about the particular dive as possible; i.e., conditions, equipment needed, potential problems. An early sign common to most panic situations is an increase in the rate of breathing—an indication of agitation. Breathing and movements are usually irregular rather than smooth. Good physical condition and adequate training appear to be major factors in a competent, safe diver.
2. Narcosis, cold
3. The ratio of sightings of sharks to actual attacks is very favorable to the diver. However, the psychological reaction to the sighting of a shark is a major factor in interrupting tasks and degrading diver performance.

Chapter 14. Drugs and Diving

1. b
2. b
3. d
4. c
5. e

Chapter 15. Hypothermia

    a. Water temperature

    b. The clothing worn by the victim

    c. The subcutaneous fat thickness of the immersed person

    d. Movement of the victim in the water or movement of the water relative to the victim

    e. The posture of the immersed person

    f. The occurrence of cold vasodilatation in the skin

    g. At great depths, loss of heat from the respiratory tract into respirate gases

2. a. Body temperature should be measured, and although it is subject to lag, rectal temperature is probably preferable to esophageal temperature because of the danger of an esophageal thermocouple precipitating ventricular fibrillation or vomiting.

    b. Arterial blood gases should be measured and corrected by gentle ventilation.

    c. The acid-base balance should be monitored and corrected for combined respiratory and metabolic acidosis.

    d. The electrolytes should be monitored and corrected where necessary.

    e. It is probably best to avoid large volumes of transfusion in the early stages of rewarming.

    f. At body temperatures below 32°C, insulin should never be given even if there is a very high blood sugar.

    g. The usual principles of nursing procedure for the unconscious patient should be used.

    h. Blood pressure and electrocardiogram will obviously be monitored continuously.

3. a. Rapid rewarming from cold water immersion is best done in a bath of water at 42-44°C.

    b. Rewarming should always be attempted even though the patient is not breathing and there is no apparent cardiac action.

4. a. A sudden cardiac arrest as a result of the cold water stimulation acting by an unknown mechanism

    b. Vigorous and violent hyperventilation immediately after immersion, causing inhalation of water.

    c. Sustained vigorous hyperventilation causing a marked reduction in arterial blood carbon dioxide tension with the result that there is a severe reduction in cerebral blood flow, possibly together with a tetanic convulsion.

    d. Rapid cooling of the limb muscles which makes it impossible either to swim or to haul the body out of the water onto a raft or capsized dinghy.

b. Yes, heated breathing gas is required with a minimum inspired temperature of 13.25°C.
4. At 1 ata the limitation is cardiovascular, while at depth it is respiratory due to the increased gas density.
5. No. If the decision is made to lock in a physician or any other attendant, the compression should not be done rapidly. Because of the HPNS problem induced by rapid compression, the person rapidly compressed will be unable to do much for an hour or more.
6. No, for several reasons. Decompression sickness does not usually occur this deep in saturation diving, and recompression of more than 2 atm which does not relieve the pain indicates that the pain is not caused by decompression sickness.
7. He is symptom free and decompression may begin since adequate time has been allowed at 30 meters (2-6 hours). Decompression should be on the original schedule.

Chapter 20. Diving Accidents

1. False
2. True
3. False
4. False
5. True

Chapter 21. First Aid and Emergency Medical Treatment

1. Number one, the major problem was the absence of a communication system between the diver and his companion, i.e., a line. Had this been available, buddy breathing could have been performed and, in any case, an unnecessary waste of time would have been avoided. He would have had assistance during the whole rescue procedure.

The second major fault was in having a carbon dioxide inflatable vest. Had he used the more appropriate air buoyancy vest he could have utilized this as an extra source of air and avoided the subsequent panic.

The third fault was one of a technique, i.e., he should have exhaled during his ascent, thus preventing pulmonary barotrauma.

2. The morbidity from jellyfish sting and the nematocysts is reduced by the application of alcohol immediately to the affected area. This will dehydrate the nematocysts and prevent further venom being injected. Only concentrated alcohol is of value, as diluted types such as beer may result in hydration of the nematocysts, with further discharge. Methylated spirits are very effective in reducing the nematocysts' discharge. Following or instead of this application, the use of local anesthetic ointment is of

immense value in alleviating pain, not only at the site, but also in the regional lymph layers.

3. A surface supply system using 100 percent oxygen can be supplied through a demand valve to the patient, by using an improvised hood or helmet. He should descend to approximately 9 meters breathing from this system and should be tendered by air-breathing assistants. After a stay of 30-90 minutes at that depth, depending on the response to treatment, the ascent should be at the rate of 12 minutes/meter, with each meter marked off on the shot rope.

4. a. One-man chambers are quite unsuitable for therapeutic use, as they result in a patient being unattended and without the ability of performing simple first aid techniques, such as mouth-to-mouth respiration, cleaning the airways of vomitus, emergency thoracotomy, etc. The minimum effective medical treatment chamber is a two-man portable and, if necessary, the total treatment can be performed within that equipment.
   b. Transfer-under-pressure capabilities should be available and be of a standardized type for all chambers within that geographical area.
   c. Recompression chamber facilities should be available immediately at the site of all free ascent training, deep diving, experiemental diving, and for surface decompression techniques.

Chapter 22. Near-drowning: Pathophysiology and Treatment

1. c
2. e
3. b
4. a
5. b

Chapter 23. Investigation of Diving Accidents

1. Shark attack.

The observation that the major lacerations were on opposing sides of the limb is consistent with the limb fitting between the shark's jaws. The smaller lacerations some distance away give some indication of the width of the open mouth of the animal, as it is mainly the lateral teeth that produce the injury when there is not a section of flesh removed. A barracuda bite would have produced a much sharper clean-cut area excised in toto. A propeller injury, which was the major differential diagnosis, usually results in parallel straight lacerations down one aspect of the limb or body.

The diagnosis was verified by an exploration of the wound with

5. a. No, the stirring effect of the swimming gives a heat loss greater than the additional heat production.

Chapter 16. Hazardous Marine Life

1. Hearing or vibration detection.
2. a. Control of bleeding
    b. First aid for shock
    d. Intravenous fluids if available
3. a
4. The diver who pokes his hand into a hole.
5. a. False. The sea wasp sting can be lethal within 30 seconds.
6. Prompt cleansing of the wound; removal of foreign particles and dead tissue; and application of antiseptic agents.
7. a
8. False. Soak the limb in hot water.
9. b

Chapter 17. Diving Adaptations in Marine Mammals

1. e
2. d
3. b
4. b
5. a
6. e

Chapter 18. The Physiology of Breath-Hold Diving

1. c
2. b
3. c
4. d

Chapter 19. Saturation Diving

1. It allows much more time for doing work or for doing intermittent tasks over several days without incurring more than one lengthy decompression.
2. There is no efficient way of removing CO from the closed environment, and even though it makes up only a small volume of gas present, the physiologic effect is a function of partial pressure and not volume percent (vol. % $\times$ absolute pressure = partial pressure).
3. a. 30.2°C - 34.6°C or range of 4.4°C

removal of triangular serrated teeth, typical of *Isuridae,* or white pointer.
2. Postmortem decompression sickness. This is due to the liberation of gas that has been in solution in tissues, which results in a gas-phase separation as the body is brought to the surface. It is an inevitable result in any diver dying from any cause after exposure to hyperbaric gas environments. Its main importance is that it is destructive to all tissues, and interferes considerably with any morbid pathology assessments and histology. It is for this reason that autopsies are best performed, where possible, at the pressure at which the subject died.
3. It was believed in the past that middle ear hemorrhage is related to drowning. It is now generally accepted that this hemorrhage is more related to middle ear barotrauma of descent, which produces hemorrhage into the middle ear as the diver descends without equalizing the middle ear pressure. Any diver who has reached his maximum depth, and subsequently dies without further descents, will not show this lesion. Any diver who submerges, either after loss of consciousness or around the time of death, is likely to have this lesion as a coincidental and nonpathognomonic disorder, unrelated to the cause of death.

   Observation of the round window may reveal a fistula, demonstrating either vestibular or cochlear damage. The former may be of etiological importance in the induction of vertigo and disorientation underwater. Histological examination of the inner ear may demonstrate evidence of either barotrauma or decompression sickness. In either case, the same effect of vertigo and disorientation may be relevant to the diving accident.
4. None. It does demonstrate that the diver has had previous exposure to hyperbaric conditions, but there is little else relevant in the investigation of the cause of death.
5. Based on the finding of air in the cortical veins following skull opening, no pathological diagnosis can be made. This is not an uncommon finding when such a procedure is performed and bears no relationship to air embolus as it occurs in divers. The correct procedure would have been to perform an infusion of the vessels supplying the brain, with the collection of the perfused fluid and an examination of this for bubbles, caught in a bubble trap. Reflecting the calvarium is a procedure that has reduced the value of the autopsy.

Chapter 24. Medical Examination of the Diver

1.	True	5.	False
2.	c	6.	False
3.	False	7.	False
4.	False	8.	False

Index